HIV/AIDS

through an Anthropological Lens

Second Edition

Tiantian Zheng
STATE UNIVERSITY OF NEW YORK AT CORTLAND

Jack Wortman
KIRKWOOD COMMUNITY COLLEGE

Kendall Hunt
publishing company

Cover image © Dave Grass.

Kendall Hunt
publishing company

www.kendallhunt.com
Send all inquiries to:
4050 Westmark Drive
Dubuque, IA 52004-1840

ISBN 978-0-7575-9041-2

Printed in the United States of America
10 9 8 7 6 5 4 3 2 1

To Dave, who has provided the aesthetic and wonderful cover for this book

Contents

Introduction

The HIV/AIDS pandemic is a global problem that has a profound impact on the world we are living in today. In many parts of the world, the calamity caused by the infection has severely eroded the political, economic, and social fabric. How should we understand the issue of HIV/AIDS in order to curb its transmission? This book provides an answer to this question. It shows that the HIV/AIDS pandemic is not merely a medical problem. It is a complex social, political, and economic problem that crystallizes class distinction, gender inequality, power hierarchy, as well as cultural beliefs.

This book underscores the social and cultural aspects of the disease that have been downplayed or dismissed by the dominant biomedical paradigm. The first three chapters lay out three different approaches to HIV/AIDS, from the perspective of epidemiology, culture, and political economy. The rest of the book employs a combined approach of culture and political economy to delve into eight case studies that include geographic studies of Asia and Africa, and topic studies of commercial sex, ethnicity, young adults, women, drug use, and prevention.

Chapter 1 discusses the fact that epidemiology is about the causes, spread, and control of contagious diseases. The cause of AIDS is the human immune deficiency virus (HIV). HIV is a retrovirus, which means that it is unique in its ability to mutate and change shape. This ability makes it difficult to develop a vaccine, and at this time there is no cure for AIDS. Acquired immune deficiency syndrome (AIDS) is the name given the disease caused by HIV. Since HIV attacks the immune system, we can say that people do not actually die of AIDS; they die of a variety of opportunistic diseases as a result of a weakened immune system.

AIDS does not transmit easily; it cannot be caught from coughs or other airborne agents, and it is not carried by insects. It is most commonly passed through either anal or vaginal sex. It is also passed from mothers to children in the womb, at birth, or through nursing. Intravenous drug users sharing dirty needles are fast becoming a major means of infection, and it can also be passed through blood transfusions.

Plagues are common throughout history, and some of the worst of them have helped bring down empires or even whole civilizations. There is great concern that AIDS will destabilize some countries around the world, especially developing countries in places like sub-Saharan Africa. Because of the global economy AIDS has spread rapidly and is now present across the globe.

Chapter 2 highlights the cultural dimension of AIDS by illustrating constructed cultural meanings of AIDS, diverse cultural understandings of AIDS, and cultural factors of HIV/AIDS transmission. First, the social and cultural meanings of AIDS are shaped by media discourses about AIDS. In the West, cultural construction of AIDS reflects a fear of homosexuality, prostitution, drugs, deviance, and a sense of xenophobia. In many parts of the world, it is foreigners that are at the center of the blame in the cultural constructions of AIDS. This chapter provides three phases of media constructions of AIDS in the United States, and points out how the media influence the language of AIDS, which in turn helps shape how people think about and deal with the pandemic. Second, cultural factors such as the meaning of sex, sexual culture, sexual practices, gender relationships, and condom use have repercussions on sexual transmission of HIV. Third, different cultures, such as the United States, Haiti, and various countries in Africa, interpret and respond to AIDS differently. Finally, a critique of mainstream media further highlights the cultural construction of AIDS. Alternative media serve as a necessary counterpoint to the mainstream media. This chapter utilizes the cultural dimension of AIDS to critique the epidemiological approach of AIDS.

Chapter 3 discusses the idea that political economy approaches the social sciences with a recognition that the various disciplines within the social sciences are interrelated; that ethnic tribes or inner-city minority neighborhoods are best studied not in isolation, but as part of a larger political economic order that greatly influences their behavior. Anthropologist Merrill Singer is critical of fellow anthropologists who fail to account for this larger context within which smaller cultures and subcultures exist. Singer believes that the influence of large, international or national entities influence the ability of smaller areas to respond to the AIDS epidemic. He sees poverty as creating the powerlessness that is critical in this issue.

AIDS began in America among male homosexuals, a minority group, but a group that included its fair share of middle-class and wealthy members. While they suffered greatly from the inaction of government, they were eventually able to organize politically and get government on their side. Today the disease is growing most rapidly among another minority group that has much less wealth and power: inner-city minorities.

The inner cities of American metropolises have been shaped by larger and more dominant historical forces that have left inner-city minorities with little wealth and little power. Inner-city minorities often lead desperate, hand-to-mouth lives with inadequate housing and little health care. Traditional family bonds have been sundered by high rates of unemployment. Drug use and prostitution have become common. Women are at the bottom of this social hierarchy, with the least wealth and power, and are now the fastest-growing group infected with AIDS. The poverty of the inner city is the result of historic prejudices against minorities that has isolated them and cut them off from employment, property rights, and adequate education.

Chapter 4 discusses the geographic case study of Asia in general, and China in particular, and pinpoints the cultural, political, and economic factors that have fueled the AIDS pandemic in this region. More specifically, these factors include authoritarian government, a colonial history, gender imbalance, intergenerational imbalances of power, migration of labor, economic disparity, and social stratification. In Asia, as a result of the global capitalist economy, unequal distribution of global income, unequal allocation of resources, and unequal access to health care have left those at the bottom of the society vulnerable to infections. Due to the drastic inequity among the sexes, classes, and generations, most of those infected are marginal to their own societies and the global economy. Moreover, due to the European colonial exploitation in Asia, wealth, resources, and treasure had been plundered away from the region, and the democratic development and modernization had been delayed for 200 years. The colonial history in Asia has a profound impact in the spread and prevalence of STDs.

Chapter 5 states that the most severe AIDS epidemic in the world is in sub-Saharan Africa. As of 2007, an estimated 22 million people were infected, including 1.9 million new infections. South Africa, with 5.7 million cases, had the highest rate of infection of any country in the world. The disease first reached epidemic proportions in the Kinshasa region of the Democratic Republic of Congo and then spread into eastern Africa and later into southern Africa. The hardest hit areas have been eastern and southern Africa.

Before the African epidemic, AIDS was considered primarily a disease of gay men and intravenous drug users. In Africa it is primarily passed on through heterosexual sex. There are several possible reasons for this difference: weak immune systems from malnutrition, genital lesions caused by a high prevalence of untreated STDs, and a pattern of concurrent sexual relations that expose a maximum number of people at a time when the infection is most virulent. The weak social and economic position of women in southern and eastern Africa is also a factor, as they are more vulnerable to the sexual demands of men. In West Africa, where women traditionally have more social and economic power, the disease has been much less devastating.

Where there has been strong government leadership the disease has been more easily contained and rolled back. Where governments have been in denial, as in South Africa, the disease has been devastating. Remnants of colonialism, including institutions such as the World Bank, have also had a negative influence on controlling the disease by insisting on such things as privatization of the health care system.

Chapter 6 illustrates the cultural, political, and economic factors that affect sex workers' vulnerability to HIV infection. The chapter begins by presenting feminists' diverse standpoints on sex and commercial sex. It then discusses different state policies on sex work around the world. Following that, the chapter examines the cultural, political, and economic factors of HIV/AIDS and commercial sex in Senegal and Asia. In Senegal, since women traditionally do not receive education, divorced women are usually unable to gain employment and are forced to shoulder the responsibilities for their children because of little or no education or skills. In this case, they turn to prostitution as a last resort and distance themselves from the community and family that were the focus of their lives. Similar to the case in Senegal, many prostitutes in Asia choose the profession because they need to support their children, siblings, and parents, or because they are divorced or disowned by their families. Some children are even sold into prostitution by poor parents. Throughout Asia, youth is an essential prerequisite for sex workers, and young girls between the ages of 10 and 16 are in high demand by clients.

Chapter 7 scrutinizes the population of women, ethnic women, and young adults in their relationships with HIV/AIDS. For each population, this chapter provides both the alarming statistics and the complex factors of culture and political economy to explain each group's specific vulnerabilities to HIV infections. Gender is a crucial factor in determining individuals' vulnerability to HIV infection. It is usually men who determine when and how often to have sex, and whether or not a condom is used. It is also men who usually have multiple sexual partners, which increases the opportunity for them to transmit HIV to their partners. Global research has proven that gender norms, gender inequality, and poverty intensify and fuel HIV transmission for women. In many parts of the world, cultural norms demand that young women maintain sexual abstinence but encourage young men to experience sexual adventures. The cultural imperative leaves young women vulnerable with inadequate knowledge about sex, STDs, and HIV/AIDS. In many developing countries, certain sexual practices such as dry sex, widow inheritance, and ritual cleansers enhance both women and men's vulnerability to HIV transmission. Due to poverty and rapid social transformations, transactional and intergenerational sex is prevalent in many developing countries. In these relationships based on power and economic inequality, young women are placed in a vulnerable position and are susceptible to abuse, exploitation, violence, and HIV. Young people are caught in a cultural milieu that valorizes virginity in girls and active sexual behaviors in boys. They also encounter a contradiction between abstinence education and a sexualized culture that is suffused with sexual images and appropriates sex in the sale of commodities.

Chapter 8 discusses the issue of AIDS being communicated between intravenous drug users through the sharing of infected needles. Those infected in this way often pass the disease to others through sexual contact. This is the major reason that AIDS is now an epidemic in American minority ghettoes, and it is the major cause of epidemics in Eastern Europe, including Russia. A solution to this problem is to provide clean needles to drug users. In the United States there are moral objections and even legal barriers to this solution. Simply informing those at risk of the dangers they face has not proven effective. The lure of drugs and sex and the human feelings attending these acts often discourage rational behavior.

Prevention of AIDS requires programs that change established cultural behaviors. This means the use of clean needles, but it also means changing sexual behaviors. Keys to reducing sexual transmission include using condoms and limiting the number of sexual partners, or "zero grazing" as it is called in East Africa. Successful programs to stop AIDS require government support and funding. Some of the most hopeful programs involve peer counseling to raise the consciousness of vulnerable youth. The goal is to give young people a sense of empowerment through helping them to understand the political, social, and economic forces that have shaped their consciousness and their behavior.

Chapter one | Epidemiology

Epidemiology is the branch of medicine that studies the causes, distribution, and control of diseases. Understanding the epidemiology of AIDS is the first step in understanding the sociology of this epidemic, and gaining some insight as to how we might begin to control its spread. Before addressing these issues, however, it is necessary to understand some of the basic biological characteristics of HIV/AIDS.

The Human Immune Deficiency Virus (HIV) is a virus that leads to AIDS. Viruses are microscopic biological materials that are so small they can only survive and replicate by attaching themselves to host cells and making use of their borrowed protein. In other words, viruses are parasites. Their use of cell proteins can cause damage to the cell and a variety of diseases, from the common cold to exotic tropical diseases such as malaria. Not all viruses damage the cells to which they attach, and there is clearly a discrepancy in the severity of diseases caused by different viruses. Different viruses attack different kinds of cells in different organs of the body.

In the case of HIV, the immune system is attacked. People do not die from HIV/AIDS; they die from a variety of opportunistic diseases after the immune system has been weakened by the HIV/AIDS virus. Commonly, people die from pneumonia or a variety of cancers. The failure of the immune system makes us vulnerable to a wide variety of viral diseases that are normally latent because they are controlled by the immune system.

HIV belongs to a particular class of viruses called *retroviruses*. What is different about retroviruses, and particularly HIV, is genetic instability. In a short period of time, within a single organism, the HIV retrovirus mutates and changes it configuration, very rapidly. This presents a serious problem for the development of vaccines. Vaccines work by attaching themselves to the virus in a manner that complements the shape of the virus, thus neutralizing it. This becomes impossible if the shape is not constant. This is the core problem in trying to develop a vaccine to stop HIV/AIDS. It is a moving target and it is not clear in what direction it is moving.

To complicate matters further, there are two main strains of HIV: HIV-1, which is the most widespread and the most dangerous, and HIV-2. HIV-2 seems to be confined to West Africa. While there is no cure for it and while it will eventually kill its host, it is not as great a threat to society because it is not so easy to catch, and, more importantly, it develops very slowly. So slowly that it usually kills people when they are older, past child-rearing age and past prime working age. HIV-1, by contrast, while latent for a long time, kills people in their prime, leaving many orphans and a devastated work force, particularly in sub-Saharan Africa. It is HIV-1 that has spread around the world and threatens social order and political stability in many countries. While recognizing the seriousness of HIV-2, and the tragedy it represents for many West Africans, it is HIV-1 with which this book will be concerned. It is HIV-1 that threatens to destroy economies and even bring about the collapse of governments.

Another complication is that HIV-1 has mutated into four major groups known as M, N, O, and P. About 90% of all infections are caused by group M viruses. However within group M there are at least nine subgroups labeled A, B, C, D, F, G, H, J, and K. In addition there are combinations of these subgroups called circulating recombinant forms (CRFs) that come about through a kind of viral sexual reproduction. So for instance there is a recombinant form called CRF-A/B. The existence of these subtypes and recombinations raises many troubling questions: How many are there? How many will there be in the future? Do they vary in geographic distribution? Are some more virulent than others? Are certain subtypes associated with certain kinds of transmission? Will it be possible to create a vaccine that will protect against all subtypes? There are tentative answers to some of these questions such as geographic distribution and virulence which we will address below.

It has also been discovered that it is possible to be infected more than once by different subtypes, presenting another potential problem for those seeking to develop a vaccine. Whether a single vaccine will protect against all of these combinations is an open question.

As it turns out the various subtypes do have different geographic distributions. Subtype A and CRF-A/G are common in West Africa and in Russia for instance. Subtype B is most common in Europe, the Americas, Japan and Australia. Subtype C, the most destructive subtype, causing about half of all infections, is predominant in southern Africa, eastern Africa, and India. There is also possibly a difference in virulence with subtype D progressing to AIDS much more rapidly and killing those infected much sooner. It is important to note that there is much controversy about the relative virulence of various subtypes and some seemingly contradictory evidence. Some subtypes do seem to be associated with certain kinds of transmission, for example, subtype B seems more common in homosexual transmission and with intravenous drug transmission. Type C which is so common in Africa, is associated with heterosexual transmission. Whether this association between subtypes and modes of transmission is more than a factor of geography is an open question.

While there are now drugs that can alleviate the symptoms of AIDS, there is no cure. To contract AIDS is to have it for a lifetime; until recently a very short lifetime. Ultimately, contracting AIDS is a death sentence, and although drugs can indefinitely delay death, they cannot cure AIDS. Given the erratic manner in which the HIV mutates, a cure seems a long way off. An interesting feature of this disease is the relationship between HIV infection and the development of AIDS. HIV has no symptoms. One can be HIV positive for a long time without any sickness, typically ten years or longer. This presents a serious problem for controlling the spread of AIDS. Being HIV positive means that you are contagious. People who are HIV infected are unlikely to know that they are dangerous to others, and are more likely to spread infection than those who have symptoms. In fact those newly infected are the most contagious. This means that a perfectly healthy appearing person is most likely to spread the disease. This particular biological characteristic of the disease is a serious problem in preventing its spread as an epidemic, especially, as we will see, in developing countries that do not have the resources to do extensive testing. Even in wealthy countries such as the United States, it is very difficult to convince people that they should be tested.

While there is little good news about this disease, it is fortunate that HIV is not easily transmitted. It cannot be transmitted by insect bites, it cannot be transmitted through the air. While there are reported cases of infection through wet kissing, and there was one case of transmission from dentist to patient through dental work, these are extremely rare instances and have not even been fully verified. Saliva has been found to be a poor carrier. The vast majority of infections have come through anal and vaginal sex, intravenous drug use, blood transfusion, and organ transplants. Much more will be said about this later in the book.

HIV/AIDS Compared with Historic Epidemics

Plagues have shaped history ever since humans have lived in communities large enough to host them. Plagues are a feature of civilizations able to support cities with dense enough populations to allow for epidemics. The Bible records the epidemic that struck the Egyptians while they held the children of Israel as captives. Later it tells the story of the epidemic that struck the Philistines after they had seized the sacred Ark of the Covenant from the defeated Israelites in 1141 B.C.E. Later still, the Plague of Athens contributed to the defeat of that city during the Peloponnesian War, leading to the downfall of the Athenian Empire.

Between A.D. 164 and 189, we have the beginning of the Galen Plague in Rome, so called because the famous physician Galen is supposed to have witnessed and described it. It had spread from the East to Rome and for the next three and one half centuries it so devastated the Roman population that it was probably a major factor in the later fall of the Western Empire, ending classical civilization in Western Europe and ushering in the Middle Ages.

The most famous plague of all was the Black Death of the Middle Ages that was carried to Europe from Asia on board merchant ships. Specifically, it was carried by fleas that lived on rats that had boarded ships in Asia and gotten off in Italy. The Black Death, or bubonic plague, spread from Italy to all parts of Europe, probably killing about 25% of the population, that is, about 24 million people. Some historians believe the death rate was higher, more than one-third of the population, and most believe that this mortality set in motion a series of economic changes that led to the end of feudalism and the end of the Middle Ages. Epidemics can have a profound influence on societies, even to the point of causing them to collapse.

As of now, the impact of AIDS, as horrible as it is for those infected, has not had that kind of dire consequence for nations or for civilization. However, the impact in one region, sub-Saharan Africa, threatens to become a politically and economically destabilizing force. Africa is a unique place for AIDS. It is the place where the disease began and where it has been most devastating. We will address this further in a separate chapter on sub-Saharan Africa. If worst-case projections were to come true, areas such as China, India, and Russia could also suffer economic difficulties and political unrest. Russia in particular has experienced a rapid increase in infection because of intravenous drug use, and it is expected that there will be a second burst of infection as the disease is passed through sexual transmission.

Certainly the American government sees AIDS as a national security issue, likely to destabilize governments around the world, particularly those with emerging economies. An obvious difference between AIDS in the twenty-first century and the bubonic plague of the fourteenth century is that modern governments have the knowledge and communications to respond. Because HIV/AIDS is not airborne or spread by insects, it should be possible to control it through appropriate social policy. This would not have been so easy with the bubonic plague, which clearly required a medical solution. This is not meant to diminish the threat posed by this disease; the right social policy requires financing and will. In many cultures it will involve confronting habits and values that are deeply imbedded. It involves confronting powerful instincts and addictions that have proven difficult even in economically developed countries such as the United States. The possibility of curbing the epidemic through social policy has been demonstrated in one African nation, Uganda. In this nation the rate of infection has dropped dramatically because the government has launched a vigorous and sophisticated education and propaganda campaign that has been based upon a clear understanding of both how the disease is spread and how people actually do behave. Even in Uganda, however, this success has been threatened by funding restrictions on money from the United States that is based upon religious and moral ideology rather than scientific evidence about the efficacy of different approaches. Whenever sex and drugs are involved it seems likely that nonrational issues will intrude on sound social policy.

One front on the war against AIDS is the attempt to find a cure, which seems a long way off. This book will focus on another and more immediate front, the attempt to understand the cultural and social patterns around the world that facilitate transmission. We will attempt to understand the varieties of human behavior that make us vulnerable, and the ways that behavior must change if we are to stop this epidemic. What makes this task both interesting and challenging is that there is no singular solution to how we can change human behavior. HIV/AIDS is now worldwide, a problem in every culture. This means that we must understand how the practices of each of these cultures either facilitates or suppresses the spread of AIDS. Then we must understand what kinds of policies can effectively change behaviors appropriately. As already noted, there is a precedent for ending the epidemic through enlightened social policy, even in poor, developing economies. Uganda is an example of this. But it is also the case that even in rich countries such as the United States, it is possible to backslide, as is indicated by the resurgence of HIV infection among gay males, a community that had formerly made gains against the disease.

How Does HIV Spread?

As noted above, earlier epidemics, such as the bubonic plague, spread easily and rapidly. There was little that people could do, short of completely isolating themselves, to prevent the spread. On the other hand, people did contract bubonic plague and survive. The opposite is true of HIV/AIDS. It is not a virus that is easily passed on. There is much we can do to prevent contagion, but once it is passed on there is nothing we can do to cure it.

So how is it spread? The most common means of transmission worldwide is through sexual contact. This can be through either heterosexual or homosexual sex. In the United States the early epidemic and the greatest amount of contagion has come through homosexual transmission, most commonly anal intercourse. In sub-Saharan Africa the most common means of transmission has been through heterosexual intercourse. As we will discuss later in this chapter, anal intercourse appears to be the most risky behavior for transmission, whether heterosexual or homosexual; however, vaginal intercourse can be made much more risky if there are other STDs present which have caused lesions that allow blood-to-blood contact. This appears to be a major factor in the spread of AIDS in Africa, where other venereal diseases are common.

Another common mode of transmission is through intravenous drug use. This has accounted for large numbers of cases in the golden triangle area of Southeast Asia, as well as in Eastern Europe. This is a spread that can be stopped by providing drug users with an adequate supply of clean needles, but this involves education and a willingness to provide funding. Here again moral concerns get in the way of efficacious policy. Politicians often argue that providing clean needles seems to be an endorsement of drug use, just as supplying condoms to teenagers seems to be an endorsement of premarital sex. In the case of intravenous drug users, they are in the grip of an addiction that dictates their actions. If we wish to stop the spread of HIV through drug use it is important to stop dangerous drug use, even if we cannot stop all drug use.

In the early 1980s in the United States, the blood supply became infected. Transfusing blood that has already been infected is obviously a very efficient way of guaranteeing the transmission of the disease. Hemophiliacs were especially hard hit, since they depend very heavily upon transfusions. The good news is that the American blood supply since 1986 has been secure. This is not the case in less developed countries; blood transfusion accounts for significant numbers of new infections in sub-Saharan Africa, and in China the practice of re-injecting blood into donors from a common supply after removing the necessary platelets has infected whole villages. Even those who view AIDS as a scourge of God and blame sexually active individuals and drug users for their behavior must recognize the innocence of those infected in this way.

Finally, there has been transmission from mother to child through both the birthing process and through nursing. The good news is that recent drug developments have reduced the risk of transmission, while not totally eliminating it. As with other good news on the HIV/AIDS front, this has not significantly changed the situation in developing countries where the expense of these drugs is prohibitive.

Before getting into the particulars of transmission, it will be useful to understand how HIV is *not* transmitted. As mentioned above, HIV does not transmit easily; it is not passed on through bug bites or through coughing or sneezing into the air. Even sexual intercourse is not a sure way to transmit the disease, although it may take only one encounter to pass infection. It is not uncommon for infected individuals to engage in unprotected sexual intercourse with partners for years without passing on the disease. The high-profile case of basketball great Magic Johnson illustrates this point nicely. He has a healthy teenage son who was conceived after he was diagnosed as HIV positive. After all these years his wife still tests negative for HIV. This should not be interpreted to mean that sexual intercourse is generally a low-risk activity, as over 30 million cases in sub-Saharan Africa should make clear. Kissing, casual touching, toilet seats do not transmit HIV. As mentioned earlier, there appears to be a case of transmission through wet kissing and one case through dental work from dentist to patient, but there is not complete verification of the cause in either case. Generally speaking, saliva does not carry that part of the virus that is dangerous; in fact there are elements in saliva that seem to inhibit HIV infectivity.

Sexual Transmission of HIV/AIDS among Homosexuals

As stated above, the most common means of transmitting HIV is from sexual activity. However, not all sex is equal in its ability to transmit this disease. The surest way to transmit HIV sexually is through unprotected anal intercourse, a common practice among male homosexuals. As pointed out earlier, the key to infection is the mixing of bodily fluids, blood in particular. The likelihood of transmission is greater with anal sex because the walls of the anus are particularly thin and easily broken, which can produce bleeding.

As mentioned earlier, HIV/AIDS in the early days in the United States was primarily if not exclusively spread through the homosexual community, presumably largely through anal intercourse. The first reported case of HIV/AIDS in a living person in the United States was reported in New York in 1979, although tissue samples have revealed an isolated case from 1959. By 1981, cases were confirmed in Los Angeles, San Francisco, and New York. Initially, HIV/AIDS was regarded as a strictly gay disease. By the late 1980s it was clear that this was not the case. As of 2007, other means of transmission had become prominent in the United States. Of roughly 42,000 new cases diagnosed in the United States in 2007, 33% were caused by homosexual contact, 30% by heterosexual sex, 19% by intravenous drug users, 4% by homosexual drug users, 1% by transfusion recipients, and 13% undetermined. The data for the United States are in sharp contrast to the rest of the world, where sexual transmission now accounts for over 90% of new cases.

It is particularly disturbing that after an initial drop in cases among American gay men, there has been a recent upsurge. The development of drugs that can control AIDS has been a factor, removing much of the fear. Between 1994 and 1998 there was an increase in unprotected sex from 35% to 55%. In San Francisco, where about 27% of the gay male population is infected, new infections had remained steady between 1999 and 2002 at about 500 per year. In 2002 the number of new cases doubled, and has continued to rise ever since. As a result, in 2007 about 27% of the gay male population is now positive.

Are there other factors leading to this upsurge in addition to the confidence now felt in the gay community as a result of new drug therapies? Does this change in trajectory tell us anything about the epidemiological pattern we might expect elsewhere in the world? Two factors working in conjunction with the new confidence inspiring drugs have been identified. The development of Highly Active Anti-Retroviral Therapy (HAART) has taken the fear out of AIDS and has led to less cautious behavior generally, with fewer gay men using protection. Two particular phenomena deserve recognition. First, the use of methamphetamines to enhance sexual pleasure has become widespread. The existence of

HAART seems to encourage reckless behavior, and the reckless use of methamphetamines leads to even greater reckless behavior, including not using protection; also, there is an increase in the amount of sex one can sustain and a subsequent increase in the number of partners. Of course, increasing the number of partners greatly increases the risk of infection, since one is exposed to the partners of all of one's partners as well.

A second new danger encouraged by HAART is intentional risk taking or even intentional contraction of the disease in solidarity with those already infected, a perverse form of gay pride. These phenomena involve universal human qualities: the excitement and adventure of risk taking and the desire to identify with a group. The need for the latter is perhaps enhanced by the sense among members of the gay community of being outsiders. There are stories of a kind of Russian roulette involving group sex, some of whose members are known to be infected. Is this just an anomaly peculiar to the American gay community, or will this be replicated elsewhere, changing the trajectory of the disease after it has appeared to be under control? Because of the unavailability of HAART in the developing world, and the seemingly lesser role of homosexual sex in spreading the disease, one might hope that it will be a phenomenon limited to the developed world.

Oral sex is common in the gay world, but it is hard to determine how important it is in spreading AIDS, since most men who engage in oral sex also engage in anal sex. It has been established that oral sex can transmit HIV, but it is not definite how important it is. One can imagine that since semen does carry and preserve HIV, oral sex is dangerous, but what percentage of infection it causes in gay men is hard to establish.

Heterosexual Transmission

As noted above, heterosexual transmission has increased dramatically in the United States, accounting for approximately 30% of transmission as of 2007. Heterosexual transmission can occur through vaginal, anal, or oral sex. There is some small evidence that it can be transmitted through deep kissing, but this is extremely rare. The most common means of transmission is through vaginal sex, where women are at much greater risk than men. It is eight times more likely that a woman will contract HIV during vaginal sex than that a man will become infected. This is because semen carries a much greater amount of the virus than vaginal fluid, and of course, a much greater amount of fluid is being injected into the woman. Studies have shown that if the man is circumcised, his degree of risk is greatly reduced, although not eliminated. Another variable that affects the chances of infection is the presence of other sexually transmitted diseases(STDs). STDs such as syphilis or gonorrhea, which can cause lesions, are thought to be a major factor in the prevalence of HIV infections caused by heterosexual sex in sub-Saharan Africa. The presence of STDs can make vaginal sex just as risky as anal sex. Exposure to blood is the key.

Finally, it should be emphasized that oral sex is not safe sex. We may not know the incidence of infection among gay men from oral sex, but we do know that semen can carry a heavy load of HIV. There has been an upsurge of oral sex among young, poorly informed heterosexuals, apparently as a means of having safe sex. Oral sex is not safe sex.

Intravenous Drug Users

In addition to its frequency in the United States, intravenous drug use is an important means of transmitting HIV in the former Soviet areas of Eastern Europe. Russia and Ukraine in particular have a rapidly growing HIV population. Initially infected through drug needles, we are starting to see a second stage of infection through sexual transmission. This is a common pattern where one contracts HIV through drug use and then passes it on to the general population through sexual contact. Now that sexual transmission has put the virus into the general population, it is expected to grow rapidly. Both countries have budgeted miniscule amounts of money to address the problem. Whether the recent prosperity from oil revenues in Russia will reverse this trend is still not clear, but Russia is one of those countries mentioned earlier, where the impact could be destabilizing both politically and economically.

Another area where drug injection is playing a major role is in the so-called golden triangle area of Southeast Asia. This includes Thailand, Cambodia, Laos, Vietnam, and laps over into southern China. The problem in countries like Thailand is that drug injection is combined with a thriving sex industry catering to tourists. In the northern region of Thailand, where grinding poverty is the norm, the drug trade and the practice of selling daughters into prostitution creates a lethal mix. Both the Northern economy and Bangkok depend on money from drugs and sex. The young girls caught up in this business are no less innocent than babies infected with their mothers' breast milk.

HIV/AIDS in China probably had its origins in the drug trade of this southern region; however, the rapid transmission of the disease now has more to do with rural poverty and prostitution than anything else. China has a "floating" population estimated at around 150 million people. Until a recent change in the law, most of these people were peasants residing illegally in the cities without work permits. This floating population has been caused by the economic boom in the cities and the excessive poverty in the countryside. Many young peasant girls find the sex trade the only, or at least the best, way to escape the countryside and survive in the city. This is likely to increase transmission greatly. This is the reason many prognosticators are gloomy about AIDS in China. This is an issue we will develop more fully in a later chapter focusing primarily on China.

Blood Transfusions and Organ Transplants

Both blood transfusions and organ transplants can cause HIV infections. As noted earlier, blood transfusions were an important and early means of transmitting this disease. Transfusion of contaminated blood is a very efficient means of passing on the disease. However, at least in the United States, getting HIV from blood transfusions is now highly unlikely. While it is true that as of 2007, 4% of infected adults and 8% of infected children may have been infected by transfusion or blood products, the blood supply has been secured and regulated in a manner that makes this nearly impossible in the future. Unfortunately, the good news from the industrialized world does not extend to the developing world, where it is estimated that 10% of the infected are being infected by contaminated blood.

Transmission from Mother to Child

HIV can be passed to babies in three ways. The fetus can be infected in the womb when the virus passes from the mother into the fetal bloodstream. Infection can also occur during the birthing process, where the child is exposed to the mother's blood and other fluids. Finally, nursing children can ingest the virus with the mother's milk. At least half of infections occur during the birthing process. How frequently infected mothers infect their babies *in utero* is not clear. One estimate is that 30% of infected mothers who are not on drug therapy pass the virus to the fetus. This can be drastically reduced to about 2% with drug therapy. Since an estimated 100,000 women of childbearing age are HIV positive, this is a serious problem and one that falls disproportionately on the children of minorities: 55% of all children infected through their mothers are black and another 20% are Hispanic. As we will see, AIDS is not an equal opportunity disease. While anyone can become infected, the proportion of minority infections from other sources in the United States is disproportional, falling heaviest on minorities, particularly African-Americans. This is mirrored around the world where the heaviest concentrations of infection are in developing countries, particularly in sub-Saharan Africa.

How Has HIV/AIDS Spread around the World?

There are things about the origins of HIV/AIDS that we are likely never to know fully. The disease apparently began in Africa with a transfer from primates to humans who were killing and eating monkeys and baboons. In other primates the disease is innocuous. It seems to have evolved in humans to become the deadly infection that it is today. As noted earlier, two strands of HIV have been identified in Africa: HIV-1 and HIV-2. Of the two it is HIV-1 that is by far the more virulent and that has spread worldwide. It is HIV-1 that we will be concerned with in this book. How long HIV has been present in humans is not clear; however, isolated cases have been identified as existing long before the epidemic began, as early as 1959 in the United States and, of course, even earlier in Africa.

The origins of the disease in the United States can be traced to Haitian workers in sub-Saharan Africa bringing the disease back to Haiti, from which it was probably brought to the United States by American tourists. The transfer to Europe can be explained by the heavy postcolonial presence of Europeans in Africa and of Africans in Europe.

Why Has the Disease Spread So Rapidly?

Certainly, this is a major question that we will be addressing though out this book, but three factors should help us begin to think about it. People have always moved about the globe, but in the period since World War II we have experienced what we aptly call globalization. In a world that has become economically interdependent, global travel has grown immensely. Air travel is particularly auspicious. Air travel means that no place is more than 24 hours away, and air travel goes from every area of the globe to every other area of the globe. Middle-class affluence in the developed world makes it possible for millions of people to visit the most remote corners of the globe, whether it's the Galapagos Islands to view interesting marine creatures, East Africa to go on safari, or sex tourism in Bangkok. This means that viruses can also travel anywhere and very rapidly. New strains of flu that develop in the hotbeds of dense populations in southeastern China can be in the United States or Europe in a day. Related to this is the economic imbalance between rich and poor corners of the globe that can lead to sex tourism going from the United States, Japan, or Europe to the poorest corners of the globe.

A second factor to explore is the development of new means of birth control since World War II. The birth control pill became widely available during the 1960s. The development of the I.U.D. followed shortly. What both these methods of birth control have in common is that they provide no protection from disease, as condoms did. The development of these methods of birth control made control of pregnancy a more sure thing. This contributed to a third factor, dramatically changed attitudes toward sexuality that were expressed vociferously during the late 1960s as a cultural revolution.

It would be unreasonable and simplistic to assume that the new methods of birth control were the sole cause of the sexual revolution. All we can say is that it was a contributing factor. Changes in attitudes toward traditional values can be traced back to the Enlightenment and perhaps even earlier. Undoubtedly the breakdown of traditional village cultural values owes much to the industrial revolution and the urbanization it spurred. Cities do not have the same ability to enforce morality that a small community does. In the less personal environment of the city it is easier to define your own moral path. Whatever the mix of causation, it is clear that today's generation sees sexuality in a very different way than their grandparents, or perhaps great-grandparents, did. For many, sex is primarily for recreation, not procreation. It appears that more people are having sex with more partners, and they are no longer, for purposes of birth control, forced to use methods that also protect them from STDs. There is also some evidence that the safety and security of the modern industrial world may cause people to take more risks, as was suggested earlier by the practice of gay men playing a kind of sexual Russian roulette. Perhaps the great challenge of the anti-AIDS campaign will be to put this sybaritic genie back in the bottle, although there seems to be no sign as yet of a new Puritanism in America.

While globalization, new means of birth control, and a more hedonistic lifestyle may explain aspects of the spread of AIDS, there are also conditions peculiar to developing economies that are important to understand. In many developing countries, notably China and the countries of sub-Saharan Africa, the separation of family members has played a part. In South Africa, for instance, men working away from their families and tribal homeland in mines, resorted to prostitutes to fill the void of sex and loneliness. In India the course of the disease can be traced along the routes of overland trucks far from home. In China, as mentioned earlier, young girls fleeing the poverty and harshness of the countryside often end up surviving by catering to the sexual needs of displaced male peasants seeking survival in the city. Quite often nationalistic pride nurtured in the crucible of past colonial exploitation causes nations to cover up embarrassments such as high rates of prostitution and AIDS infection. This has been evident in China, where data on subjects like prostitution and AIDS are considered state secrets, with penalties for disclosure. What is frightening about AIDS in places like China is not the percentage of infection, which is still relatively low, but the fear that it will get out of control because it is not being adequately addressed while the numbers are still manageable. In places like Russia, the weak economy of the 1990s meant there was very little money to address the problem. Because of the oil boom, Russia now has money, but still maintains a low budget to deal with HIV/AIDS. If the current downturn in the world economy persists, driving down the price of oil, it is likely that the budget will remain small or even shrink further. Indeed, the failing economy is bad news for the war on AIDS everywhere, but especially in the developing world, because it takes money to develop social programs. It also takes lots of money to provide testing and anti-viral drugs for those who are infected. In the following chapters we will examine all of these issues in detail and take a very close look at specific conditions in places such as China and sub-Saharan Africa.

Hopeful Developments

Since the first edition of this book certain positive trends in the fight against AIDS have become apparent. It now appears that the disease peaked world wide in 1999 and that as of late 2010 new infections had fallen by over 19%. AIDS remains a major threat to social and political stability and to economic development, especially in the developing world, but the over all trends, for now at least, appear to be in the right direction. sub-Saharan Africa is part of the good news. Eighteen African countries have reduced their infection rates and other sub-Saharan African countries have at least stopped the increase in rates. Social programs such as those instituted in Uganda seem to have been successful. However, the region is still experiencing 1.3 million new infections annually, More than the rest of the world combined. Several countries in southern Africa still have infection rates exceeding 20% of the population, and in spite of the World Health Organizations ambitious plan to supply all in need of anti-retroviral drugs, as of 2009 only 3.2 million, less than half those in need, were receiving the drugs.

To continue the success of the last several years will require resources from outside of Africa, and here the news is not so good. The slow economic recovery in the United States and the debt crisis in Europe will likely have a negative effect on near-future funding.

While the over all picture has improved there are troubling signs in West Africa, which until now has been spared the severity of the epidemic in eastern and southern Africa. In Nigeria, the continents most populous country, there are three million known cases, a small percentage of the population, but the lack of attention by the government during the early period of the epidemic leads many to suspect that there may be many more in the latent stage of HIV. President Obsango finally launched an anti-AIDS program in 2001, which focused on testing, and providing anti retroviral drugs to prevent transmission to children. As of 2007 it was estimated that only 7% of mothers with HIV were receiving these drugs to prevent transmission to their children. Obsango's goal is to have 100% coverage of children by 2015. If followed through with adequate funding, this could head off a crisis greater than the current crisis in Southern Africa. What contributes to skepticism about a positive outcome in Nigeria is their ranking in the United Nation's Development Program's human poverty index of 158th out of 177 nations. In the past, corruption has kept Nigeria's considerable oil wealth from reaching those in most need.

Another exception to the good news about Aids is the former Soviet Union, especially Russia. While prevalence rates in sub-Saharan Africa have dropped from a high of 5.8% to 5.2% Rates in Russia have nearly doubled. This comparison is even more stark when you consider the rapid growth of population in Africa compared with a static or declining population in Russia. In the mid-90s when Russia and Eastern Europe were in Chaos from the breakup of the Soviet Union, Drugs began flowing from Afghanistan. In Russia and Ukraine as well as much of the rest of eastern Europe, HIV has been spread by drug users sharing needles. It is now being spread out of the drug users circle into the general population, initially by prostitutes who were themselves often drug users or had clients who were drug users. As we will discuss later in chapter eight, infection from needle sharing is a problem with a solution, government dispensed clean needles. However, as we will also discuss in chapter eight, there are powerful objections to these seeming endorsements of immoral behavior. In Russia much of the objection comes from a revitalized and powerful Orthodox church.

The crisis in Russia illustrates the importance of government action in the fight against AIDS. It also reminds us of the importance of having wealth to apply to the problem. The collapse of the Soviet Union caused a precipitous fall in the Russian economy, accompanied by chaos in government as Russians attempted to institute a free market economy to replace the failed command economy. Along with this came relatively low oil prices which were good for much of the world but devastating for a major producer of oil like Russia. Today there is a stable, if less than democratic, government in Russia. With about one million AIDS cases and the fresh entry of AIDS into the general population, Russia must act quickly. President Medvedev has publicly committed to funding a battle against AIDS, but has been slow to take specific measures. It is not too much to say that the fate of Russia may hinge on whether he follows through. Russia with about 145 million people occupies by far the largest land mass in the world. It already faces a staggering demographic crisis with a birth rate of 1.4 children per woman. A disease that not only kills many people, but especially devastates the most productive age group is not something that Russia could likely survive in tact.

Good News for Treatment

The development of anti-retroviral drugs to slow and arrest the development of the disease has been the biggest victory in the AIDS war. There is no cure; AIDS is for a lifetime and as we have said before, until the development of anti-retroviral drugs that was a very short lifetime. During the past year more hopeful news has come from the medical front. There is still no pill, vaccine or other means that will provide perfect protection from AIDS, but recent breakthroughs may provide protection that improves the odds.

Perhaps most intriguing is the development by Gilead Sciences of a pill, Truvada. This pill was administered to 2499 men in Brazil, Ecuador, Peru, South Africa, Thailand, Boston, and San Francisco over a three year period. While the pill did not prevent infection, it did reduce the rate of infection by 44%. An interesting problem emerged when testing to see how much of the drug was actually in the participant's systems. It was established that of the 36 infected people who were on the drug, two had been infected before the trial began and of the remainder only three had any of the drug in their system. This suggests that most of the infected participants had not taken the pill or at least had not taken it consistently. This means that the pill may have been over 90% effective. Follow up showed that a high percentage of participants had lied about taking the pill. Side effects seemed minor, although some men stopped taking the pill when they experienced headaches or nausea.

There are now follow up trials to try to replicate the success of the Initial study. The big problem, if the current trials confirm the efficacy of the pills, is the cost. Truvada, patented by Gilead sciences, cost $12,000–$14,000 per year. When considering that this pill is for prevention not treatment, the question is who will pay for it? Globally, of the 33 million infected with HIV only about five million are receiving anti-retroviral drugs. These are people already infected, what are the chances of poor governments in sub-Saharan Africa or Eastern Europe spending this kind of money on people who are not infected? Even in rich countries like the United States medicaid and medicare do not provide preventative drugs. Given the current health care debate that is not likely to change.

Another breakthrough is the development of a vaginal gel that has been tested in South Africa. The gel reduced infection rates by almost half at the end of a one year follow up study. Because humans are involved, the studies are not perfect. Just as with Truvada, participants were not all consistent in using the gel. There does seem to be a correlation between those using the gel most consistently and reduced infection rates. An added bonus was the reduction by half of genital herpes infections.

It is important to remember that these hopeful developments are tentative. This is illustrated by another breakthrough based upon tests of a vaccine in Thailand. Over a six year study the vaccine RV144 reduced infection rates by about a third. However, it seems to not work as well over time, and it does not protect a high enough percentage to be licensed. It may be that the vaccine simply wears out and must be renewed on a regular basis. These developments have a common problem; they require human behavioral changes to be effective. In the case of the vaccine, users must not become reckless because it provides only partial protection. The danger is that reckless behavior will become more common, negating the statistical advantage provided by the vaccine. This is also true of the gel and the pill, with the added problem that users must become disciplined to use these products on a regular basis.

For a long time there has been evidence that circumcision reduces the vulnerability of men to infection. This was confirmed by trials in Uganda and Kenya. The trials showed that circumcised men were 60% less likely to become infected. This has lead to an aggressive campaign in Botswanna to circumcise 500,000 men by 2012. Zambia, Lesotho, and Swaziland, areas with extremely high infection rates, have made it official government policy to encourage circumcision.

As encouraging as these developments are, they do not represent a solution to the AIDS problem. As stated earlier, AIDS is a very difficult disease. Because no one has ever recovered from AIDS, there is no natural mechanism to study and replicate. As we have suggested, the above breakthroughs may create new problems for social scientists fighting the AIDS epidemic. How do we get people to apply gels and take pills on a regular basis? A more serious problem is that all of the above breakthroughs do not provide 100% protection, but may encourage risky behavior. As seen in the gay community in the United States after the development of anti-retroviral drugs, there was a significant increase in risky behavior.

This is not to belittle these scientific breakthroughs which besides offering improved protection may be steps on the way to a 100% effective drug. In the long run the answer will be a scientific breakthrough that will provide 100% protection at a price affordable by everyone. That breakthrough appears to be many years in the future. In the meantime there is a major role for social scientists and policy makers to create the kind of change that will reverse the horrifying trends of this disease. That problem will be the concern of the next seven chapters of this book.

Summary

In this chapter we discussed the basic biology of HIV-AIDS and some of the characteristics of the disease: how it spread and how it did not spread. As we saw, the disease is not airborne; you cannot get it from people sneezing or from mosquitoes. It is spread through both heterosexual and homosexual sex, through tainted blood, intravenous drug injection and from mother to child through birthing and nursing. There is no cure and finding a cure will be difficult because of the dynamic nature of the virus which has mutated into several different forms. The global economy is a major factor in the rapid spread of the disease which now exists on every inhabited continent, although Africa remains by far the worst affected area. The are two hopeful developments: progress in developing vaccines, gels and pills that have some protective benefits, and progress in educating and changing behaviors that seem to have caused some decline in new infections in the worst hit areas of Africa. However, the disease is growing in some areas, notably Russia.

Study Questions

1. Where does the evidence suggest that AIDS began?

2. Why is it so difficult to develop a vaccine for AIDS?

3. True or false: AIDS is often transmitted by mosquitoes in Africa.

4. Why is homosexual sex generally more of a risk factor for AIDS than heterosexual sex?

5. What is the difference between HIV-1 and HIV-2?

6. How does male circumcision affect the transmission of HIV?

7. How does intravenous drug use spread HIV?

8. What is the difference between HIV and AIDS?

9. Is it true that no one dies of AIDS? Explain.

10. What are problems with the new AIDS pill?

11. How has AIDS achieved a foothold in Russia?

12. How are rising and falling oil prices likely to influence the fight against AIDS in Russia?

13. Why is a vaccine a better solution than a pill or gel?

Chapter two | Cultural Construction of HIV/AIDS

Cultural Meaning of HIV/AIDS

Although AIDS is a real disease syndrome, the very meaning of AIDS is constructed through language. The disseminated discourse and knowledge on AIDS forms and formulates the social and cultural meanings of AIDS. In other words, we understand and interpret AIDS "through" language. Hence AIDS is not only an epidemic of a transmissible fatal disease, but also an epidemic of meanings or signification (Triechler 1987).

In the United States, upon the outbreak of HIV/AIDS, AIDS was constructed in such a sensational way that it caused much of the U.S. population to believe that they could catch AIDS through casual contact, such as shaking hands with an infected person or sitting next to an infected person on a bus. Because AIDS was first named as GRID—Gay-Related Immune Deficiency—in the epidemiological reports, AIDS was referred to as a "gay plague." The Centers for Disease Control referred to AIDS as a "4 H disease," linking AIDS with homosexuals, Haitians, heroin users, and hemophiliacs. By December 1986, the major U.S. news magazines were reporting on the danger of AIDS to heterosexuals as their cover stories (Triechler 1987).

This social construction of AIDS is not based upon objective science, but upon social discourses generated within biomedical science (Triechler 1987). It was committed to categories based on stereotyped identities rather than human behaviors. It was perceived and constructed as alien and exotic by scientists, physicians, and journalists. The gay population, who were conceived as promiscuous and perverted, made it convincible that AIDS was an out-of-ordinary disease. The connection between sex, death, and homosexuality made AIDS a story of cultural metaphor.

In the "geography of blame" (Farmer 1992), the origin of AIDS was constructed as the "exotic" and "promiscuous" African culture, and the Haitians were listed as a high-risk population. Doctors Seigal and Seigal implicated Haiti as the origin of AIDS on the basis of three cases of transfusion-related transmission and the case of a former nun whose sole sexual contact was said to have been in Haiti. From this "compelling" evidence, they extrapolated that "the disease is quite prevalent in Haiti; that it predates AIDS in the United States; and that it may be endemic there."

As Farmer contends, the U.S. public and medical doctors were so willing to classify Haitians as a high-risk group because of the stereotypes of Haitians, and Africans in general, as the Exotic Other. North American scientists linked the spread of AIDS with a panoply of exotic behaviors allegedly related to African culture. For instance, they claimed that Haitian women added menstrual blood to the food and drink of partners to prevent them from straying. Haitians contracted AIDS from monkeys as part of bizarre sexual practices in Haitian brothels. They also claimed that other sources of infection included ingestion of sacrificial animal blood, the eating of cats, and ritualized homosexuality. However, none of these are actual social practices among Haitians! In 1987, the Collaborative Study Group of AIDS in Haitian-Americans released a report titled "Folklore rituals have been suggested as potential risk factors for HTLV-III/LAV transmission in Haiti. Our data do not support this hypothesis" (Farmer 1992).

The epidemiologists' identification of the Haitians as the risk group, according to Farmer, has led to an epidemic of blame and accusation. The cost to the Haitian community included loss of jobs, eviction from rented housing, and violence against the Haitians, bringing about pain, suffering, and even death to the Haitians. In 1984, the prejudice against Haitians mounted. The AIDS Discrimination Unit of the New York City Commission on Human Rights described the effect on Haitian communities as devastating: "Haitian children have been beaten up (and in at least one case, shot) in school; Haitian store owners have gone bankrupt as their businesses failed; and Haitian families have been evicted from their homes." Graffiti on the walls of a predominantly Caribbean Brooklyn neighborhood read: "Haitians = Niggers with AIDS."

The Public Health Service recommended that Haitian-Americans refrain from donating blood. School blood drives openly excluded Haitian adolescents. In April of 1985, under mounting pressure from Haitian communities and activists, the Centers for Disease Control removed the term "Haitian" as a risk-group designation. However, community leaders were quick to point out that the stigma remained. In particular, the FDA (Food and Drug Administration) continued to bar Haitians from donating blood. In February of 1990, the FDA expanded restriction on Haitian blood donation. Previously, only Haitians who had come to the United States after 1977 were prohibited from donating. A *New York Times* article headline read, "Now, No Haitians Can Donate Blood." In March, more than 5,000 Haitian-Americans marched outside of the FDA office in Miami. In April, 50,000 people marched in New York City to protest the FDA's discriminatory decision to exclude Haitians from the list of potential blood donors. In December, the FDA formally rescinded its ban of Haitian blood.

Sontag noted that "It has been common to associate dreaded diseases with foreignness" (Sontag 1989: 54), and "There is a link between imagining disease and imagining foreignness,"—the alien, as "an exotic, often primitive place" (Sontag 1989: 48, 51). Sontag states that epidemic disease usually elicits a call to ban the entry of foreigners and immigrants. "Xenophobic propaganda has always depicted immigrants as bearers of disease" (Sontag 1989: 62).

In the West, including the nation of Australia, cultural construction of AIDS reflects a fear of homosexuality, prostitution, drugs, deviance, and a sense of xenophobia (Lupton 1994). To get AIDS is to be revealed as a member of a certain "high-risk group"—"a community of pariahs," who indulge in delinquent and deviant behaviors (Sontag 1989: 24–25).

Similarly, in other parts of the world, it is the foreigners that are at the center of the blame in the cultural constructions of AIDS. The Soviet Union attributed AIDS to American biological warfare research and hence deemed AIDS a "foreign problem" (Stine 2007). In the Caribbean, AIDS was widely believed to result from U.S. biological testing (Triechler 1987).

In Malawi, the discourse on AIDS blames an unspecified cabal of wealthy countries that intend to wipe out the African population. Due to the colonial history, many Africans disbelieve foreign governments. They believe that condoms from overseas bring the disease with them, and that free condoms are filled with germs so that they can spread AIDS. According to them, foreign governments that donate condoms put holes in them so that Africans will die (Stine 2007).

In India, facing the onslaught of HIV infections at the end of the 1980s, the director general of the Indian government's Council for Medical Research declared, "This is a totally foreign disease, and the only way to stop its spread is to stop sexual contact between Indians and foreigners" (Sontag 1989: 80). Media in South Korea also invoked the menace of AIDS from the outside and the fear of foreign sexual contamination (Cheng 2005a). Their neighbor nation Japan has construed AIDS as a foreign disease because it was introduced from the outside, primarily the United States, through infected blood products, and hence they blamed foreigners, especially migrant sex workers, for sexual transmission of HIV (Buckley 1997). Since the emergence of AIDS in China, discourses have also targeted foreigners and immoral Chinese women as vectors and transmitters of the disease. Other countries such as Taiwan, Thailand, Nepal, and the Philippines also echoed this pattern (Hsu 2004; Pigg 2001; Smyth 1998).

Blaming foreigners and immoral women as vectors and transmitters of HIV/AIDS confirms Paul Farmer's theory of "geography of blame," and Carol Vance and Leclerc-Madlala's argument about the danger of women's sexuality and women as the agents of pollution (Farmer 1993; Leclerc-Madlala 2001b; Vance 1982).

Construction of AIDS as a disease of certain "high-risk groups" rather than high-risk behaviors has led to marginalization, essentialization, and stigmatization of the "deviant" groups as both the culprit and the object of blame (see also Porter 1997). A focus on risk groups rather than risky behaviors not only carries the wrong message to the public, making people outside of the categories believe they are not at risk, but also serves to demonize, blame, and stigmatize certain groups (see Lyttleton 1996; Parker 1987). As illustrated above, in the United States, in the history of HIV/AIDS, gay men, Haitians, and Africans were placed in the "high-risk" category, stripped of other identities, discriminated against and dehumanized. Such a construction helps maintain the social hierarchy of the mainstream and the marginalized, and leaves the risky behaviors of the "general population" unchallenged.

Cultural Reaction to HIV/AIDS

In the United States, after AIDS first emerged in 1981, the nation was not ready to talk about subjects like anal sex, needles, and condoms. Because health officials and journalists used the phrase "bodily fluids," which did not specify semen, blood, and vaginal secretions, many people feared that they could contract AIDS from toilet seats, drinking fountains, eating at restaurants, or going to school.

Many gay men were heavily in denial in the 1970s because they were enjoying sexual liberation to subvert social marginalization for their sexual identity. Blood banks, in view of economic considerations, rejected the extra precautions of blood screening that were necessary to prevent transmission. Progress was also thwarted by scientists who withheld information from health officials in order to compete with one another to be first to publish articles in medical journals with exclusive information. AIDS was buried deep inside newspapers and seldom mentioned on television. President Reagan did not deliver a formal speech on AIDS until 1986. The death of movie star Rock Hudson in 1985 finally put AIDS on the front pages. Still, three young hemophiliacs, Ricky, Robert, and Randy Ray, were driven out of their home in Florida when their neighbors learned they were HIV positive. Even when there was convincing evidence that AIDS could not be transmitted by casual contact, HIV positive people were still fired from their jobs across the country, because of fear of a potential threat to co-workers.

In South Africa, where millions of men, women, and children were infected with HIV, in 2000, President Thabo Mbeki proclaimed that he supported a discredited view that challenged the role of HIV as the cause of AIDS. This alternative view originated from scientist Peter Duesberg, who was certain that the scientific community was investigating the wrong causative agent. According to him, HIV is not the cause of AIDS. Duesberg believed that the disease did not result from a single causative agent, but from a person's lifestyle, especially related to drug use, malnutrition, parasitic infections, and other specific risks. Along with Duesberg, a physician named Robert Willner also claimed that no scientific evidence supported the fact that HIV causes any disease.

As a new form of public denial, President Thabo Mbeki took up this alternative theory and declared that HIV was harmless and that AIDS was a phony epidemic. To the chagrin of doctors and scientists in his own country and around the world, he announced that there was no such epidemic or deaths from AIDS. He believed that it was a conspiracy among international pharmaceutical companies propelled by political and medical self-interest that led to this mass hysteria. Rather than the AIDS epidemic, Mbeki claimed that it was poverty that constituted the only endangering element to the health of Africans. As a result of his denial of an AIDS epidemic, the country suffered from massive numbers of death and orphans.

Three years later, in 2003, Mbeki proclaimed public withdrawal from his previous stand on the cause of AIDS. He shifted his position and announced that his cabinet would lead the fight against AIDS.

It is the alternative theory of AIDS—another cultural construction of AIDS that was led by scientist Duesberg and physician Robert Willner—that fueled the political and scientific uproar and commotion denying the existence of AIDS in South Africa. This alternative theory continues to undermine the constructive public health interventions put forward by this government. It confuses and obfuscates public health workers and activists who have committed themselves to the cause of eradicating and ending the epidemic. It also exerts a negative impact upon the morale of HIV positive patients and families. The influx of such an alternative theory also has a dangerous and harmful repercussion on the scientific development in a developing country, especially while the developing country is still on the route to establishing a strong scientific research base. It also dissuades investors from providing funding in the country and hence leads to a dire and more dreadful financial and economic situation (Stine 2007).

Cultural Understanding of HIV/AIDS

United States

In the United States, when the AIDS news broke out, religious people described it as a means of punishment from God. According to them, because the victims engaged in immoral sexual behaviors, they were targets of God's wrath. In the story, Jesus punishes them by striking down the unjust and showering arrows on them from heaven.

Haiti

In Haiti, people blame AIDS on the supernatural force of witchcraft and sorcery (Farmer 1992). Witchcraft could work in numerous ways. For instance, you have done something bad and have been bewitched. Your neighbor's jealousy has invaded you. You have not appeased your ancestors, so they have cursed you. Some believe that it was introduced by the white population as a way to control black Africans after the history of apartheid.

The following story will help illustrate how sorcery works (Farmer 1992). Etienne, a poor farmer on the brink of starvation, experienced a tragedy: his only pig died. Etienne determined that someone had given his pig *kola*, a poison. Other villagers were unconvinced, believing that his pig had died of natural causes. Nevertheless, Etienne fingered his wealthier neighbor across the road, Rezima. Later, three of Rezima's six pigs died. Etienne was suspected of foul play. Then, one morning, he discovered a gourd with his wife's kerchief tied to its stem placed in the front room. The gourd was marked with strange symbols. Etienne later succumbed to AIDS and died. The villagers unanimously agreed on the etiology of his illness: Etienne died of sorcery-induced disease (Farmer 1992).

Belief in sorcery is shared by most rural Haitians, in the social backdrop of a fierce competition among powerless people with scarce resources (Farmer 1992). Farmer notes that in a field of great scarcity and a zero-sum setting, one person's fortune is manifestly another's ill fortune, and the price for wealth is poverty for another (Farmer 1992).

Africa

In the Central African Republic, the immune system is shown surrounding the human figure like a rope. Viruses are pictured as beaked and bat-like birds, eating through the protective boundary.

In 1987, a Brazilian magazine graphic portrayed HIV attacking cells that looked like Caspar, the Friendly Ghost. This was a popular way of illustrating the immune system in 1950s medical textbooks.

In Malawi, gossip about AIDS revolves around wealthy men who purchase the favors of schoolgirls and thereby infect them, and well-dressed and conceited urban women who enjoy a number of admirers and sexual partners.

In Botswana, people describe AIDS as the radio disease because it is widely publicized but not yet experienced. Though it is associated with violation of sexual proprieties, traditional healers proclaim that they have to wait until the disease becomes more common to decide whether it should be diagnosed as a traditional Tswana disease or as a modern disease.

Cultural Factors of HIV/AIDS Transmission

There has been a growing focus in anthropological works on the impact of cultural factors as central and crucial to fully understanding sexual transmission of HIV (see Micollier 2004a; Parker 2001). The meaning of sex, sexual culture, sexual practices, gender relationships, condom use, and so on all constitute the cultural factors that have repercussions on sexual transmission of HIV.

Sexual Cultures

In many parts of the world, the culturally prescribed sex roles allow men to have multiple sex partners and encourage women to be virgins before marriage. Studies have shown that in countries such as South Africa, Mexico, China, and Brazil, girls are inculcated with moral values about the perils of sex and the need to wait until later in life, preferably until marriage, to be sexually active (Inciardi 2000). This is a cultural effort to protect women's virginity, and social order as a whole.

Men in Mexico describe themselves as hunters by nature—"A man could be sexual with little consequences" (Carrillo 2002: 46). Research of men in Mexico has also revealed that men favor the excitement of sexual transgression (Carrillo 2002). Sexual transgression is special because of the background of sexual silence in their society—the prevalence of a social environment not conducive to open, formal communication about sexuality among adults or sexual partners (Carrillo 2002: 149). In Mexico, it is the culture of sexual silence that contributes to an excitement associated with transgression, as it "flavors cultural scripts about seduction, sexual passion, and the enactment of sex itself" (Carrillo 2002: 149).

In Brazil, a virgin is defined solely by her lack of sexual experience, innocence, and her intact hymen. The unbroken hymen is testament to the control her male relatives exercise over her. Upon marriage, the breaking of the hymen symbolizes that the control of her sexuality is transferred from her father to her husband (Inciardi 2000). The Brazilian definition of masculinity embodies the characteristics of the male role of force, power, violence, aggression, virility, and sexual potency (Inciardi 2000). In the context of sexual culture in Brazil, it is not uncommon for macho men to have sex with their wives, mistresses, female and male prostitutes, and male transvestite sex workers (Inciardi 2000).

Research in South Africa has also pointed out that social constructions of masculinity promote the norm that men need sex and women should refuse sex outside of committed relationships (Campbell 2001; Moore 1992; Ramazanoglu 1993; Wilton 1991). Women are brought up to be subservient to men (Stine 2007). In matters related to sex, men are always in charge and women feel powerless. Even when a woman wants to protect herself, she is usually not able to do so, because it is not uncommon for men to beat partners who refuse intercourse or request a condom. According to the cultural belief, a real man does not use condoms. For a woman, talking to her partner about condom use will invite accusations of infidelity, abuse, or abandonment (Stine 2007).

In South Africa, society classifies "normal" men as having multiple partners and power over women. Young men are expected to adopt this masculine sexuality and overcome emotional vulnerabilities in order to be accepted as masculine in the society (Holland 1994a). In schools, male teachers can pick sexual partners easily, and female students are aware that they can profit from a teacher's favor with a good grade. Female students also consider it an honor to sleep with teachers.

As Linda Gordon contends, "It is easier and more 'normal' for men to be lustful and assertive, for women merely to surrender, to be carried away by a greater force" (Gordon 1979: 126). Scholars have argued that male violence and coercion with condom-less sex is more prevalent in developing countries (Campbell 2001). Entrenched in such a cultural environment—coercive and obligatory sex for women, and multiple sexual partners for men—increases their risk of sexual transmission of HIV.

Sexual Practices

Studies of parts of Africa have shown that condoms are seen to disrupt the underlying value of sexual exchange because condoms preclude the semen from entering the vagina (Kalipeni 2004: 65). In northern Tanzania, sex is like a market transaction for the young men because it is a woman's bargain to take a man's semen (Kalipeni 2004: 65; Setel 1999). Using a condom in this context is "like getting cheated in a deal" (Setel 1999: 1175).

Other culturally defined sexual practices also enhance risks for HIV transmission. For instance, women in parts of sub-Saharan Africa practice painful dry sex to please men. Women try to dry their vaginas by sitting in basins of bleach or salt water, or stuffing astringent herbs, tobacco, or fertilizer inside their vaginas. Some women use drying agents such as soil mixed with baboon urine obtained from traditional healers, while others use detergents, salt, cotton, or shredded newspaper. As a result, the tissue of the lining swells up and natural lubricants dry out. The resulting dry sex is painful and dangerous for women. The drying agents that are used to suppress natural friction easily lacerate the tender walls of the vagina and suppress the vagina's natural bacteria. The extra friction caused by dry sex also makes it easy for condoms to break and tear.

Research of the Bulawayo women has revealed that to satisfy men with dry sex, women suffer lower abdominal pain and internal infections. Other side effects include sores on female genitals, bruised skin, vaginal swelling, cuts and abrasions. Women are reluctant to use condoms because condoms would block the "love potion" effects of the agents and stop their magic. Despite these health sacrifices, women continue to use drying agents because of the positive effect on men's libido. They believe that the effects of drying agents attract and keep a sexual partner (Civic 1996).

In Zimbabwe, a woman explained that it was not her choice to use dry sex to please her man. Rather, it was because men enjoyed it. She said, "Our African husbands enjoy sex with a dry vagina" (Stine 2007). She used herbs from the Mugugudhu tree. She ground the stem and leaf, mixed a pinch of the powder with water, wrapped it in a piece of nylon stocking, and inserted it into her vagina for 10 to 15 minutes. The herbs swelled the soft tissues of the vagina to dry it out. This makes sex very painful (Stine 2007).

Many African women admit that dry sex hurts, but it is a common sexual practice throughout southern Africa. According to researchers on dry sex in Zimbabwe, it was very difficult to find a group of women who were not practicing some form of dry sex (Stine 2007).

Dry sex increases the incidents of HIV infection for women, who are already twice as likely as men to contract the virus from a single encounter. In southern Africa, women are unable to negotiate sex, and they find it imperative to risk infection to please the man. The stark gender inequality in sexual practices contributes to the spread of HIV. Because the cultural practice of dry sex enhances the likelihood of HIV infection, it is not surprising that southern Africa is plagued with the AIDS epidemic.

Trust and Unprotected Sex

It has been proven on a global scale that the nature of the relationship influences condom use. Condoms are much less acceptable to couples involved in cohabiting or romantic relationships, and non-condom use is justified by trusting relationships (Blecher 1995; Campbell 1995; Campbell 2001;

Cohen 1996; Worth 1989). In fact, condom use decreases as a relationship grows more stable and more intimate over time.

Studies in South Africa, Cameroon, and Zambia have demonstrated that interviewees exhibit strong negative attitudes toward condom use in these kinds of relationships (Agha 1997; Calves 1999, 2004a; Maharaj 2004b). In Zambia, trusting partners is the most commonly cited reason for non-use of condoms (64%) (Agha 1997). In London, Manchester, Tanzania, and Khutsong, interviewees classified their new relationships as serious and incorporated issues of trust to justify their non-condom sex (Campbell 2001; Holland 1990, 1991, 1994a, 1994b; Klein 1999).

Research in Tanzania has revealed that the extent to which one trusts one's partner can explain the lack of protective behavior (Klein 1999). The focus groups in the research centered on the meaning of trust and how it interfered with condom use. Young people in the group referred to their partners' general characteristics and behaviors such as church attendance and dress to determine whether their partners were deserving of their sexual trust. As a result, although they lacked concrete knowledge of their partners' sexual history or HIV status, the generalized interpersonal trust in their partners reduced the sense of risk associated with unprotected sex. Partners felt safe from infection because they generally "trusted" that their partner had goodwill toward them and would not intentionally infect them (Klein 1999).

Trust is defined by Moim et al. as "expectations that an exchange partner will behave benignly, based on the attribution of positive dispositions and intentions to the partner in a situation of uncertainty and risk" (Klein 1999). Most often, trust develops when one exposes oneself to a small amount of risk. Over time, as partners repeatedly behave benignly toward each other, they increase not only the trust they have developed for each other, but also the risk they are willing to take with each other.

In the focus group in Tanzania, young adults found it hard to address their sexual history and expectations for their partners because such discussions could potentially leave them open to rejection (Klein 1999). They assumed that their partners would reciprocate their sexual health and monogamy. This reciprocal trust was made possible because of the lengthy latent period of STD and HIV that had led partners to assume that they were free from infection.

Research in Baltimore, Maryland, has also shown that a number of low-income African-American women were reluctant to request condom use from their male partners (Wiutehead 1997). Their reluctance was based on their need or desire to maintain their ongoing relationships, and the fear that men would leave them because of their strong dislike of condoms. Women were also very cautious about initiating condom use in their sexual practices because they feared that men would associate such practices with a woman being "sexually loose." If a woman initiated discussions of condoms, she ran the risk of being suspected of promiscuity. Men interpreted this action as an insinuation that the women had been sleeping around and carrying diseases (Wiutehead 1997). Therefore, women were afraid to bring up condom use for fear that it could threaten the survival of the relationship. Research in Greece (Paxson 2002: 319) has also shown that for a woman to introduce condoms into marital relations could be seen as shedding doubt on her own or her spouse's sexual fidelity.

Research has also shown that people rely upon their intuition and cultural stereotypes to judge whether a person has STDs or HIV. People are ready to drop their guard in the absence of any intuitive red flags. Those red flags would have risen if a partner had evoked the person's stereotypes about who has STDs or HIV (see Carrillo 2002: 253). In South Africa, young men in Khutsong rely on appearance and reputation to make decisions about certain women being safe and therefore not requiring condoms for sexual intercourse (Campbell 2001). Men in Mexico were reported to trust a clean, respectable, nice, and healthy person, and mistrust someone who is dirty, poor, and badly educated (Carrillo 2002: 248–249). People in Tanzania (Klein 1999) refer to a person's general characteristics and behaviors such as church attendance and dress to determine whether s/he is deserving of sexual trust (Longfield 2002). Young people in South Africa also believe that they can filter out partners dangerous to their health through categories of "clean" or "unclean" based on their social interactions and appearance (Waldby 1993).

Studies conducted in sub-Saharan Africa have reported high levels of infection in committed sexual relationships. This is because cultural meanings associated with condoms have thwarted the acceptability and use of condoms in married and cohabiting relationships. People in general believe that committed relationships do not pose any risks for HIV/STD infections. Condoms are less acceptable in these relationships because of people's strong negative attitudes toward the use of condoms within committed relationships. Condom use is strongly related to lack of trust. For this reason, both men and women interpret condom use as offensive and suggestive of infidelity. People are not willing to jeopardize their relationships with condom use because introducing the idea of condom use would raise suspicions of infidelity. Studies have shown that in many regions of east Africa, condoms are seen as symbols of promiscuity. Asking one's partner to use a condom is tantamount to accusations or admissions of sexual promiscuity (Kalipeni 2004: 65).

Researchers have revealed widespread resistance to condom use, especially within marriage, because condom use is perceived as representing a lack of trust between partners and suggests that one partner might have an STI. Suspicions arising from condom use will create tensions, anger, and confrontation between partners. Insistence on condom use is perilous and ominous as it conveys infidelity, disease, and mistrust to their partners.

Pursuit of Sexual Pleasure

Research around the world has revealed that unprotected sex arises from people's worry that condoms inhibit sexual enjoyment. There is a great deal of concern about the reduction in pleasure with condom use from both men and women. For instance, studies have shown that both men and women perceive condoms as impeding sexual pleasure (Kalipeni 2004: 65).

In countries such as Thailand, China, and Greece, wives are considered responsible for contraception. The prevailing gender norms and expectations of masculinity make it difficult for many men to accommodate condom use, especially because they believe that condom use interferes with sexual pleasure. For instance, research in China (Qu 2002) has found that the notion of preserving male comfort is a recurring theme in the focus-group transcripts. Many men complain about the attenuation of pleasure due to condom use.

It was reported that there was a surge of unprotected sex among gay men in large American cities, because of the pursuit of absolute sexual pleasure (Stine 2007); and it was reported that unsafe sex among gay men increased from 35% in 1994 to 55% in early 1999. The 1999 statistics also showed that 66% of gay men surveyed had unsafe sex during the previous 18 months. The *San Francisco Chronicle*, in 1999, reported a story about an $8 admission for a night of communal sex, with no clothes, no condoms, and no discussion of HIV (Stine 2007). The article also mentioned an Internet link that offered gay men an extreme sex party where the erotic allure was to become infected or infect another with HIV. It was also reported that three uninfected men had sex with five others, one of which was HIV positive, in a Russian Roulette Party (Stine 2007).

An empty blister pack of Viagra was discovered in a gay sex club during a health inspection. It was said that the drug use might have fueled the unsafe sexual behavior and an increase in HIV and other diseases. It was also speculated that it might have something to do with the success of the therapy of HAART (Highly Active Anti-Retroviral Therapy). Because HAART decreases mortality and improves the quality of the HIV infected people's lives, it has increased the number of people living with HIV who are engaging in sexual activities. As a result, gay men were less concerned about contracting HIV, and HIV-positive gay men were less concerned about transmitting HIV. Therefore, both groups were less cautious and were more likely to engage in unsafe sex (Stine 2007).

Despite the fact that the use of HAART reduced possibilities of HIV transmission by 60%, it was reported that the increase in unsafe sex rose from about 6% in 2000 to 25% in 2003 during the same time period. It became worrisome that the behavioral change from protected to unprotected anal sex had counteracted the benevolent effects of HAART (Stine 2007). As researchers point out (Stine 2007), the photos of buff HIV-positive men in the ads were deceiving because they dismissed and concealed the real struggles and sufferings of the HIV-infected people. The fact is, most HIV-infected people on drug cocktails hardly had any time on their own. Their daily routines were preoccupied with dealing with the HIV virus by responding to negative side effects of the drugs and meeting with medical doctors. In the mornings, they stayed in the bathroom, suffering from the side effects of the drugs with vomiting or diarrhea. In the afternoons, they headed to the doctors' appointments, clinics, and pharmacies. In the evenings, they were busy working and trying to survive financially due to their ill health and the high price of the HAART.

Migration and Unsafe Sex

Research has suggested that migrant labor is central to the HIV/AIDS epidemic in Africa (Kalipeni 2004; Setel 1999). Migrant labor was established in eastern, central, and southern Africa to support the mining, agricultural plantations, and other economic activities (Kalipeni 2004: 54). As a result, a large number of migrant laborers, mainly young men, left their families and hometowns to work under a long-term contract of one to three years. During these years, their wives in the rural home were responsible for raising children and taking care of the old in the absence of their husbands. The women's limited ability sometimes led to declining fecundity of the land, and eventually a shortage of food and malnutrition. As a result, such women often ended up migrating to the city. Among the few options available to them, some engaged in prostitution for economic survival, which exposed them to high-risk behaviors for possible HIV transmission.

Male migrant workers usually resorted to alcohol and visits to prostitutes to attenuate their loneliness and regain the lost manhood that they had enjoyed back in their rural hometowns (Campbell 2000). Male workers had easy access to prostitutes or a town wife with whom they formed a second family, and from whom they contracted a STD or HIV. Without knowing that they were carrying the virus, they went back home to their wives and girlfriends and transmitted the virus to them.

Research has shown that male migrant workers in underground mines viewed "flesh to flesh" sex as necessary for a man's good health (Campbell 2000). In other words, flesh-to-flesh sex could maintain balanced levels of blood and sperm within the body. Male informants contended that the accumulated sperm would lead to a range of mental and physical problems. They regarded flesh-to-flesh sex as the only pleasurable way of meeting male sexual desires, and they perceived condoms as cold and unpleasant. The kind of masculinity associated with physical strength and bravery through flesh-to-flesh sex served as a key coping mechanism for miners to deal with the harsh, dangerous, and lonely working conditions of underground mining (Campbell 2000).

For men and women in eastern, central, and southern Africa, long-term separation and dire economic conditions have fostered dislocation of families, instability of marriages, increased sexual partners for men and women, and engagement of high-risk sexual behaviors. In short, it is migration and economic and labor markets that put both men and women under increasing risks for HIV transmission.

Sex Education in the United States

It is reported that around 4 million new STD infections occur among teenagers in the United States each year. Currently, there is no federal program dedicated to supporting comprehensive sex education that teaches young people about both abstinence and contraception. While it is abstinence that state curricula emphasize and teachers cover the most in the classroom, other topics are less likely to be covered, such as sexual identity and orientation, sexual response, masturbation, and abortion.

Studies have shown that teachers fail to meet students' needs due to the restrictions and requirements imposed on sex education.

In the United States, sex education is not required in 32 states. Ten of these 32 states demand that if sex education is taught, it must include abstinence. Yet there is no requirement to include information about contraception: 86% of the public school districts require that abstinence be promoted in teaching sex education; 35% require that abstinence be taught as the only option and prohibit the discussion of contraception, and 51% demand that abstinence be taught as the preferred option.

Abstinence-only sex education has become more common in the United States over the past ten years because of the federal government funding initiatives. Between 1996 and 2006, the U.S. government directed more than a billion dollars to abstinence-only education programs via direct funding and other financial initiatives. In 1996, the federal government issued a provision to a welfare reform law, which initiated a special program to fund the states for abstinence-only-until-marriage programs. This special program was called Title V. It dedicated $50 million annually to participating states who were recipients of the grant.

Title V clearly stipulated specific requirements for grant awardees. Once funded, the programs were prohibited from advocating or discussing contraceptive methods unless the purpose was to emphasize their failure rates. According to this Title V, Section 510 programs, "abstinence education" means an educational or motivational program which:

- Has as its exclusive purpose teaching the social, psychological, and health gains to be realized by abstaining from sexual activity;
- Teaches abstinence from sexual activity outside marriage as the expected standard for all school-age children;
- Teaches that abstinence from sexual activity is the only certain way to avoid out-of-wedlock pregnancy, sexually transmitted diseases, and other associated health problems;
- Teaches that a mutually faithful monogamous relationship in the context of marriage is the expected standard of sexual activity;
- Teaches that sexual activity outside of the context of marriage is likely to have harmful psychological and physical effects;
- Teaches that bearing children out of wedlock is likely to have harmful consequences for the child, the child's parents, and society;
- Teaches young people how to reject sexual advances and how alcohol and drug use increase vulnerability to sexual advances; and
- Teaches the importance of attaining self-sufficiency before engaging in sexual activity.

Research conducted by the Kaiser Family Foundation in 2002 revealed that by 2002, about one-third of the U.S. secondary schools adopted the abstinence-only approach. In 2000, the federal government initiated another large program to fund abstinence education, which was called Community-Based Abstinence Education (CBAE). CBAE became the largest federally funded abstinence-only program, receiving $115 million for the year 2006. The awards went directly to state and local organizations that offered abstinence-only education programs in local public and private schools and local communities. Many were faith-based or small nonprofit organizations such as crisis pregnancy centers.

In 2004, U.S. President George W. Bush proclaimed his Five-Year Global HIV/AIDS Strategy. Among the $15 billion to be donated over a five-year period for AIDS relief in 15 countries in Africa and the Caribbean, and in Vietnam, one-third of the $3 billion prevention funding was designated specifically for abstinence-only-until-marriage programs. The United States also supports a foreign policy that discourages condom use and promotes abstinence-only education.

AIDS prevention activists have criticized this funding restriction. In 2006, this criticism was supported by a report by the U.S. Government Accountability Office, prodding Congress to lend more thought to the ways in which this funding should be spent.

According to the proponents of abstinence-only sex education, this approach is superior to comprehensive sex education for the following reasons. First, sex education, as they contend, should emphasize morality that confines sex within the sanctuary of marriage. Sex outside of marriage and sex at a young age can spawn physical costs and emotional stress. Comprehensive sex education, according to the proponents, would encourage premarital sexual activities among teenagers. Premarital activities, as they argue, have a deleterious effect on teenagers as they account for the phenomenon of teen pregnancy and widespread incurable STDs and HIV/AIDS.

Opponents and critics of the abstinence-only approach comprise eminent professionals in the fields of medicine, public health, and psychology. They argue that abstinence-only programs leave young people uninformed of the ways in which they can protect their health. They point out that religious beliefs should not impinge upon school education, and question the claim that comprehensive sex education encourages teens to engage in premarital sex. They also put forward the idea that, for people who are not interested in marriage or cannot get married because of legal and social implications that might apply to gays and lesbians, sexual intercourse should be an option available to them.

The federal funding of over $1 billion has made abstinence-only sex education more prominent in the United States over the last decade. This cultural context has an overriding effect on the kind of sex education young people receive in the United States. The abstinence-only approach limits the amount of knowledge young people can receive and hence mitigates their capability to protect themselves. As critics point out, the abstinence-only sex education stimulated by the federal funding has failed to delay the onset of sexual intercourse. Nor has it succeeded in its goal of increasing abstinence. Rather, it has led to a lack of adequate knowledge and information that has put teenagers at high risk for STD and HIV infections. As a result, as the statistics show, the United States has the highest rates of STDs and teen pregnancy in the developed world (Hunter 2005).

The following facts and diagrams are cited from "In Brief: Fact Sheet. Facts on American Teens' Sources of Information About Sex," February 2011, Guttmacher Institute.

In 2006, 87% of public and private high schools in the U.S. taught abstinence as the most effective method to avoid pregnancy, HIV and STDs in a required health education course.

65% of high schools taught about condom efficacy and 39% taught students how to correctly use a condom in a required health education course.

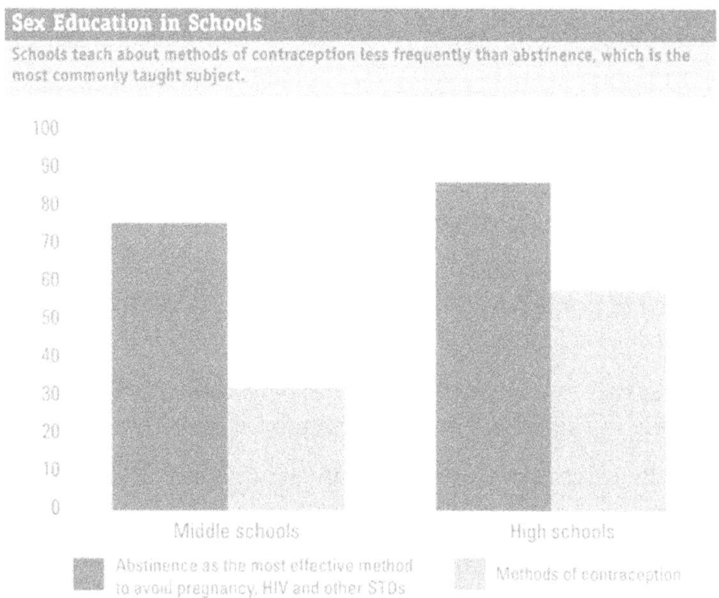

Source: Guttmacher Institute, Community health centers and family planning, In Brief, New York: Guttmacher, 2001, http://www.guttmacher.org/pubs/ib_6-01.html, accessed February 2, 2011.

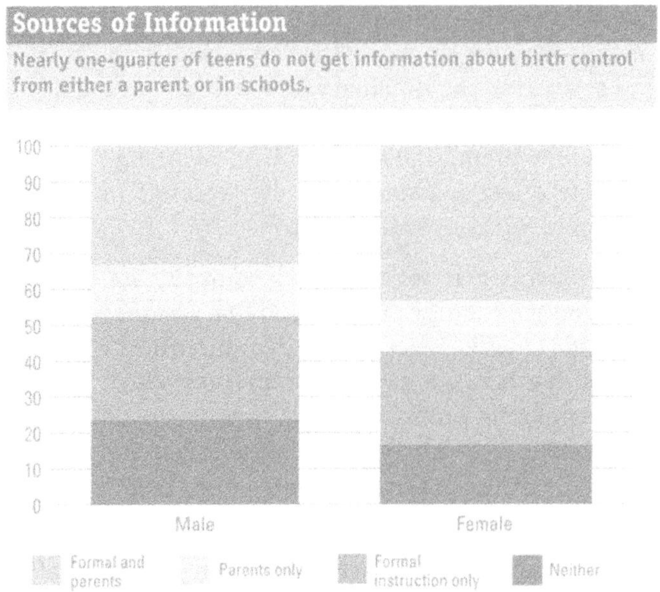

Source: Guttmacher Institute, Community health centers and family planning, In Brief, New York: Guttmacher, 2001, http://www.guttmacher.org/pubs/ib_6-01.html, accessed February 2, 2011.

In 2006, public school districts were more likely to require teaching of pregnancy prevention in high schools than in elementary or middle schools (86% vs. 27% and 70%, respectively).

Public school districts were more likely to require teaching of STI prevention in high schools (87%) than at the elementary and middle school levels (33% and 77% middle, respectively).

Parents, peers and the media are ranked important sources of sexual health information by adolescents.

70% of male teenagers and 79% of female teenagers reported talking with a parent about at least one of six sex education topics (how to say no to sex, methods of birth control, STIs, where to get birth control, how to prevent HIV infection and how to use a condom).

Girls were more likely than boys to talk with their parents about birth control or "how to say no to sex."

Even when parents provide information, their knowledge about contraception or other sexual health topics may often be inaccurate or incomplete.

More than half (55%) of 7th–12th graders say they have ever looked up health information online in order to learn more about an issue affecting themselves or someone they know.

The Websites teens turn to for sexual health information often have inaccurate information. For example, of 177 sexual health Websites examined in a recent study, 46% of those addressing contraception and 35% of those addressing abortion contained inaccurate information.

Exposure to high levels of sexual content on television has been shown to be associated with an increased risk of initiating sexual activity, as well as a greater likelihood of involvement in teen pregnancy.

Currently, 20 states and the District of Columbia mandate sex and HIV education; another 12 states only mandate HIV education.

A total of 36 states require that sex education include abstinence: Twenty-seven require that abstinence be stressed, while nine require simply that it be included as part of the instruction.

18 states and the District of Columbia require that sex education programs include information on contraception; no state requires that it be stressed.

Three Federal Programs For Teens, FY2010

Teen Pregnancy Prevention Program	Personal Responsibility Education Program	Title V Abstinence-Only Program
run by the Office of Adolescent Health	run by the Administration on Children, Youth and Families	run by the Administration on Children, Youth and Families
$114.5 million	$75 million	$50 million
• $75 million to public and private entities for proven programs	• $55.25 million to states for proven programs.	• $50 million to states for abstinence-only-until-marriage programs
• $25 million to public and private entities for innovative strategies	• $10 million to public and private entities for innovative strategies	
• $14.5 million for program support and evaluation	• $9.75 million for program support, evaluation and Indian tribes	

A recent review of 13 commonly used abstinence-only curricula found that 11 had incorrect, misleading or distorted information.

In December 2009, Congress replaced the rigid Community-Based Abstinence Education Program with a new $114.5 million teen pregnancy prevention program to support evidence-based interventions, as well as others that have demonstrated promise.

In March 2010, Congress created through health care reform a five-year Personal Responsibility Education Program (PREP). Its stated purpose is to educate adolescents on both abstinence and contraception and to prepare them for adulthood by teaching such subjects as healthy relationships, financial literacy, parent-child communication and decision-making.

Congress also renewed (per another provision in the health care reform legislation) the Title V abstinence-only program for five years. This funding stream makes available $50 million annually for grants to the states to promote sexual abstinence outside of marriage.

Assessment of Sex Education Program

Strong evidence suggests that comprehensive approaches to sex education help young people both to withstand the pressures to have sex too soon and to have healthy, responsible and mutually protective relationships when they do become sexually active.

A November 2007 report found that "two-thirds of the 48 comprehensive programs that supported both abstinence and the use of condoms and contraceptives for sexually active teens had positive behavioral effects." Many either delayed or reduced sexual activity, reduced the number of sexual partners, or increased condom or other contraceptive use.

There is no evidence to date that abstinence-only-until-marriage education delays teen sexual activity. Moreover, research shows that abstinence-only strategies may deter contraceptive use among sexually active teens, increasing their risk of unintended pregnancy and STIs.

A 2007 congressionally mandated study found that federally-funded abstinence-only programs have no beneficial impact on young people's sexual behavior.

Leading public health and medical professional organizations, including the American Medical Association, the American Nurses Association, the American Academy of Pediatrics, the American College of Obstetricians and Gynecologists, the American Public Health Association, the Institute of Medicine and the Society for Adolescent Health and Medicine, support a comprehensive approach to educating young people about sex.

Critique of Epidemiology

Epidemiology has been portrayed as hard science that is detached from human culture. However, research has shown that culture permeates medical diagnosis and treatment (Hans et al. 1997).

Scholars have argued that biomedicine is part of a cultural system because epidemiologists use the cultural mentality to describe the disease of AIDS. Biomedicine deploys cultural terms such as "war on AIDS" or "war on cancer." In the description of the "war on AIDS," the war is portrayed as an attack against a deadly and evil internal growth, led by the T-cells—courageous soldiers in a battle. The main imagery employed in popular and scientific descriptions of this immune system portrays the body as nation-state at war over its external borders, containing internal surveillance systems to monitor foreign invaders. Hans, Singer, and Susser describe this as "frontier mentality" that continues to live on in an urbanized and industrialized society. They point out that "the war on drugs" is a symbolic cultural continuation of the war against Native Americans that cleared the frontier for white settlement (Hans et al. 1997).

According to Hans, Singer, and Susser (Hans et al. 1997), corporate and government interests also permeate biomedicine. Doctor–patient interactions mirror class structure in society and reinforce hierarchical structures in the larger society by stressing the need for the patient to comply with a social superior's or expert's judgment. Social scientists use the word "medicalization" to refer to the process of biomedical treatment through pathological terminology. What is wrong with medicalization? It contributes to increasing social control on the part of physicians and health institutions over behavior. It demystifies and depoliticizes the social origins of personal stresses. It transforms a problem in the social structure—stressful work demands, unsafe working conditions, and poverty—into an individual problem under medical control (Hans et al. 1997).

Hans et al. assert that the profit-making orientation caused biomedicine to evolve into a capital-intensive endeavor heavily oriented to high technology, the massive use of drugs, and the concentration of medical services (1997). The state legitimizes the corporate involvement in the health arena and reinforces it through support for medical training and research. "Medicine has from the beginning functioned in the service of imperialism, supporting logically the voracious search for ever widening markets and profitable deals" (Hans et al. 1997: 35). The ruling elites control Third World countries by collaborating with international agencies to determine health policies.

Ideologically, biomedicine is based on dualism—the idea that reality is made up of two opposing forces: mind and matter, soul and body, good and evil, and so on. Dualism is interconnected with ideas of good and evil in Christian tradition. Dualism is deeply rooted in European thought, as Plato divided humans into Mind (higher and finer, belongs to celestial realm of ideal forms) and Matter (lower, cruder, corruptible, belongs to earthly realm) (Hans et al. 1997). That is, despite the fact that human beings have physical bodies, their true, fine, and high nature is spiritual. The soul seeks God, whereas the body is subject to base, evil, material temptations. In reality, patients suffer from mental stress because of society's stigmatization and patients' self-struggle. However, biomedicine operates on the idea of dualism and is only concerned with the physical body, not the mind (Hans et al. 1997).

Scholars such as Hans, Singer, Susser, and others also argue that the primary sense of medicine is drugs. Other senses are concerned with diseases and body. The central concern of biomedicine is "not general well-being, nor individual persons, nor simply their bodies, but their bodies in disease" (Hans et al. 1997). While patients suffer "illness," physicians treat "disease."

Physical reductionism is a central tenet of biomedicine. Biomedicine radically separates the body from the mind, and the body is thought to be knowable and treatable in isolation (Hans et al. 1997; Kleinman 1980, 1988). As Hans et al. state, the object of internal medicine and the core of biomedicine is "physiological integrity." To biomedicine, the body is a mindless body. It operates like a machine. It requires periodic repair to ensure that it performs all assigned tasks productively and effectively. The body is compared to a battery-driven machine or a drainage system with engines and hollow cavities connected with each other and orifices by pipes and tubes. The major cavities are identified as chest and stomach, and the pipes are defined as intestines, bowel, and blood vessels. Any blockage of an internal pipe induces illness and the pipe can be replaceable (Helman 2000). Birth is seen as the control of laborers (women) and their machines (their uteruses) by managers (doctors) often using other machines to help (Hans et al. 1997).

Hans et al. point out that biomedicine represents individual patients as passive or impersonal objects (1997). In reality, however, individuals respond to the material conditions they face and challenge the medical hegemony. Hans et al. argue that social scientists should study how they suffer from illness and how they respond to sickness. For instance, when a patient experiences job-related stress that manifests itself in various symptoms, the physician may prescribe a sedative to calm the patient. The sedative may temporarily help the patient cope with an onerous work environment, but it leaves the power of an employer or supervisor untouched and unchallenged (1997).

Social scientists have demonstrated that many factors play a role in initiating a sexually transmitted HIV epidemic. Among the behavioral and social factors are (a) condom use, (b) proportion of the adult population with multiple partners, (c) overlapping sexual partnerships—individuals are highly infectious when they first acquire HIV and thus more likely to infect any concurrent partners, (d) sexual networks, (e) age mixing, between older men and young women, and (f) poverty and, in particular, women's economic dependence on marriage or prostitution, robbing them of control over the circumstances or safety of sex. Among the behavioral factors are (a) high rates of sexually transmitted infections, especially those causing genital ulcers, (b) low rates of male circumcision, (c) high viral load HIV levels in the blood stream that are typically highest when a person is first infected and again in the late stages of illness.

In addressing the epidemic of AIDS, the current dominant biomedical model explains health as stemming from individually chosen lifestyles. Following the rational choice model, epidemiologists tend to assume that people engage in dangerous behavior because they either fail to recognize or underestimate the risk involved in such behavior. By the same token, it is assumed that if individuals are informed of these risks, they will recalculate and abstain from such behavior.

However, studies throughout the world have discovered that increased knowledge of AIDS did not translate into widespread protection and that interventions based on information and reasoned persuasion had apparent limitations. This dominant biomedical approach dismisses the fact that human behaviors are related to social conditions and shaped by cultural systems, and therefore, are unable to deal concretely with the lived social realities.

Because different societies and different subcultures within the same society exhibit different understandings of sexual expression, it became apparent that a far more complex set of social, structural, and cultural factors that mediate the structural risk in every group need to be taken into account to fully explain sexual conduct.

Role of Media and Media Construction of HIV/AIDS

Our comprehension of HIV/AIDS stems from media construction of HIV/AIDS. In China, for instance, in the late 1990s when the issue of AIDS was introduced into the public discourse, it was almost universally portrayed as a "foreign" disease brought into a formerly healthy Chinese public. More specifically, the gateway for AIDS' entry into China is pinpointed at the nexus between foreign men and Chinese women. One Chinese television-movie creatively uses this media-generated perception to create a strong sense of drama and suspense. The movie tells the story of how a young, attractive, Chinese woman doctor contracts AIDS from a foreign man. The mother of the woman (and the audience) is kept in the dark about the details of the young woman's relationship with the foreign man until almost the very end, and we of course can only assume the worst: she had sex with him! Finally, she tells her story, and we (and the concerned mother) are relieved to discover that she contracted the AIDS virus while performing an emergency surgical operation on her foreign friend, thereby removing her moral culpability.

Other women are not so lucky. Newspaper articles recount stories of Chinese women who—in the pursuit of sexual pleasure, a quick buck, or because they worship the West—have sex with foreign men only to later discover that they have contracted the dreaded AIDS disease. Without denying that sex with foreigners is one possible avenue of contracting AIDS, the amount of attention that is poured on the topic is completely out of proportion to its significance as a source of transmission. In fact, it is negligible when contrasted with the number of Chinese peasants who have contracted AIDS through the selling of blood—in some areas so severe that entire villages have been devastated. The emphasis on the Chinese women–foreign men nexus, in other words, is mostly sensationalist and distracts people from the real issues.

Role of Media: Information or Education?

Should journalists play the role of educator, carrying a responsibility for bringing education vital to the prevention of the AIDS epidemic? Is there a real distinction between the concept of information and education in the process of bringing information about AIDS to the broad general public?

In most cases, journalists and even scientific writers who supposedly have expertise in this area are not trained as educators. It seems that in general, health educators play the role as educators and journalists play the role as informers. The role of media is to report and update the public with the most recent information about AIDS, including medical facts, scientific understanding, and social and public policy.

Many scholars have commented on the limitation of media. For instance, Garrett states (2007: 23), "If the mass media were an excellent source of public education, nobody in the U.S. would smoke cigarettes. Nobody would misuse pesticides. Nobody would be eating cholesterol-rich foods as a steady part of their diets. And probably nobody would inject heroin or smoke crack. If all it took was to hear something was dangerous, behavior would change. No media has received the volume of press coverage than AIDS has, and by and large that press coverage has stressed the most crucial points the public needs to know to decide if they personally need to be afraid or change their sexual or drug-abuse patterns. The press is very good at raising the level of fear and concern. But it takes more than fear and concern to move people to take rational, pragmatic action".

Despite the limited function of media, they still maintain the power to keep the issue of AIDS before the public eye, and help set both the tone and agenda of AIDS prevention activities. Mass media can become a vital conduit for providing information that is educational to the public, and can help people prevent HIV transmission and understand the AIDS issue. It is essential to integrate health education with media to ensure the widest possible impact of health education and help establish media as an educational tool.

Surveys found that the most common way people heard about HIV was on TV news, followed by newspapers and television programs, radio programs, magazine articles, and so on. Television was rated first in public attention. TV has played a significant role in helping enhance people's awareness of HIV and responding to people with HIV/AIDS in a sensitive and informed fashion. Newspapers came in second, and the medical profession was third. It would be easier for public health professionals to convey prevention messages and harm-reduction techniques so long as the media put AIDS in the forefront of society's consciousness.

Media should be able to initiate, foster, and strengthen a sensitive and responsible dialogue on HIV/AIDS and the underlying social causes that fuel the epidemic. Media have a central role in bringing change at all levels of society, particularly among leaders. They can call for and encourage a commitment from leaders to strive to curb the HIV spread and transform the society's HIV epidemic in their own countries. The World Health Organization Global Program on AIDS is strongly committed to working with the mass media to enhance public knowledge about AIDS and to help implement the WHO global strategy against HIV/AIDS.

Historical Development of Mass Media and AIDS in the United States

Scholars such as Phyllida Brown have illustrated three phases of mass media construction of AIDS in the United States. Brown pointed out that mass media developed in parallel to the development of AIDS, as illustrated below. It developed in three phases, which could be described roughly as initial reactions of fear and ignorance, followed by development of experience and understanding, with a third phase moving into concentration on precise scientific and policy developments.

First Phase: Fear and Ignorance

Like other countries, the media in the United States experienced fear and ignorance in its first phase during its first contact with HIV/AIDS. The media exaggerated AIDS infection through casual contact and infused the public with fear and prejudices by displaying morbid images and photos. Media were suffused by pictures of authorities burning the automobile of an HIV carrier who was the victim of an accident, and of the police wearing yellow rubber gloves while arresting protesters. The frightening images and sensational stories only enhanced public fear of AIDS and discrimination against people who were infected with HIV.

Media consistently underscored rare and bizarre ways of the spread of HIV, instead of focusing on the common modes of transmission. Such a trend illustrated that the primary concern of media was to sensationalize stories to attract attention. Sepulveda, Fineberg, and Mann (1993) referred to a press room term for riveting stories: "sexy news." They pointed out that the story did not have to be about sex to fulfill the necessary criteria for a hot headline, as long as it was grabbing news. When American movie star Rock Hudson died of AIDS, it was considered a sexy story in the press room.

Similarly, rare incidents, such as a patient getting infected in a dentist's office in Florida, received an incredible amount of coverage, whereas one million HIV-infected people in the United States did not receive any comparable media attention. The media made an enormous scene about the peril at the dentist's office, but at the same time left the topic of safer sex untouched and unexplored. Similarly, in Zimbabwe, Phyllida Brown recounted that stories about injection drug users appeared in the media much more frequently than stories about blood screening or pregnancy.

Sepulveda et al. (1993) revealed the negative impact media had on the public. The survey unraveled the fact that people were confused about the meaning of body fluids, whether body fluids meant sexual fluids and blood, or other fluids such as urine or saliva. Sepulveda et al. noted that such vague terms could make individuals feel more vulnerable to HIV infection. They also asserted that the public was deluged with conflicting press information about AIDS until 1988. As a consequence, polls show the American public continued to harbor dangerous misunderstandings about AIDS. In 1988, three-quarters of the American people said they had no sympathy for homosexual and intravenous drug using people with AIDS. Over one-third were unaware that the disease was caused by a virus, and 40% thought one could get AIDS from a toilet seat.

Media also influenced people's perceptions of HIV-infected people by sympathizing with innocent victims of HIV such as infants and recipients of infected blood or blood products through health care, and stigmatizing others who allegedly deserved their own infection and were thus seen as an ominous threat to society. Media stigmatized people living with HIV/AIDS with insensitive wording that insinuated that people who were infected were punished for their immoral lives. Stigmatization not only led to much misery for people who were infected with HIV; it also discouraged people from getting tested. After all, people feared being stigmatized should they test positive for the virus.

Phyllida Brown noted that media described people with AIDS in terms such as "AIDS-ravaged," "heavily emaciated with the killer disease AIDS," and "AIDS sufferer." These terms not only sensationalized media stories, but also fueled panic, discrimination, and hopelessness. Such stigmas could lead people to deny rights and services to people who were infected with HIV. Early reports on AIDS were characterized by misconceptions, misunderstanding, and prejudice. Articles on AIDS cases and infections with HIV unanimously referred to AIDS as the "gay plague." The problem with the term was that it dismissed forms of transmission of HIV such as through blood or blood products, or from mother to fetus or child.

Media also carried a multitude of false and sensational information on the modes of transmission such as casual contact. As *And the Band Played On* illustrates, medical authorities at the time often concealed crucial information such as the number of AIDS cases and HIV infections (Shilts 1987).

While AIDS was first identified as the gay plague in the United States, it was defined as a product of a Western lifestyle in many developing countries. Phyllida Brown has illustrated that in Ghana, AIDS was labeled as "white man's burden." In Brazil, the media portrayed AIDS in the United States as the disease of white, rich gay men.

As research discovered that heterosexual people were also victims of HIV infection, media portrayed AIDS as a problem of the Other, and started blaming other countries or regions as the source of AIDS being introduced into the United States. Africa was the first region the media placed the blame on. Coverage about exotic cultural practices in Africa that generated HIV and the origin of HIV in Africa was ubiquitous, to the extent that media portrayed the African continent as analogous to the disease. As Phyllida Brown has contended, this media coverage induced negative reactions from many Africans, triggering a counterblame of the West.

Phyllida Brown offered examples of Kenya and Haiti to illustrate the fact that around 1988, health ministers in some African countries were compelled to waste time rebutting exaggerated reports by Western media instead of building up their own AIDS programs. For instance, since the Kenyan economy relied upon tourism, the Kenyan government faced extensive pressure to take urgent measures to terminate the destructive news headlines about Kenya. Haiti too, suffered from long-lasting damage to its tourist industry due to the adverse media reporting. Brown pointed out that many governments in African countries were preoccupied with mitigating the media damage, which hampered their ability to cope with the disease at this crucial early stage in the epidemic.

In a nutshell, early reports on AIDS reflected journalists' own cultural prejudices. AIDS was portrayed as a problem of others—gay men, foreigners, drug users—rather than an urgent threat to all. Media construction of AIDS not only crystallized homophobia, but also highlighted racism, ethnic hierarchy, nationalism, hatred of or disdain for drug addicts, class stratifications, and the exaggerated fears of disease held by many reporters.

Sepulveda et al. (1993) intimated that sensationalist reporting of AIDS led to high levels of stigmatization. They observed that one of the reasons why journalists sensationalized AIDS stories was because they harbored a narrow understanding of the pandemic themselves. This was also a result of the dearth of specialized AIDS desks in the newsrooms, which could effectively tackle the issue. Just as Phyllida Brown noted, the initial reactions to AIDS were irresponsible, generating hysteria and fear, and associating AIDS with sinful activities, promiscuity, and the bizarre Other. Media insensitivity and sensationalist reporting during the first phase led to unfounded and prejudicial reaction to AIDS.

Second Phase: Accurate Information

Phyllida Brown marked the second phase of media reporting on AIDS around 1987 and 1988, characterized by the media's shifted attention to accurate information and the effort to acknowledge the fact that AIDS is a new health issue for society to face, rather than fear. In the second phase, as Brown argued, most journalists made an effort to report news accurately, responsibly, and fairly.

Third Phase: Declined Interest

Phyllida Brown noted that the third phase of media reaction began around 1989, demarcating the time when AIDS was treated as a public issue for serious treatment and policy review. There appeared to be a trend toward greater understanding not only of AIDS as an issue, but for those who were HIV-infected or had AIDS. During the third phase, as Brown stated, it was apparent that the intensity of media interest and reaction that marked the early days of the AIDS epidemic was over. In the early days, any and every story on AIDS could attract a press conference or press attention. That era was gone. There was a slight decline in the volume of reporting. As Brown intimated, many journalists were reluctant to report on issues concerning AIDS, as it was regarded as a soft beat. Indeed, for those who did, they were often ridiculed or even questioned by their colleagues over their allegiance to the issue.

Brown pointed out that despite the fact that many journalists were better informed about HIV/AIDS, they still allowed their cultural judgments to affect the media coverage. For instance, in 1991, the British press explained the nation's gradually rising levels of heterosexual infection by blaming foreigners.

Critique of Media

Sepulveda et al. (1993) offered a critique of mass media in their book. First, they argued that in the production of mass media, editors and reporters might or might not have basic scientific knowledge or background about AIDS. They shared drastically different criteria from public health workers in judging the newsworthiness of a story. Because media workers had little access to accurate, timely, or relevant information about AIDS, there was a consistent discrepancy between the mass media and public health–related institutions and organizations. As a result, the media tended to be imprecise, which could potentially lead to people's vague and inaccurate understanding about AIDS.

Second, mass media played a negative role by disseminating false information about AIDS, making facile comparisons with the Black Plague, exaggerating the risks for transmission of casual contact, and seeking to put blame on a specific region or group. In this way, media induced stigmas against HIV-positive people and disrupted prevention of further infection.

Third, media reporters were not updated with developments about HIV/AIDS and wrote in an ad hoc manner. As Sepulveda, Fineberg, and Mann (1993) contended, there was no serial documentation of the history of the country's struggle against HIV/AIDS.

Fourth, Sepulveda et al. (1993) argued that media reporters easily succumbed to the manipulation of top government. For instance, San Francisco journalist Randy Shilts in 1989 expressed his dismay over what he described as a rather cozy relationship between the U.S. press and government officials. "AIDS had spread because indolent news organizations shunned their responsibility to provide tough, adversarial reporting, instead of basing stories largely on the official truth of government press releases." Hence, to avoid sacrificing news' objectivity and to evade compromising media journalists' independent judgment, media must maintain their independence and shy away from being integrated into any government or any nongovernmental organization.

Last, according to Sepulveda et al, (1993), officials deluded themselves by believing that the press had reached all the nooks and crannies of the society. In the United States and Europe, a significant number of individuals who were at a high risk for AIDS were alienated from mainstream press sources due to a combination of reasons such as language difficulties, illiteracy, and cultural differences.

Sepulveda et al. ascertained that educational efforts other than mainstream media must be targeted at the vulnerable, marginal population that included foreign immigrant workers, unemployed drug users, semi-literate homeless women, and recent immigrants, who were at risk of infection by HIV. They contended that public health officials should not rely solely upon the mainstream media to disseminate such vital information as modes of transmission, methods of protection, and reasons for not fearing particular social groups.

Alternative Media about HIV/AIDS

In general, cultural production of the standardized, profit-oriented, and commercial network is called mainstream media. The works of videomakers who work outside of commercial television are usually referred to as the alternative AIDS media.

Martin Foreman, former Director of the Panos London Global AIDS program, noted, "Whether they actively seek to do so, the media either fuel the epidemic through sensationalism and poor or unethical reporting, or help to restrain it by promoting information, understanding and behavior change." As illustrated, mainstream media furthered stigmatization and reinforced prejudice through establishing the association between AIDS with immoral behaviors and the pariah population such as prostitutes and drug users. Under such circumstances, alternative media emerged.

The incentive of alternative media is not only to challenge the mainstream media, but also to provide a forum where a plurality of voices, including the voices of the people living with HIV, can be heard. In this sense, alternative media constitutes a form of activism, resisting against the inadequate and belated government responses and the stigmatizing and negative reports in the mainstream media. By telling the story of AIDS from the perspective of the people living with HIV, alternative media depict these people as neither victims nor pariahs, but as empowered human beings actively taking charge of their lives and health in political and social arenas. This portrayal of the people infected by HIV, hopefully, can counteract the denigrating reports of them in the mainstream media.

As early as 1987, in response to the nonchalant attitude by the government toward AIDS, AIDS activist videos emerged. The first activist show was "Living with AIDS," which was broadcast through cable regularly. It was operated by Jean Carlomusto, who was hired by the organization of Gay Men's Health Crisis (GMHC) into its Audio-Visual Department. In 1987, another video titled "Testing the Limits" started documenting and archiving the burgeoning AIDS movement.

AIDS activist videos went hand in hand with a sharp increase in political activism. For instance, in New York, ACT UP was established in early March and launched its first large-scale demonstration on Wall Street on March 24. In 1989, ACT UP organized a videomaking group called Damned Interfering Video Activist Television (DIVA TV). DIVA TV was responsible for producing three videos within a year.

The period from 1988 to 1993 witnessed a deluge of AIDS-activist video produced and broadcast to the public. Among the hundreds of produced videotapes, the vast majority were made in New York City. The main reason that most tapes were made in New York was because New York was the epicenter of AIDS and the predominant center of political activism. New York City provided an enormous amount of supportive mechanisms, including art schools, media access centers, free classes, and inexpensive access to equipment that greatly facilitated the production process of alternative videos. New York City also has a well-established community of videomakers who can secure some small grants and tap into available graduate programs such as the Whitney Independent Studies Program, which offers sophisticated, theoretical thrust for filmmaking.

The mushrooming production of AIDS-activist videos waned in 1994, concomitant with street activism. It is worth noting that there was one exception: "AIDS Community Television" by

James Wentzy. From 1993 through 1996, James Wentzy continued his ties with New York ACT UP and made over 150 half-hour programs on AIDS and various responses from communities.

In the new era of globalization and internationalization of media, people living with HIV and activists deployed the Internet as a forum to break the silence and voice their opinions about their lives, society, and survival strategies. They were intent in representing themselves rather than being represented. Framing themselves as active agents rather than passive victims and outcasts, they articulated their critique of the extant mainstream's depiction of themselves and created an open space to construct their collective identity.

AIDS in the Barrio is one example of such an alternative AIDS video (1990). This film was shot in the Latino barrios of Philadelphia. Like many other activist tapes, this video imparted the authority to the interviewees—the Latino community. This posed a stark contrast with the mainstream media that invited scientists and doctors to speak and recognized their expert knowledge and full authority. *AIDS in the Barrio* offered a space for the Latino community to speak out and for their voices to be heard. From the stance of the community members, the video unraveled the social, cultural, and political complexities of AIDS. *AIDS in the Barrio*, through the voices of those living with HIV and Latino community members, argued that the issue of AIDS in Latino communities in the United States was inextricably intertwined with racial hierarchy, prejudice and discrimination, unemployment, and illegal drug use. Instead of blaming the individuals' immoral lifestyles, the video showed deeper social and political issues that framed and shaped individuals' behaviors and in turn, fueled the AIDS epidemic.

In addition to exposing the political and social intricacy of the AIDS issue, *AIDS in the Barrio* also articulated the cultural values entrenched in the Latino community that helped increase the spread of HIV. Twelve of the 36 people interviewed were women, and only three exhibited accurate knowledge about HIV/AIDS. The cultural values demanded women to be pure prior to marriage and required men to be machismo and sexually adventurous. Such latent cultural ideals were deleterious and harmful, leading to both women's and men's vulnerability to HIV infection.

Like *AIDS in the Barrio*, other activist videos allowed various communities to speak, and evinced the cultural, political, and social nuances revolving around the disease of AIDS. These activist videos were generally made by members of communities affected by AIDS. Like *AIDS in the Barrio*, the videos targeted and spoke to a specific community in its own language.

Other alternative AIDS videos include the following:

1. *Women and AIDS:* Interviews with female activities, educators, and health care providers who present the issues of women and AIDS.
2. *Living with AIDS:* Half-hour show devoted to people living with AIDS.
3. *All People with AIDS are Innocent, We Care: A Video for Care Providers of People Affected by AIDS:* calling for collective action.
4. *Reclaiming Desire: How to Have Sex in an Epidemic.*
5. *Speak for Yourself.*
6. *Constructing Community in the Age of AIDS.*
7. *From Witness to Subjects: Women in the AIDS Crisis.*

Summary

Chapter 2 highlights the cultural dimension of AIDS by illustrating constructed cultural meanings of AIDS, diverse cultural understandings of AIDS, and cultural factors of HIV/AIDS transmission. First, the social and cultural meanings of AIDS are shaped by media discourses about AIDS. In the West, cultural construction of AIDS reflects a fear of homosexuality, prostitution, drugs, deviance, and a sense of xenophobia. In many parts of the world, it is foreigners that are at the center of the blame in the cultural constructions of AIDS. This chapter provides three phases of media constructions of AIDS in the United States and points out that the media influence the language of AIDS, which in turn helps shape how people think about and deal with the pandemic. Second, cultural factors such as the meaning of sex, sexual culture, sexual practices, gender relationships, and condom use have a repercussion on sexual transmission of HIV. Third, different cultures, such as the United States, Haiti, and various countries in Africa, interpret and respond to AIDS differently. Finally, a critique of mainstream media further highlights the cultural construction of AIDS. Alternative media serve as a necessary counterpoint to the mainstream media. This chapter utilizes the cultural dimension of AIDS to critique the epidemiological approach to AIDS.

Name: ______________________________ **Date:** ____________________

Chapter 2 Cultural Construction of HIV/AIDS

Exercises

Exercise 1 Discuss with your partner your previous readings about HIV/AIDS from the media. If you have not been exposed to discussions about HIV/AIDS in the media, find an article in newspapers or on a website. List the key topics/issues raised in the media and discuss your overall impressions of how AIDS, people with HIV/AIDS, and causes of HIV are represented in the media.

Exercise 2 Reading Comprehension:

1. How was AIDS constructed upon the outbreak of HIV/AIDS in the United States?

2. What impact did the cultural construction of AIDS have on the U.S. population upon the outbreak of HIV/AIDS?

3. What does "geography of blame" mean?

4. Please list two to three examples to illustrate the "geography of blame."

5. How do you compare the U.S. and South Africa's cultural reactions to HIV/AIDS?

6. Please illustrate the cultural factor of migration and HIV/AIDS transmission.

7. Why is epidemiology criticized?

8. What kind of role do you think media should play?

9. What are the three phases of mass media and HIV/AIDS?

   1st phase:

   2nd phase:

   3rd phase:

10. What are the cultural practices that influence HIV/AIDS transmission?

11. Please list and explain three cultural factors that affect HIV/AIDS transmission.

Exercise 3 Discussion Questions:

1. Have you seen public education programs on smoking? Do you think people who smoke know that smoking is dangerous to their health? Why do you think individuals who are well-informed about the medical facts may still engage and persist in harmful behavior?

2. In your opinion, why is unprotected sex so appealing to people, even at the expense of their lives? What do you think are the most effective methods to persuade people to jettison unsafe sex and start performing safe sex?

3. What is your position on the enforcement of abstinence-only education? Support your position with factual information—not just opinion.

4. What do you think today's media should do to contribute to the global combat of AIDS?

5. What is your opinion on the alternative theory of AIDS?

Exercise 4 Test Your Knowledge:

1. The social construction of AIDS is based on objective science.

   a. True

   b. False

2. The epidemiologists' identification of the Haitians as the risk-group has no impact on the Haitian community.

   a. True

   b. False

3. Once the Centers for Disease Control removed the term "Haitian" as a risk-group designation, the stigma disappeared.

   a. True

   b. False

4. In the West, cultural construction of AIDS reflects a fear of homosexuality, prostitution, drugs, deviance, and a sense of xenophobia.

   a. True

   b. False

5. Construction of AIDS as a disease of high-risk behaviors rather than a disease of high-risk groups has led to marginalization, and stigmatization of certain groups.

   a. True

   b. False

6. Different cultures construct AIDS differently.

   a. True

   b. False

7. Different cultures define normal sexual activities differently.

   a. True

   b. False

8. This chapter focuses on medical facts of HIV/AIDS transmission.

   a. True

   b. False

9. This chapter discusses attitudes toward sex education in the U.S.

   a. True

   b. False

10. This chapter discusses cultural factors of HIV/AIDS transmission.

    a. True

    b. False

Chapter three | Political Economy

This chapter is concerned with the politics and the economics of AIDS. We are using the old term political economy because we believe you can't do economics apart from politics. Economic policy is made by politicians and it is seldom free of political considerations. The term is also reminiscent of Marxist analysis where it is assumed that the social, political, and intellectual nature of society, which Marx calls the superstructure, reflects and reinforces the economic interests and control of a dominant class, those who control the means of production. Marx believes that the means of production, which he calls the base, determines the nature of the superstructure. For instance, agrarian medieval Europe produced a political and economic system known as feudalism. In feudal society the land (means of production) was controlled by an upper class aristocracy who enjoyed the benefits of ownership without having to labor, which was performed by the vast majority of society, the peasants. This exploitive system, the base, was maintained and justified by a superstructure that included the church which taught the subordination of individual striving to a vision of society as an organic whole. This was explained through an "organic metaphor" which proclaimed the Monarch as the head of the body of society, the aristocracy as the strong arms of society who defended it, and the peasantry as the feet of society who performed the work. As this metaphor suggests, there is little room for individualism. The system works because each part performs its assigned role. Supporting this is a religious value system that emphasizes loyalty to one's superior, acceptance of one's place in society as divinely ordained, and looking to the afterlife for reward and justice. This explains why Marx referred to religion as the opiate of the people.

This changed as commerce and then industry developed and a new class emerged that controlled a new and more efficient means of production. Eventually the old system was overthrown by revolution and replaced by a new base, industrial capitalism, and a new superstructure, republicanism. The new superstructure posited a new set of values appropriate to the new base; affirming the importance of private property, a free and mobile work force, individual initiative, competition and a strong work ethic. Sociologist Max Weber has pointed to the role of Protestantism in shifting the value system to emphasize individualism and the "Puritan" work ethic, which are keys to individual success; something not valued in the old organic metaphor. As republics evolved into democracies in the 19th century, much was made of the myth of social mobility; the notion that anyone can become a financial success is critical to the stability of this system. We do not use the word myth here in the sense of something that is necessarily untrue but rather in its traditional sense of a story that embodies powerful values. The new superstructure rejects the metaphor of society as an organism and instead emphasizes the autonomy of the individual.

Marx rejects all of this, insisting that both feudalism and industrial capitalism succeeded by producing false consciousness where medieval peasants and modern industrial workers accepted the perverse values of the superstructure. For Marx, the good news was that false consciousness could not survive in the face of greater and greater exploitation. An inevitable revolution, he believed, would usher in the final stage of society, a kind of worker's paradise.

As we now know, the societies that claimed to be based upon Marxist principles, were anything but a paradise. Marx predicted that a worker's revolution would sweep away capitalism in the most advanced industrial societies. Instead, Marxist revolutions were only successful in societies that were still largely agrarian, such as Russia, China, Cuba, and Angola. The most advanced industrial societies, such as The United States, Germany and Britain, proved adept at liberalizing and adapting to the needs of workers. Marx recognized this danger to his mission. As we will discuss later, liberal reform was the great threat to Marx's vision.

While we are clearly not advocating Marx's vision of revolution, we believe that Marx makes an important point about the myth making power of the superstructure. In America we can see the power of myths about the infallibility of the free market, and the benevolence and wisdom of those who have made a lot of money, and the hopeless misery of people in societies like Sweden who have adopted elements of socialism as part of basically capitalist societies. In fact the superstructure teaches us to automatically shut off our brains and respond with fear when we hear buzz words such as socialism. The power of these myths has allowed a democracy where 1% of the population controls over 25% of the wealth, and where a modest attempt to cease being the only remaining industrial society to not have universal health care, causes a gigantic populist response that throws out much of a congress that has voted for this measure. As we explore the relationship between politics and economics and the AIDS epidemic, we do not mean to suggest that citizen and worker advocacy groups are without power, but a brief look at the history of the union movement, for instance, will show that it has operated within the comfortable confines of capitalist ideology ever since Samuel Gompers and the rise of the American Federation of Labor (A.F. of L.) and the decline of the International Workers of the World.

Gompers, leader of the AF of L focused upon getting workers better wages and working conditions within the capitalist system; he did not challenge capitalism. The IWW did challenge the system, but was a small union that disappeared under heavy government persecution in the 1920s. Today there are many NGOs challenging industry and government on many fronts; however, like the AF of L, they seldom challenge the virtues of a market-based economy. The focus has consistently been on finding solutions to problems without disruption of the prerogatives of business.

Defenders of capitalism have historically contended that economics and government should, as much as possible, be separated from each other. They have believed that the economy is governed by a natural law that is self–correcting, and that government interference with this natural law will be destructive of the economy. While this notion has been successfully challenged both in theory and in practice since the Progressive Movement of the early twentieth century, it still holds considerable sway in both business and government. What has followed from this is a rejection of macro analysis in the sense of a social science that looks at the interconnections between culture, economics, and politics and a division of the social science into economics, anthropology, political science, and sociology, each presumed to work best while looking at their corner of the world in isolation from other social science disciplines. This is being challenged by social scientists today, and in this chapter we will be agreeing with that challenge as we look at the political economy of AIDS.

Economists like to create "ideal" models as though politics need not be considered, but in the real world economic policy is made by governments and governments are influenced by interest groups. As we said above, these interest groups in America may represent various minority groups, but successful advocacy almost always operates within the confines of the market system. The most powerful of these interest groups, representing business interests, are usually able to modify the market system to suit their needs, but insist upon the market system when it is to their advantage. A good example of this is the pharmaceutical industry that is able to spend millions lobbying government to prevent competition from foreign drugs and to even create government programs to provide their drugs to seniors at very high prices, yet rail at attempts to fix prices for drugs critical to people's lives. But pharmaceuticals are only a part of the health policy picture in America, although a good example of the general principle that emphasizes free-market individualism as the primary principle governing health care. It is also a good example of the fact that within this free-market system those that have wealth and power can use the rules of the market or bend the rules to suit their own interests. It is within this context that we will examine the epidemic of AIDS in America and, because of the influence and power of America, the AIDS epidemic elsewhere in the world. It is within this context that AIDS takes place, and as we will see AIDS (as well as many other diseases) follow poverty. As we will show later in this chapter, both political power and economic power, hand in hand, set the parameters for AIDS infection. While anyone can display behavior that puts them at risk, those in poverty are at much greater risk, both because of certain behaviors that poverty encourages, but also because of the lack of health care that is a consequence of a lack of wealth. For instance, those with non-HIV sexually transmitted diseases are much more vulnerable to HIV infection. Genital lesions from diseases such as gonorrhea allow fluid transfers that cause the infection. Those with these lesions are many times more susceptible than those without. Relative power within impoverished communities is also an issue. Women are particularly vulnerable because of their lack of power relative to men. Women who are economically and/or emotionally dependent upon men may not be able to control basic health guards such as the use of condoms.

To fully understand the nature of the ideas undergirding our political economy, it will be useful to look briefly at the history of this ideology. Both British and American capitalism were heavily influenced in the late nineteenth century by Herbert Spencer's philosophy of Social Darwinism. Social Darwinism asserted that life was naturally a struggle for survival among competing elements. Through that struggle we are constantly weeding out the unfit and improving the qualities of the human race. Industrialization removed humankind from the jungle, but the principle of a healthy struggle for survival still applied. The new beasts in the jungle were the entrepreneurs and businessmen who struggled in the workplace for survival and hegemony. This was seen as embodying a natural law, and therefore, ironically, carried moral implications. The Medieval and Biblical injunctions to charity were stood on their head. Spencer himself was fond of saying: "We must be very cruel in the short run to be kind in the long run." In other words, we must let the weak and defenseless perish as part of the evolutionary process that is inevitable in nature. Through this philosophy Dickens' character Scrooge from [*A Christmas Carol*] becomes a hero of capitalism rather than the villain we all know him to be.

Because the actual practices of industrial capitalism were extremely brutal before Spencer invented a philosophy to justify these practices, one can say that Spencer's ideas were contested before they were in existence. Besides novelists like Dickens, the great British social scientist John Stuart Mill saw the ravages created by unfettered free markets, or perhaps more accurately, unfettered capitalists. Mill gave us our most recent interpretation of the word "liberal" by arguing that while the system had virtues, humans also had to be considered. There must be a safety net for those who failed in competition and there must be some reasonable regulation of the market system; there must be a balance between market needs and human needs. Today this is still the battlefront.

Orthodox Marxists argue that the liberal followers of Mill are a greater danger to long-run social justice than the Social Darwinists. Marx taught that greater competition in business and the inevitable worsening treatment of workers would forge a class consciousness among workers that would inevitably lead to revolution and the creation of a socialist system.

Liberalism, with its patchwork of remedies for human suffering, would mitigate the anger of workers and stifle class consciousness, delaying or even heading off the revolution. This has put liberals in a position to be attacked as traitors by both the Left and the Right. For better or worse, liberalism basically accepts the principles of the free market while attempting to soften its impact on people, and modify and control its instability. But it works best in a system where people are able to organize and exert pressure through interest groups. Those who are not able to organize to flex political muscle do not fare so well in this system.

The fragmentation of the social sciences into micro disciplines such as political science, and economics preserved the core concept, especially in economics, that there is a natural self-correcting law that must be respected. It is interesting that we have retained much of the language that accompanied this assumption. Even today we speak of creative destruction and moral hazard. Creative destruction refers to the natural process of the market system destroying what has proved to be unfit. Moral hazard refers to the danger of unnatural intrusion (government) into the free workings of markets. The argument is that entrepreneurs who are rescued from failure by government will be reinforced in their unfit methods thereby weakening the economy. It is worth noting that the class prone to making these arguments, the capitalist class, have not been averse to using the considerable political power that accrues with wealth to shield themselves from adverse market forces without any reference to moral hazard or creative destruction in their own cases. The well-documented history of powerful economic entities (such as the automobile manufacturers) protecting themselves, whether through high tariffs on imported automobiles or government bailouts, is clear evidence of the connection between economics and politics. Economies always exist in a political context.

As we have seen, besides Social Darwinism and Mill's liberalism, there existed also the specter of Marxist socialism. Marxism accepted many of the assumptions that capitalism is based upon: materialism, the inevitability of conflict, and a belief in the inevitability of progress. However, it differed in its core values. Locke, one of the fathers of capitalism, had invented a "labor theory of value" to justify private property as the basis of capitalism. His argument against the biblical injunction to "share the world in common" (socialism) argued that God intended that we had a right to the fruit of our own labor. Since we own our own bodies we have a natural right to the fruit of that labor our body performs. For Locke this was an argument against common ownership that was controlled by the church and aristocracy, which denied access to property by the new middle-class entrepreneurs. Marx takes this idea of the labor theory of value and uses it to show how the relationship between property and labor had become so distorted that those who worked most owned least. The moral center of this materialistic philosophy was that labor had the right to the wealth it created. By accepting Locke's evaluation of nature as having no intrinsic value, he argued that only labor was responsible for transforming nature into useful commodities and therefore having value. Those who gained wealth because they owned the means of production were simply leeches. Key to his analysis was the relationship between ownership and power. This was true in an agrarian society where the aristocrats controlled the land and now it was true in industrial society where capitalists controlled the new means of production, the factories and mines and railways. The class that controlled the means of production exploited those who worked for them, whether peasants or industrial workers.

Marx reconnects the fragmented social sciences; his analysis sees economic power inevitably linked to political power. As we look at the health care system in America in general and as it relates to AIDS, it will be useful to understand how the realities of our political economy influence the spread of this disease and the care for those who have contracted it.

We will begin by tracing the beginnings of this disease in the gay community and observe how the gay community was able to organize to influence their local government, but were unable to push their agenda at the national level. We will next trace the disease as it explodes into the minority communities, particularly in the inner city. Here we will see how the powerlessness attending poverty influences the progress of the disease.

The Beginning of AIDS in America

AIDS was first recognized in the gay community in America in 1980. What was noticed was that gay men were catching and dying from diseases that were not usually fatal and not usually caught by young men. For instance, a common cause of death was Karposi's Sarcoma, a cancer that typically struck older Italian or Jewish men and was seldom fatal. Gay men were also dying of pneumonia and from taxoplasmosis, a disease of cats. Medical authorities were confused by the strange diseases and failed to understand the common problem contributing to these very distinct and different maladies. As we saw in Chapter 1, nobody dies of AIDS, but AIDS does facilitate a host of other opportunistic diseases that do kill people. By destroying the immune system, AIDS allows these other usually latent diseases free range to destroy the body.

In order to understand the political economy of AIDS in the gay community it is necessary to trace that community's history. The gay movement began in June of 1969 in Greenwich Village in New York, at the Stonewall Inn. Gay men turned on police who had been harassing them and fought back. This was a turning point. Out of this a new gay identity was born, based on gay pride. In order to fully understand this movement one must place it in the larger context of the 1960s counterculture. The Civil Rights Movement had been asserting itself since 1954. The women's movement was emerging. A strong anti-war movement was in full stride and many Americans were deeply suspicious of government and even more so of that broader concept "the establishment." A deep pride in more specific and usually oppressed identities was being expressed and gays fit this category. It was a time of youth rebellion and for questioning traditional attitudes toward almost everything; without this context it is hard to imagine a gay liberation movement.

Even though the gay movement had begun in New York, it was San Francisco that came to be at the forefront of the movement. In fact, as large numbers of gays descended into the Castro District of San Francisco it became the radical cutting edge of gay liberation. During the 1970s activists began organizing the gay community politically. Since tens of thousands of gay men had immigrated to San Francisco by the early 1980s, two out of five males in the city were homosexual.

Gay political strategy was to build a power base at the local level. This power base had allowed Harvey Milk to be elected as a district supervisor and after he was assassinated along with liberal mayor Moscone by anti-gay supervisor Dan White, his gay successor, Harry Britt, was easily elected to succeed him. The key to political success was door-to-door organizing that not only won seats and political sympathy at the local level but voted ten-to-one for liberal Senator Cranston, giving the gay community a foothold on the national level.

Door-to-door organizing served two purposes: first, it made clear to people the importance of support for the Democratic Party, and second, it greatly increased turnout. The gay community showed further sophistication by reaching out and forming coalitions with other groups such as San Francisco's Chinese community. In 1980 they won the support of Ted Kennedy, who challenged Carter for the Democratic nomination. In contrast to the inner-city minority community we will discuss later, gays had the advantage of representing an economic cross section of the population that included the well educated and affluent. This provided the leadership that allowed considerable success at organizing.

The organizational success of gay activists in San Francisco became a model for activists in other gay centers, notably in New Orleans and New York City where grassroots, door-to-door organizing turned out large numbers for the Democratic Party. However, the situation in New York and elsewhere required a less radical, less ambitious agenda. The gay community outside of San Francisco did not have the high ratios of San Francisco. Lesser numbers meant compromise with the straight community. Gays in New York City, reflecting their minority status, were less likely to come out of the closet, and more content with a less aggressive posture. Their hope was to be left alone and they were leery of arousing the hostility of the straight community. This created tensions in the national coalition and a divided strategy.

San Francisco had become a hub for male homosexuals. As we have seen, huge numbers migrated to the city from every part of the United States. Their numbers naturally emboldened them, but the fact of migration had created a mythology. San Francisco had become, for many, a Utopia, an ideal place where they could practice their sexuality without restraint or apology. The annual gay pride parade had become a demonstration of this. By the late 1970s, over 350,000 people were participating in the parade that became a radical expression of a wide variety of desires, sure to inflame much of the non-gay population across the country. In San Francisco, people who had endured humiliation and suppression of their desires found an outlet, and many if not all were determined to give full vent to their unique feelings.

It is easy to see why gays in places such as New York City, who represented a considerable minority, were worried that there would be a backlash. The movement in San Francisco had created a large target for those who regarded homosexuality from a less benign perspective.

The Rise of the Religious Right

The emergence of the counterculture in the late sixties had scared a lot of normally passive Americans. Richard Nixon gave a name to these people, the "silent majority." Nixon and Republican strategist Kevin Phillips recognized an opportunity and began calculating a strategy to turn the Republican Party into the majority party. During the 1960s, Republicans had relied upon their traditional base in the business community, plus citizens worried about the threat of global communism to hang on to political power. The New Deal coalition had made the Democratic Party the majority party and only the Cold War rescued the Republicans from completely marginalized status. As the Democratic Party moved to the left following the election of 1968, culminating in the nomination of George McGovern in 1972, they created a new opening for the Republicans.

One part of this opening was race. It was not lost on Nixon or Phillips that Barry Goldwater's few electoral victories in 1964 were in the deep Southern states of the old Confederacy where Civil Rights legislation still rankled. It was also clear from the primary success of Alabama governor George Wallace in Northern states such as Indiana and Wisconsin that the electorate was changing. They understood that rapid changes and the counterculture had scared people and they set out to take advantage of that fear.

The key in coalescing that fear required that the enemy have a face. Until the debacle of the Vietnam War, communism had provided that face. Now came the angry black man, feminists, hippies, and homosexuals. This was the new face of terror that would drive the moral majority into a new, safe refuge in the Republican Party. Up until the end of the Vietnam War, the electorate was driven by political and economic issues. The new politics would trump this with a third issue, culture. Of course the moral majority was not a unitary body. Within its ranks were many kinds of unrest. The new Republican majority would include the business community, with their concerns about taxes and government regulations, and the defense hawks, still concerned about the Cold War. These groups merged together on one side, as a huge business opportunity had been created by the defense needs of the Cold War, what former general and president Dwight Eisenhower had called the military industrial complex. Finally and importantly, there was the new group, the cultural conservatives. The core of this group was Evangelical Christians who were mobilized around the issue of abortion in 1971 when the Supreme Court handed down the *Roe vs. Wade* decision. Later homosexuality, and particularly gay marriage, would be mobilizing issues for this group. In fact, three issues would be paramount: abortion, teaching evolution in the schools, and homosexuality, particularly gay marriage. Certainly concern about abortion was not limited to the religious right, as they came to be called. It became a connective issue with less radical groups such as the Catholic Church.

Just as the AIDS epidemic was beginning, the country was on the eve of an election that would bring to power the new Republican coalition. The Kennedy challenge had failed, Carter was in the midst of the Iranian hostage crisis, and Ronald Reagan swept to victory even though an independent Republican, John Anderson, had siphoned off some of the moderate Republican vote (as well as a respectable amount of the gay vote). This was a big victory for the anti-gay forces, but San Francisco's gay leaders consoled themselves that most decisions affecting them were local and they continued to show their muscle in the local elections. It was too early to understand the importance of federal funding for gay health issues.

The Bath Houses

The bath houses were privately run clubs where gay men could meet, fraternize, and have uninhibited sex. They were immensely popular among repressed young men who could fully vent pent-up sexual repression. They represented liberation from puritanical standards that young men had experienced in the places they came from: small towns in the Midwest, the Southern countryside, and virtually every other place in America. The bathhouses came to be about more than sex; they came to be a symbol of gay liberation. In the bathhouses one could have sex with dozens of partners, most of whom might be strangers, and one could experience the most exotic of sexual practices. One person, testifying later to how many partners he had in a year, began saying about 250 and then upon reflection insisted that that was a very conservative estimate.

Male gay sex commonly involves both oral and anal intercourse. In the bathhouses a combination of these practices became common. It was called rimming and involved oral anal sex. Even before the outbreak of AIDS this had contributed to a dramatic increase in venereal diseases associated with the bathhouses: this included syphilis, gonorrhea, and hepatitis B. Given the principle that intercourse with a partner is, from a health point of view, intercourse with all of his partners, it is not hard to understand why sexually transmitted disease (STDs) rates were soaring.

By 1983 there was evidence that the activities in the bathhouses were spreading AIDS, and yet, remarkably, much of the gay community refused to recognize this. While some of San Francisco's gay leaders, such as Bill Kraus, were urging the community to exercise sexual moderation, the rank and file of those who used the bathhouses were in denial. Calls for moderation were met with anger and scorn. Many were convinced that this was just a ploy to restrict their sexual freedom. To make sense of this one must remember that the bathhouses were not just places to have sex. As sexual havens they came to symbolize freedom. People who had come from all over the United States to escape repression of their sexuality, and were enduring nationwide attacks from the likes of Anita Bryant and Jerry Falwell, clung to the bathhouses as fortresses of freedom in the storm of national attacks. Protestors claimed that they would rather die than give up the bathhouses. Many of them would get their wish.

In June of 1983 the issue came to a head. Bill Kraus headed up the faction calling for sexual restraint; on the other side were members of the Alice B. Toklas Democratic Club. San Francisco health director, Dr. Merv Silverman, was being urged to close the bathhouses or at very least put up warning signs. The Toklas Club regarded even the posting of warnings as the beginning of infringement on their freedom and as an attack on gay businesses. Silverman was politically sensitive to the gay community. As he remarked, "all public health policy was basically political." In a tense meeting with the concerned parties he called for a vote. The vote was overwhelmingly in favor of the bathhouses. With that vote the fate of many of San Francisco's gays was sealed.

Posters were put up, although not in prominent places. The posters advised use of condoms, avoiding exchange of bodily fluids, limiting use of recreational drugs, and urged men to "enjoy more time with fewer partners." It did not make clear that just one encounter with an infected needle or partner could mean death. Even this mild warning provoked the wrath of the Alice B. Toklas Democratic Club. They charged Bill Kraus and his supporters with attacking the social and economic viability of their community, and of suffering from an internalized homophobia. In the end the democratic politics achieved were fatal to the gay community as were the economic interests of the bathhouse owners.

Politics, Economics, and Science

Meanwhile, scientists were searching frantically to identify the cause of the disease. As it was determined that a retrovirus was probably responsible for destroying the immune system, scientists turned to Dr. Robert Gallo at the National Cancer Institute. Gallo was a leading expert on retroviruses and he now threw himself into the search to identify the cause of AIDS. At the same time, the Pasteur Institute in Paris was close to discovering the retrovirus that caused AIDS. Luc Montagnier headed the French team that shortly did discover the culprit virus, but nobody believed them. Having two first-rate scientific teams pursuing a cure should have been a good thing, but as it turned out competition did not necessarily work well in this case. While some of the American scientists cooperated and shared discoveries, some did not. Large egos of eminent people were involved and this got in the way of good science. Gallo in particular was later criticized for his lack of cooperation.

Meanwhile, it was becoming apparent that a crisis was happening to the American blood supply. Here too economic interests would get in the way of prudent science and would cause many unnecessary deaths. In July of 1982, the case histories of three hemophiliacs who had died of AIDS were published. However, instead of assuming that the blood supply was tainted, which would have cost various institutions such as the Red Cross a great deal of money, leaders of these organizations chose to listen to scientists who believed that AIDS in homosexuals was caused by an overload of the immune system because of their numerous infections, and assumed that the same was true of hemophiliacs. This hypothesis, which was hotly debated, turned into a tragedy. The cost of monitoring the blood supply would have been astronomical and every excuse not to make it secure was seized upon. The decision not to test the blood supply turned into one of the many tragedies of the epidemic. As a result, there were tens of thousands of deaths from blood transfusions.

Up until this time AIDS had been assumed to be a gay disease. It had been labeled Gay Related Immune Deficiency and went by its acronym GRID. But now, besides cases in the hemophiliac community, two other groups were identified with AIDS. In early 1982 it was confirmed that a number of non-hemophiliac heterosexuals had contracted the disease; most of them were intravenous drug users. Finally, at about the same time, 34 cases of AIDS in Haitian immigrants were documented. It was assumed that there were more, since these largely illegal immigrants kept a low profile and did not often seek medical treatment. That they were impoverished was undoubtedly an additional factor discouraging them from seeking medical help.

Now the disease came to be associated with the four Hs: Homosexuals, Hemophiliacs, Haitians, and Heroine users. Unfortunately, with the exception of the hemophiliacs, none of these were sympathetic categories. The Reagan administration was determined to cut all nondefense spending and the health budget was hit especially hard. The politics of funding was nicely summarized by Tim Westmoreland, council for Representative Henry Waxman's subcommittee on health and the environment, in an opening statement he wrote, for Waxman to kick off hearings on the health budget cuts: "I want to be especially blunt about the political aspects of Kaposi's Sarcoma [a common cause of death due to AIDS]. This horrible disease affects members of one of the nations most stigmatized and discriminated against minorities. The victims are not main street Americans. They are gays from New York, Los Angeles and San Francisco. There is no doubt in my mind that if the disease had appeared among Americans of Norwegian descent, or among tennis players, rather than gay males, the response of both the government and the medical community would have been different.

Legionnaire's Disease hit a group of predominately white, heterosexual, middle-aged members of the American Legion. The respectability of the victims brought them a degree of attention and funding for research and treatment far greater than was made available so far to the victims of Kaposi's Sarcoma.

I want to emphasize the contrast, because the more popular Legionnaire's Disease affected fewer people and proved less likely to be fatal. What society judged was not the severity of the disease but the social acceptability of the people affected with it. . . ." He went on to say that he would fight any effort to base health policy on prejudice against other people's sexual preference or lifestyle. Yet this is exactly what happened for a long time, in spite of Waxman's efforts.

Reagan came into office determined to build up the American military and cut other spending. It was also a factor that a sizable part of his coalition regarded AIDS as a judgment of God against homosexuals. Waxman and Westmoreland had high hopes for the hearings, which they thought had gone very well, but they were disappointed to find that the press's response to their hearings mirrored the Reagan administration's response. Without the press it was nearly impossible to pressure the Reaganites.

Science and Politics

While the Reagan administration was ignoring the AIDS epidemic, by 1984 it was becoming apparent in the scientific community that a serious epidemic was in progress. Tragic though this was, it also represented an opportunity. Whoever solved the problem of AIDS would be in line for a Nobel Prize, and both the National Cancer Institute under Robert Gallo and the Pasteur Institute under Luc Montagnier joined the hunt. There are many real heroes in the AIDS story, selfless doctors who shared information with other scientists and the Pasteur Institute, which also cooperated with American researchers, especially Robert Gallo, to whom they sent samples of the retrovirus they had discovered. But, in the context of a political economy that emphasized individual accomplishment as opposed to cooperation, perhaps it is not surprising that cooperation was not consistent.

In 1984, in a conference in Park City, Utah, a visiting French researcher, Jean-Claude Chernon, was scheduled to present discoveries made by the Pasteur Institute. To begin with, much of his time was co-opted by colleagues of Dr. Gallo, who was rumored to be close to a breakthrough in identifying the AIDS virus. When Chernon did finally get a chance to speak, he stunned the audience with news that the "French team had made the breakthrough that Gallo was on the verge of making." Bob Gallo appeared shaken. One New York scientist described the scene this way: "Look, Bob Gallo is speechless, he's just figured out that the other guy is going to get to go to Sweden to get the Nobel Prize." Gallo recovered quickly, attacking and downplaying the French discovery. In spite of Gallo's skepticism, most of the scientists left convinced that the French had won the race.

In February 1984, samples of the retrovirus arrived from France at the Center for Disease Control in Atlanta. This allowed the Center for Disease Control to test and confirm that the French retrovirus was the same virus inhabiting AIDS patients in the United States. Bob Gallo, ever alert to the politics of the disease, was concerned that the infectious nature of the disease would cause it to be moved to the National Institute for Allergy and Infectious Diseases, costing his group its central role in research. He was also concerned that the French would get all of the credit for discovering the virus, which of course they had discovered. This later played out with a legal suit against Gallo, who had applied for and received a patent on "his discovery." The suit was settled in favor of the French. Meanwhile, the lack of cooperation on the part of the Americans slowed work on the disease. One can look at the scientists' squabbling over who gets credit, and failing to cooperate in the fight against the disease and blame individuals for their selfishness, but these individuals operated within a system that encouraged competition rather than cooperation. The emphasis in the American system on individual competition and striving may not justify the actions of some of the scientists, but it does help to explain it.

Reagan Comes on Board

In July of 1986, it was announced that movie actor Rock Hudson had contracted AIDS. Although Hudson was a closeted gay, in his public persona he represented something else entirely. In the movies he was the ultimate masculine American male whether playing the Hemmingway hero in *A Farewell to Arms* or the Texas oilman in *Giant*. The response to his announcement was a triumph of image over reality and shocked the nation. Instead of thinking that AIDS had just struck another gay they saw that this was a disease that could strike the rich and famous, their own personal idols. Up until this time conservatives had held sway over the budget for AIDS, actually stopping funding for AIDS education and limiting funds for research. They continued to successfully limit funding until October of 1986. However, they had now lost the press, and in October, C. Everett Koop, the Surgeon General, issued his report on the AIDS epidemic. Koop, a religious fundamentalist and anti-abortion advocate who was a favorite of the religious right, issued a call to arms against the epidemic that insisted upon AIDS education for children, and urged use of condoms. He also called for voluntary, not mandatory testing, recognizing that people would be tested only if guarantees of confidentiality were in place. Basically he came down in support of everything that the gay community had been advocating since the early 1980s. Koop became the hero of the AIDS advocacy groups and was suddenly anathema to the conservatives. Phyllis Schlafly, conservative anti-feminist, spoke out against him and various anti-abortion groups also spoke out against him.

These two events, the death of Rock Hudson and the leadership of the Surgeon General, changed the balance of power nationally. The newspapers took up the story and it became a political juggernaut. By the spring of 1987 the disease had spread to 113 countries, reporting a total of over 51,000 cases. The World Health Organization warned that we could expect 3 million cases by 1991. Europeans rushed to institute education programs. Only the United States, among developed countries, failed to launch an education campaign, but this was about to change.

By late spring, public pressure forced the Senate to push a resolution demanding that Reagan appoint an AIDS Commission. Koop continued speaking out, calling for action against the disease.

Reagan finally agreed to appoint a commission to advise him on the epidemic. However, it was not until 1987 that he finally addressed the nation and recognized the AIDS epidemic. By this time 36,058 Americans had been diagnosed with the disease and 20,849 had died. Reagan's acknowledgment of AIDS did not mean he was willing to do much about it. His speech called for testing of those getting wedding licenses, an insignificant part of the population likely to get AIDS, and made no mention of the hard-hit gay community. The speech was primarily a political response to a growing political problem, not the beginning of a new health policy. As we have seen, a key part of the Reagan coalition was the so-called religious right, made up primarily of Evangelical Christians. Leaders such as Jerry Falwell had declared the AIDS epidemic as God's judgment against homosexuals. It was not until the AIDS epidemic was perceived as a threat to the general population and the Surgeon General stepped forward to articulate that threat that Reagan responded. Even then, as we have seen, the Reagan response was designed to co-opt the political problem, not address the health problem. Valuable time had been lost both in terms of funding scientific research on a sufficient scale and on addressing educational issues.

By the end of the Reagan administration the epidemic was spreading beyond the four H categories into the mainstream of heterosexuals. In November 1991, basketball great Magic Johnson announced that he was HIV positive. This symbolized the movement of the epidemic into the mainstream, and helped change the public attitude toward the disease. However, the psychological cost to HIV/AIDS- infected people had been severe. Health professionals had refused to treat AIDS patients. Infected students had been sent home from school, ministers had refused to counsel infected parishioners. The failure to provide adequate public education had allowed rumors to spread and had created panic. Misinformation was the rule. Sex researchers Masters and Johnson reported that there was a chance of casual transmission from such things as toilet seats, while, at the other end of the spectrum, *Cosmopolitan Magazine* insisted that there was very little chance of women catching AIDS, even through having intercourse with an infected male. Both were wrong. There is no evidence of casual transmission and women are vulnerable to AIDS through heterosexual sex, in fact, much more vulnerable than men.

It was not until 1990, after the death of 120,000 Americans, that a serious care act was passed by Congress and signed into law by President George H. W. Bush. The Ryan White Care Act, named after a courageous young hemophiliac who had been horribly discriminated against and died in April 1990, finally provided federal aid for an extensive care program for those suffering from HIV/AIDS. The Ryan White Act is still in place, although it must be renewed periodically. Initially, AIDS had been a disease associated with marginalized groups, homosexuals, Haitians, and drug users. Now mainstream people like Ryan White, who was white and straight (he was infected because of his hemophilia), were marginalized because of the disease. The failure to provide adequate public information about the disease caused additional unnecessary suffering on top of the distress caused by the disease itself.

As we have seen, AIDS was early defined as a gay disease, its first name, GRID, reflected this. We have also seen how by 1983 it had spread to include new groups such as intravenous drug users, hemophiliacs, Haitians, and finally ordinary, mainstream heterosexuals. As the disease spread to heterosexuals, a new consensus emerged that demanded government action.

News of the disease from other countries confirmed that it was not just a gay malady. As AIDS was redefined as mainstream, the political and economic issues changed, as signified by the Ryan White Care Act. During the nineties better funded research did not produce a cure, but did produce drugs that could inhibit the progress of the disease in some cases and control the symptoms. Those with access to these drugs like Magic Johnson can sometimes remain symptom free for long periods of time (although not always). Those with access to education about AIDS and STDs can protect themselves. Those from middle-class homes that have fostered self-confidence can make better judgments about activities that will put them at risk. However, this leaves a lot of socially and economically disadvantaged people still vulnerable.

AIDS among New Minorities

While AIDS began in America as a disease afflicting a particular minority, gay men, by the 1990s it had moved into other minority communities. Today the fastest-growing demographic for AIDS infection is African-Americans. The second-fastest is Hispanics. While the gay community had a fairly typical distribution of wealth, including lots of professionals and other educated people who were natural leaders, this is not true among the new minorities with AIDS. AIDS is a disease of inner-city African-Americans and inner-city Hispanics. While many African–Americans and Latinos have made the transition into the middle class, they are still as a group on average poorer than white Americans. It is the poorest members of these communities that are suffering the ravages of the epidemic. Gays were able to organize, and, after much tragic loss of life, make the system work for them. In inner-city black and Hispanic communities this has not been the case. In the United States and around the world, AIDS has become a disease of powerlessness and poverty. It now strikes the most disadvantaged elements of the world's population and the very worst of the epidemic is in sub-Saharan Africa, the poorest region in the world. In the Western world the hardest-hit country has been Haiti, the poorest country in the Western Hemisphere.

Anthropologist Merrill Singer has written persuasively of the relationship between inner-city poverty and minority communities. While his research has focused on Puerto Rican immigrants who have the highest incidence of AIDS infection of any Hispanic group, his analysis sheds light on inner-city minorities generally. His general thesis is that poverty equals powerlessness, and those who are powerless in our political system do not have their problems addressed. As we have seen in looking at the gay community in the 1970s and 1980s, political power requires organization that in turn requires leadership. But as is also shown by the fate of the gay community in the eighties, there is a limit on the power of even well-organized people when they are the victims of majority prejudice, and stereotypes.

The Inner City

What we call the inner city has existed almost since the rise of big cities during the nineteenth century as a result of industrialization. First, native-born Americans and Irish and German immigrants, and then Italian, Polish, and other immigrants from southern and eastern Europe occupied the city. There was a push-pull to their immigration. Industrialization was transforming agriculture in both Europe and the United States, turning small-scale, half-subsistence farming into large-scale market farming. In the United States the depression of 1873 drove about 6 million people from the land as corn, wheat, and cotton prices dropped below the cost of production. In southern and eastern Europe, where the land was often in the hands of big land owners, the industrial revolution had created big cities with rich markets for large-scale, efficient production. New market crops and mechanization drove millions of peasants from the land, providing the push.

The rapid growth of the American economy following the Civil War provided the pull. The cities had to be built, railroads and canals had to be built, and people were needed to work in the factories and mines. But there were problems. The rapid growth of the city meant crowding and the crowding created high demand for a limited number of dwellings that in turn increased crowding as people with large families shared small tenement apartments. During a later immigration of African-Americans from the South, it was common to criticize multiple families who shared a single dwelling, as though their lack of good taste had caused them to do this. Of course, the cause was poverty combined with high real estate prices, and it was a practice pioneered by their nineteenth-century white predecessors. Desperation, not a lack of taste for the amenities of life, was the cause. Crowding meant overloading the infrastructure for sewage disposal, clean water, and fire protection. The result was fires and disease. In one year about 15% of the population of Chicago succumbed to cholera. In another year the city burned down in the famous Chicago fire of 1871. Initially, all classes of people shared the city, but as trolley lines appeared in the late nineteenth century, the middle class began forming a suburban ring around the cities. It was now possible to live in a healthier, more spacious environment and commute into the city, if you were prosperous enough.

The possibility of suburbs created the inner city. The movement of the more affluent middle class to the suburbs changed the political and economic dynamics. Poor immigrants, often not able to speak English, were powerless. Without the leadership of affluent neighbors, conditions, particularly health conditions, declined rapidly. The response to this problem was the rise of the big city political machines. Political bosses organized the immigrants into voting blocks to gain power. There is much misunderstanding about the machines that were regarded as corrupt and self-serving. They were corrupt and self-serving, but they flourished because the lack of government response to real problems had created an opening for them. Besides disease, pollution, and fire hazards, the new immigrants had to deal with a roller-coaster economy that saw big depressions in 1873 and in 1893. People out of work could not live off the land in the middle of New York or Chicago. The machine bosses used some of their ill-gotten gains to provide relief for these desperate people.

The Progressive Movement, led by Anglo-Protestant Americans, cleaned up the machines and reformed city government. However, their analysis of the problem did not lead to full understanding of the dynamics at work. Racial, ethnic, and religious prejudice played a big part in their understanding of the problems of the inner city, just as it did after World War II when African-American immigrants from the South came to occupy the cities. Americans of northern European descent regarded the Jewish or Catholic religious beliefs of many of the new immigrants with suspicion, and looked down on various cultural practices, particularly immigrant attitudes toward alcohol. The prohibition movement was to a large extent directed at the new immigrants. While the Progressives brought important and needed reforms to government and industry, their failure to understand the underlying causes of urban problems and their inclination to blame the victims left a popular residue of mistrust of urban people, of the poor, and of immigrants.

One final point about traditional American attitudes toward the city will be helpful in understanding the current attitudes toward the inner city. Until the end of the nineteenth century, America was a largely rural and frontier country. American identity had been shaped by this fact. The archetypal American heroes, from Natty Bumpo to Roy Rogers, had been frontiersmen or cowboys. America defined itself in opposition to Europe, especially Britain. They were the urban people crowded, congested, and unfree. We were the people of the land, unfenced and free. Freedom itself was seen to be a function of space. As an old cowboy lament says: "give me land lots of land under starry skies above, don't fence me in. . . ." Even today many American males define their masculinity in terms of the wilderness: fishing, hunting, or even crowding into national parks in an RV and with a color TV. Until the 9/11 tragedy New York City itself was despised as an almost un-American city. Undoubtedly this attitude was enhanced by the events of the late nineteenth century alluded to above, and continues to color many Americans' attitudes toward the urban.

AIDS in the African-American Community

The story of African-Americans in the city is similar in many ways to the story of earlier European immigrants. Immigration began in the post–Civil War period as African-Americans escaped repression in the post-reconstruction South. As with European immigrants they were initially integrated into the community. Certain trades such as barbering were more or less reserved for black males. Besides the rise of the suburbs, a new attitude toward African-Americans was emerging in the national consciousness. Reconstruction had been rife with corruption. Most of the benefits of this corruption had gone to Northern carpetbaggers or white Southern collaborators. Never-the-less, as white Southern governments were reestablished in the South (the so-called Redeemer governments that had "redeemed" the South from black Republican rule), Northerners basically accepted the South's story that the corruption showed blacks unfit to participate in government. Blacks were largely stripped of voting rights through violence, literacy tests, and a variety of other means. What followed was a period of extreme repression that was only marginally better than slavery for African-Americans in the South.

During the 1890s the Southern narrative about African-Americans was established as the law of the land by the Supreme Court. The most prominent and farreaching of the Court's decisions on race was *Plessey-Ferguson*, handed down in 1896. *Plessey-Fergusson* established that it was legitimate to establish segregation so long as blacks in their segregated accommodations were treated equally. Of course the accommodations were not equal, but until *Plessey-Ferguson* was overturned by *Brown vs. Board of Education* in 1954, this fact was ignored.

White Southern landowners had a problem to solve following the end of slavery. The Southern economy depended upon labor-intensive crops such as cotton and tobacco. How were they to survive without slaves? The answer was found through a system known as share cropping. The old plantations were divided into small plots of land allotted to poor whites and blacks. These sharecroppers would farm the land and give half of the crop to the owners to pay their rent. The system was such that sharecropping families were put into permanent debt to the owners. This created a situation of semi-bondage, since Southern states passed laws binding people in debt to the land. What this created for poor white and black families was essentially Third World conditions of poverty, malnutrition, violence, and ignorance. It did not prepare them to function easily in the urban settings to which many were driven during the twentieth century.

During the Great Depression of the 1930s, African-Americans fled the South in large numbers, seeking nonexistent jobs in Northern cities. Following World War II the number of immigrants became even greater. They were driven by new agricultural technologies that made them obsolete. As they poured into the Northern cities, they replaced an earlier generation of white immigrants who, benefiting from training from the G.I. Bill and the postwar boom, were moving to the suburbs, although there was considerable conflict with ethnic whites who had remained behind, unable to take advantage of the improved economy.

Earlier immigrants to the city from southern and eastern Europe had also experienced discrimination from the Anglo-American middle class, and had struggled with hard conditions to make their way in this new environment. However, by the early twentieth century they were able to find jobs in the booming factories that had undergone a dramatic change in organization. Frederick Taylor, an industrial engineer obsessed with efficiency, was finding ways to take the skills of craftsmen, who had been essential to the industrial process, and break them down and mechanize them so they could be accomplished by unskilled workers. He encouraged the invention of "smart machines" that could allow "dumb workers," that is, unskilled workers, to replace skilled workers. This drove down wages, but provided work for new, unskilled immigrants.

During the 1950s, the new African-American arrivals were finding a different kind of change in the workplace. New technologies developed during and after the war led to automation, which required fewer unskilled workers. In addition, industry was giving way to a service economy that was staffed with more educated employees. The result was that by the late fifties and sixties black male unemployment in the cities was sometimes over 50%. This took a horrible toll on the black family. Going all the way back to the late nineteenth century, African-American males had found it difficult to find employment. Black females by contrast, were in demand as nannies and maids. This reversed the traditional family relationship of the time, where males were expected to provide a living and women were expected to stay home and take care of the family. The damage to black male pride was devastating. The black family that had survived slavery now found itself faced with a new threat and one that they would not fare so well with.

What developed from this was a new kind of family relationship, a kind of serial monogamy. The instability of African-American men's economic situation made permanent relationships difficult. Illegitimacy soared, sometimes reaching over 80% in the inner city, and we had a new-style family emerging, the single-parent family. Mothers existed on support from welfare, sometimes a series of men, and low-level work. Children were often left on their own in a dangerous and deteriorating environment. The normal hopes for the future that allow most children to mature and achieve in a normal way did not exist for these children. They faced a bleak future. What existed was a situation rife for exploitation, and during this time organized crime began to move into the community with drugs.

The drug culture of the inner city has received a lot of attention by journalists, TV cop shows, and film, most of it very sensationalized. What is missing for most Americans is an understanding of the dynamics that have created this tragedy. As we have seen, the lack of employment for black men has been key to the problem. The subsequent collapse of the black family complicated the problem, creating a hopeless environment that made black youth particularly prone to grasp short-term pleasures in the absence of long-term hope. The introduction of drugs into the community provided both a respite from pain and a means to income. Entrepreneurial skills that with appropriate education might have allowed success in the mainstream economy found expression in the drug trade. Competition between large numbers of drug entrepreneurs led to extreme violence. It became so bad that violence became the leading cause of death for young black males. It also led to incarceration rates for black men that filled half the prisons, even though African-Americans, at this time, represented only 12% of the American population.

Drug dealers targeted teenagers. Addiction to drugs spawned other crimes. Women, to support themselves and their families as well as their drug habits, turned to prostitution. Theft became more common as a means of survival and to pay for drugs. This downward spiral of crime made an already difficult environment nearly impossible.

While all of this was going on in the inner city, largely invisible to white middle-class Americans, great progress was being made in passing national Civil Rights legislation. Lyndon Johnson was able to pass the Civil Rights Act that Kennedy had introduced but was unable to get through Congress, in 1964. The next year, in 1965, he was able to pass the Voting Rights Act, which transformed politics in the South, giving African-Americans rights to political participation that they had not had since Reconstruction. By 1965, the white middle class in the North had largely embraced Civil Rights after witnessing a number of atrocities committed against African-Americans in the South. And then things changed very suddenly.

In the summer of 1965, at the height of national euphoria about the progress made in Civil Rights, a riot broke out in an inner-city enclave of Los Angeles known as Watts. Before it was over, much of the area had been devastated by fire and 26 people were dead from the violence. The nation was shocked. How could this have happened when so much progress had been made in the Civil Rights cause? The Watts riots were followed over the next three years by even greater riots in all the major cities of America, the most devastating of which was the Detroit riots of 1967 that destroyed downtown Detroit and killed 48 people. While the war was going on in Vietnam, American National Guard troops were being deployed in open gun battles with black rioters.

What had gone wrong? Lyndon Johnson was aware of the potential dangers in the inner cities. Shortly after coming to office, he had announced his Great Society programs and his war on poverty initiative that targeted economic development in the inner city. White Americans were well aware of these programs and during this high tide of liberalism, many supported them. But now, an apparently ungrateful population was ignoring what had been done for them. The result was a severe backlash. This feeling among the white middle class was further exacerbated by the emergence of a more general counterculture movement among youth that seemed to threaten the stability of the Republic. In 1968 they went to the polls and elected Richard Nixon, who had run on a not-so-subtle anti-black platform and promised to restore order for the "silent majority" of Americans.

What had gone wrong was that the National Civil Rights Bills passed in 1964 and 1965 had done little to relieve the situation in the inner city. Johnson's war on poverty undoubtedly created rising expectations among inner-city blacks, but those expectations were soon dashed when funding for the Vietnam War superceded funding for the inner-city programs. The objective situation of urban African-Americans had not changed; in fact it had gotten worse in spite of all of the rhetoric. Rising expectations combined with deteriorating reality is a dangerous combination. The results were a disaster.

The Civil Rights era produced positive changes. It allowed a rising black middle class to prosper and integrate into the economy, and often geographically into the suburbs. But in doing so it created a problem for inner-city African-Americans. The integration of upwardly mobile African-Americans into the mainstream of American life took much of the energy and leadership out of reform. The result has been a sizable minority population left behind and soon joined by new minorities, primarily Hispanic. The backlash against liberal politics has also been part of the problem. The commitment to a more laissez- faire economy and so-called welfare reforms during the 1990s have not helped. To the problems of poverty, drugs, violence, and crime there is now the AIDS epidemic that threatens to be the biggest problem facing this already devastated community.

AIDS, once the scourge of one kind of minority community, leapt into the mainstream during the late eighties and nineties. Now it is fast becoming the disease of a new minority community consisting of inner-city African-Americans and Hispanics. Access to information and anti-viral drugs have slowed the advance of the disease in gay and mainstream straight communities, although there are disturbing signs that the existence of drugs has tempted risky behavior once again in the gay community. In the inner city we have seen the creation of social and economic conditions that have made that community much more likely to engage in behaviors (drugs and sex) that make them vulnerable to AIDS infection. We have also seen their growing powerlessness as the Civil Rights Movement has ebbed and middle-class blacks have moved on. These are exactly the conditions that Merrill Singer described as a precondition to an epidemic in the inner city.

Data from 2006 show clearly the new trends. The majority population, white non-Hispanics are now only the second-largest demographic for AIDS infection, and they are heavily represented by gay men. In 2006 they numbered 394,024. Blacks, who now represent only 13% of the population, have the most cases of AIDS infection with 409,982. Hispanics, who are only slightly more than 13% of the population, have 161,505 people infected. What is particularly troubling are the data on new infections diagnosed during 2007; 10,929 whites were diagnosed as HIV positive, 6,907 Hispanics were diagnosed, but 17,960 African-Americans were diagnosed as newly infected. This is an astonishing and disproportionate rate of increase for both Hispanics and African-Americans. If this continues it will soon be a minority disease once again. Looking further into the statistics, the results are even more disturbing: 72.9% of all infected intravenous drug users are either black or Hispanic. As of the end of 2006, the number of people infected through injection drug use had risen to 244,589, over half the number infected through male-to-male sex.

Why should there be this growing disproportion in infection rates? The answer lies in the history of the inner cities that have created the social conditions encouraging sexual promiscuity and drug use, but also in the condition of economic and political powerlessness that characterizes the inner city today. We have seen the importance of political organization in the San Francisco gay community that, although in the short run was counterproductive, in the long run helped stem the tide of infection. The lack of what we might call middle-class leadership in the inner city represents a big difference.

Rather than addressing the problems in a manner that would benefit entire communities, the conditions in the inner city have encouraged energetic people to solve their own problems through a criminal entrepreneurship that has further devastated the community. The enduring nature of the inner-city problem tends to nourish a cynicism that makes positive social action unlikely. Ironically, African-American youth have been encouraged to adopt a Social Darwinist attitude out of their cynicism, putting them in philosophic agreement with the same power structure that created the problem in the first place, although for very different reasons.

Merrill Singer and Political Economy

Singer calls for closely examining AIDS in terms of social class, ethnic relations, and gender politics. We see this as relevant to the growing epidemic in the United States, and in subsequent chapters we will argue that this is also true around the world, although different regions all have their unique histories that have created the conditions fostering the epidemic. Singer goes on to critique the methodology of his own discipline, anthropology, which he charges has erred in regarding inner-city communities as "exotic tribes" with their own cultures and therefore free from the influence of the larger society. Citing Eric Wolf's work, he argues that: "Increasingly, human groupings come to be seen and understood as concrete, independent wholes when they were in fact like peasants, part and parcel of larger social units brought into being and shaped continually by wider fields of power."

Singer acknowledges that there are advantages to approaching these groups from an ethnographic perspective, but the disadvantages are also very real. Inner-city ethnics as well as exotic tribes operate within a larger social, political, and economic context that they have little power to shape. They are only able to react to it, not to significantly influence it. Unlike San Francisco gays, they cannot represent themselves to the larger world.

Singer's research documents the way in which the inner city is influenced by outside political and economic forces. The starting point is the vulnerability created by racial discrimination and lack of education. As we have seen in this environment, drugs and sex come to play a disproportionate role in the community, partly, as he notes, because the Mafia has targeted the area for drug distribution; but also, as we have noted, because of the lack of parental guidance and the general hopelessness about the future that pervades the area. Drugs, as Singer points out, offer temporary escape from the harsh economic realities of life in the ghetto. As one of his informants says: "You grow up in a place where everything is a real mess. Your Father is a thief, your Mother is a whore, your kid sister gets herself some new clothes by fucking the landlord's son. Your brother is in the joint, your boyfriend gets shot trying to pull down a store, and everybody else around you is either smokin' dope, shooting stuff, taking pills, stealing with both hands, or workin' on their backs, or all of the above. All of a sudden you find that you are sweet sixteen and doin' the same things . . . it all comes on kind of naturally." Drugs and sex are clearly interrelated, first because both represent escape from the horrible reality of the ghetto, but also because one way of paying for drug habits is through prostitution or pimping.

There is a chain of vulnerability in the inner city. Besides drugs and sex there is poor health care and poor nutrition, both products of poverty. Poor nutrition leads to weakened immune systems. Poor health care means one is less likely to have treated non-AIDS sexually transmitted diseases (STDs) among other things. It has been established that STDs are a major contributing factor to AIDS, especially in heterosexual sex. Genital lesions from STDs can make vaginal sex more dangerous than anal sex. The prevalence of STDs in the sub-Saharan African population is assumed to be a major factor in the prevalence of heterosexual sex as a transmitting agent on that continent. Singer documents the role of non-AIDS STDs in the inner city, showing rates of infection for syphilis 3 to 7 times higher for African-Americans as for whites. Gonorrhea was especially prevalent in the African-American community, accounting for 82% of the cases by 1991. Herpes Simplex was 2–3.4 times higher for

African-Americans and Hepatitis B was 4.6 times higher for African-Americans than for whites. Given these conditions, HIV/AIDS can be seen as an opportunistic disease that follows poverty and powerlessness.

Within the African-American community the fastest-growing infected group is women. African-American women are 23 times more likely to be diagnosed with HIV-AIDS than white women. This is further confirmation of the principle that AIDS follows poverty and powerlessness. While the minority community as a whole is powerless in relation to the larger community, black women have a further degree of powerlessness. In their relations with men they are frequently either economically dependent or emotionally dependent. As women they are usually physically disadvantaged and frequently subjected to the rage and abuse that conditions impose on African-American men. In a community where the institution of marriage has broken down, or at least under serious stress, control of sexual encounters is problematic for women. The principle referred to before that having sex with someone is, from a health perspective, like having sex with all of that person's sexual partners is particularly relevant in the black community. The one thing other than abstinence that provides reasonable if not perfect protection from STDs, including AIDS, is prophylactics. The problem is that they get in the way of the full, unfettered joy of sex. They also signify a lack of trust. Since there are other means of birth control it is hard to argue that they are being used solely for contraception. Women worry that insistence might suggest that they have been unfaithful and might be infected, or that they do not trust the man they are with to be clean. The women can be threatened both emotionally and economically with abandonment or even physically with violence. The results are rapidly increasing rates of HIV/AIDS among African-American women that has already made it their leading cause of death. Only a recognition of the problems in the underlying social and economic system in the ghetto, and appropriate action, are likely to solve that problem; action that seems less likely as the economy moves into recession.

Recent Political Developments

The election of Barack Obama in 2008 at the start of the worst recession since the 1930s seemed to be a repudiation of the movement to the right represented by the Bush administration. During the Bush years the federal deficit had risen to nearly $12 trillion. Tax cuts, the biggest going to those in the upper one per cent of the income distribution, were supplemented with borrowing from overseas. Two costly wars were exacerbating the debt crisis. The recession and unemployment pushed down tax receipts and in addition to the federal debt problem, most states also found themselves heavily in debt. Meanwhile Obama doggedly pursued his promise to universalize health care to include 45 million uninsured Americans. After a year of intense political battle, he was able to pass a watered down bill. However, it turned out to be a costly victory, it not only galvanized opposition on the right, but the sacrifice of a single payer option angered Obama's liberal supporters. Other Americans were angered by the perception that Obama had focused too much on health care and not enough on job creation. As the jobless rate hung around 10%, voters went to the polls in 2010 and elected a Republican house and lots of Republican governors. Although the recession was officially over, joblessness persisted and therefore tax receipts remained low.

The political scene was complicated by the emergence of a grassroots conservative movement taking the name "Tea Party". Like the original Boston Tea Party they were protesting high taxes and intrusive government. The word socialist was bandied about, applied to Obama's health care bill and to Obama himself, this movement not only targeted the new health care bill, but threatened both the medicaid and medicare programs. Republican representative Ryan from Wisconsin introduced a new plan that would get rid of both the medicare and medicaid programs as we know them, substituting fixed payments to insurance companies for medicare and block grants to states for medicaid. Neither proposal adequately anticipates continuing inflation in health care costs leaving shortfalls to be made up elsewhere, by individuals or states. Gutting the medicaid program would cause considerable difficulty in the war on AIDS, since it provides health care for the poor. As we have seen, AIDS gets a foothoid where there is poverty and inadequate health care. The new health care bill should improve care in the inner city where minorities are bearing the brunt of the epidemic. But not only is the health care bill at risk of being defunded, repealed, or overturned by the courts, but even the status quo is being rolled back with the attack on medicare and medicaid.

The threat to American health care is not just at the federal level. New tea party backed governors are cutting budgets at the state level also. Beginning in Wisconsin with Governor Walker, new governors are cutting back on insurance benefits and a variety of outreach programs that provide health care and family counseling. As part of the small government mantra, there is an attack on anti-poverty programs such as head start that aim to raise disadvantaged children out of the demographic that is so vulnerable to AIDS, and an attack on public education which historically has allowed the poor some possibilities of social mobility. Considering our discussion earlier in the chapter of children growing up in the inner cities, what is needed are resources that will provide some hope if we are to address the despair felt by children that leads to destructive behaviors.

If one listens to the rhetoric of the new right it sounds a lot like the rhetoric of 19th century conservatism. This affirms the enduring power of the superstructure. The myths of the past continue to shape our values and political discourse. During hard times we seem to forsake reasoned discourse and turn to familiar and emotionally powerful myths to guide our actions.

Political Economy and the Rest of the World

In subsequent chapters we will be examining the political economic influence on AIDS in a variety of communities, in Africa, Asia, and elsewhere. Each community has its own story. What is shared is that every community in the world is now, and has been for some time, tied into the larger world economy, and to some extent has been influenced by political forces greater than themselves. Certainly colonialism is one of those forces that we will be looking at. It is a cliché, but still true that the world is shrinking. All areas, whether weak Third World countries or global powers, are influenced heavily by everyone else. As we look at these areas, especially in sub-Saharan Africa and Asia, we will be exploring how these influences and connections are shaping the contours of the AIDS epidemic.

Summary

This chapter looks at the creation of political and economic values that have shaped our attitudes towards government action to address economic, social and health problems. It argued that American attitudes towards government were shaped by powerful interest groups that have not always followed the principles they have set forward. We discussed the beginning of the AIDS crisis in the gay community and the success of that community in organizing at the local level. We also saw that hostility towards this minority prevented a forceful federal intervention until much damage was sustained. We noted that politics is often a problem in the scientific community and can hinder cooperation and thereby slow progress. We saw that the middle class gay community was able finally to gain the political support it needed to stem the disease, but that other minorities have not been so successful. We discussed the historic development of a racially defined underclass in the inner city and the economic blight and despair that has made African-Americans and Hispanics the new center of the AIDS epidemic in America. Finally we looked at the political and economic events of the past two years and saw a resurgence of anti-government conservative values that we believe will make it more difficult to address the AIDS epidemic particularly among the poor in the inner city.

Name: ______________________ Date: ______________

Chapter 3 Political Economy

Exercises

Exercise 1 Test Your Knowledge:

1. Both political power and economic power set the parameters for AIDS infection.
   a. True
   b. False
2. Herbert Spencer's philosophy of Social Darwinism asserted life was naturally a struggle for survival among competing elements.
   a. True
   b. False
3. Creative destruction refers to the natural process of the market system destroying what has proved to be unfit.
   a. True
   b. False
4. The gay movement began in June of 1969 in San Francisco, CA.
   a. True
   b. False
5. Bath houses were privately run clubs where gay men could meet, fraternize, and have uninhibited sex.
   a. True
   b. False
6. Ronald Regan addressed the nation and recognized the AIDS epidemic immediately when AIDS first hit gay American community in 1980.
   a. True
   b. False
7. Today, the leading and fastest growing demographic for AIDS infection is Hispanics.
   a. True
   b. False
8. The Civil Rights era allowed a rising black middle class to prosper and integrate into the economy, and often geographically into the suburbs.
   a. True
   b. False

9. AIDS is a disease of powerlessness and poverty.
    a. True
    b. False
10. *Roe v. Wade* provided federal aid for an extensive care program for those suffering from HIV/AIDS.
    a. True
    b. False

Study Questions

1. How did the American Federation of Labor (AF of L) approach capitalism?

2. How does Social Darwinism regard the problem of social justice?

3. How does John Stuart Mill advocate modifying the market system?

4. What is the attitude of orthodox Marxists toward Mill's ideas? Why?

5. Why are gay men in San Francisco more militant than gay men in New York City?

6. Explain the importance of the bathhouses to gay men in San Francisco? What is their symbolic meaning?

7. How did politics impede scientific research on the causes of AIDS?

8. What technological changes led to the isolation of the inner city?

9. What drove blacks North into the inner cities after World War II? What changes caused such high rates of unemployment in the inner city during this time period?

10. What group of people in America today (gender and race) has the highest rate of increase in HIV infection? What are the reasons for this?

11. What is the relationship of the superstructure to the base according to Marx?

12. Why did the success of the Civil Right Movement create problems for the inner city?

13. Why has Obama's health care bill angered people on both the right and the left?

14. Why is medicaid important in the struggle against AIDS?

Chapter four | HIV/AIDS in Asia

Until the late 1980s, no Asian country had experienced a major AIDS epidemic. By the late 1990s, however, all of Asia was faced with a complex and devastating epidemic of AIDS. According to the UNAIDS (United Nations Program on AIDS), in 2007, an estimated 5 million people were living with HIV in Asia, including 380,000 people newly infected in that year (UNAIDS 2008).

Due to the stigmatization of the HIV infected and the conservative number provided by many governments, the HIV/AIDS epidemic in this region is much more severe than what the public statistics show. Some governments deliberately reduce the number to hide the severity of the epidemic. Due to stigmatization and marginalization, intravenous drug users, commercial sex workers, and same-sex behavior remain clandestine, and some of the infected go underground. Consequently, the epidemic could suddenly surge without any warning.

In Asia, it is the cultural, political, and economic factors that have fueled the AIDS pandemics. These factors include authoritarian government, a colonial history, gender imbalance, intergenerational imbalances of power, migration of labor, economic disparity, and social stratification.

FIGURE 4.1 HIV Prevalence (%) in Adults in Asia, 2007

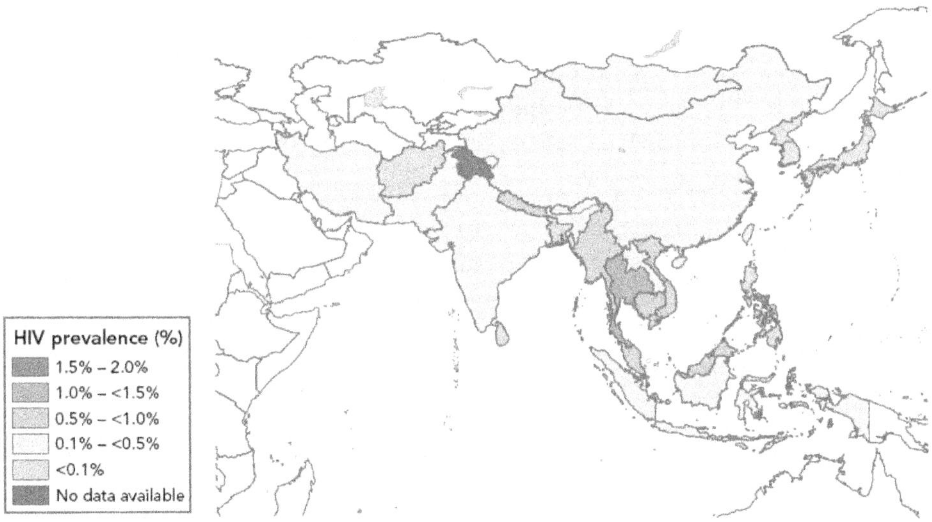

As a result of the global capitalist economy, unequal distribution of global income, unequal allocation of resources, and unequal access to health care have left those at the bottom of the society vulnerable to infections. Due to the drastic inequity among sexes, classes, and generations, most of the infected are marginal to their own societies and the global economy.

In this chapter I will first elaborate on a wide array of factors leading to the AIDS epidemic in Asia, and then explore the situation of the AIDS epidemic in several countries.

Colonial History

Due to the European colonial exploitation in Asia, wealth, resources, and treasure had been plundered away from Asia and the democratic development (Hunter 2005). Colonial countries utilized the resources of Asian countries to carry their own economies to high standards of living, leaving the economies in many Asian countries stagnated (Hunter 2005). The educational and economic systems in many colonial countries were financed through the opium trade in Asia in general, and the opium war in China in particular. For many Asian countries, the history of being colonized has profound political and economic implications. It has created entrenched poverty, illiteracy, violence, and polarized social stratifications (Hunter 2005). While the elite have reaped the fruit of the colonial disorder, the lower echelon of the society has not been able to taste the sweetness of the economic growth. Rather, they were left behind, disenfranchised and marginalized.

Colonization has also led to the wide spread of STDs. In many colonized areas, colonizers demanded that the colonial state provide women for the sexual needs of its military forces. The supply of comfort women for the Japanese colonizing military groups is one example. The British in India, the Dutch in the East Indies, the French in Indochina, and the Spanish in the Philippines, all helped with the growth of regulated prostitution and generated spread of STDs associated with prostitution. Until the twentieth century, the sexual health of the colonized was almost entirely neglected (Lewis 1997: 3).

For instance, the Japanese colonial war in China during the early twentieth century promoted the spread of STDs in Republican China, due to rampant rape, displaced populations, poverty, rural to urban migration, and recruitment of comfort women for the Japanese military troops. Furthermore, the Japanese invasion of China drove more than half a million refugees into Hong Kong, precipitating the growth of prostitution for economic survival (Lewis 1997). The Japanese not only forced women into prostitution, but also closed civilian venereal disease clinics. As a result, "a large population of the community became infected" (Lewis 1997: 9).

Similar situations occurred in Korea, Singapore, Malaysia, the Philippines, and Indonesia (Lewis 1997). In the Philippines, from 1942, Japanese economic policy destroyed the sugar industry and produced a great rice shortage. Many rural people migrated to the urban areas looking for survival, where some women became prostitutes. Some Filipinos were also forced to work as comfort women for Japanese troops. During the Japanese occupation throughout East Asia and parts of Southeast Asia, not only Filipino women, but also Chinese, Korean, Indonesian, and European women were drafted and forced to work as comfort women for the Japanese troops (Lewis 1997: 9).

After the United States entered the Vietnam War in 1965, more than 10 million civilians were displaced in the South and at the end of the war in 1975, more than 1 million South Vietnamese were infected (Lewis 1997: 9). The U.S. military base expanded to Thailand where thousands of American servicemen arrived on "Rest and Recreation"—so-called "Intoxication and Intercourse," from Vietnam. It was reported that in 1968–1969, the number of prostitutes increased from 151,000 to 300,000, according to the sources such as the World Bank. Along with it, prevalence of STDs soared during this time (Lewis 1997: 9).

This part of the colonial history in Asia had a profound impact on the spread and prevalence of STDs in the region.

Gender Inequality

Gender-based political and economic disparities have played a significant role in the spread of HIV in Asia. In this region, for women, one of the highest risk factors for HIV infection is often marriage, or what the woman perceives as a monogamous relationship. This is because men are more likely to engage in extramarital sex. Even if some women suspect that their husbands are HIV positive, they still have little power to insist on condom use. Most often, low levels of education and poor access to information impede women from procuring the knowledge they need to protect themselves.

In 2007, women accounted for 29% of adults with HIV in Asia. In Thailand, though the epidemic has diminished, more and more people traditionally believed to be at lower risk of infection get infected. About 43% of new infections in 2005 were among women, most of whom were infected by husbands or partners. In India, a significant proportion of women with HIV have probably been infected by regular partners who have paid for sex (UNAIDS 2008).

In many parts of Asia, religious and cultural beliefs have led to gender inequality. Men have most of the political, economic, and social power. Politically, men held 85% of the seats in Asian parliaments (Hunter 2005). Economically and socially, men amassed more wealth and held more positions of power than women in many Asian countries. Also, because cultural mores prescribe that women be sexually pure and do not engage in sex unless married, they are expected to be ignorant about sex prior to marriage. In China, for example, girls are inculcated with moral values about the perils of sex and the need to wait until marriage to be sexually active. This is a cultural effort to protect women's virginity, and social order as a whole. However, for men, in many Asian countries, cultural norms recognize men's biological need to engage in sex without considerations of feelings or love. Men are not expected to be faithful. Culturally prescribed gender norms aim to preserve male comfort and accommodate masculine sexual urges.

Research has revealed that from 5 to 20% of adult men in Asia visit sex workers at least once a year, among which the subsidiary rates are 7% in the Philippines to about 11% in Japan to 15–20% in Cambodia (Brown 2003). In Thailand, the figure fell in 1993 from 20% to 10% due to intense prevention campaigns. In Indonesia, since only 14% of men who buy sex say that they use condoms with sex workers, it is not surprising that 14–16% HIV infection rate has been found among sex workers in parts of the Papua province (UNAIDS 2008).

As a result of such gender norms, women in general are less informed about sex than men, whereas it is commonly accepted that men have multiple sexual partners. For instance, in Southeast Asia, only 13% of young women could identify two ways to protect themselves from HIV. In Laos, a 2003 survey revealed that 70% of women had never heard of HIV/AIDS. In Cambodia, 30% of women thought they could get HIV upon being cursed. In Central Asia and Eastern Europe, half of young women believed a healthy person could not be carrying HIV (Hunter 2005). As men have the power to decide whether condoms are used or not, many women are infected by their husbands or their sexual partners.

Religion produces and reinforces gender inequality in political leadership and social and economic entitlement. Certain religions such as Hinduism exhibit a misogynist viewpoint. Hinduism, for instance, defines feminine without the masculine as destructive and fierce. It is believed that women are unclean and impure, and can be so powerful that they can nullify men's sacred mantras. Thus it is the religious decree that women must be dependent on men. Furthermore, women are classified as the lowest caste in the caste system. Many instances have occurred in India, such as female infanticide; sati (the cultural practice where a wife is obliged to die on her husband's funeral pyre), or widow burning; dowry-related murders; and crime against women.

In many parts of Asia, women are treated as property and they are expected to achieve a livelihood and social status through marriage. In Thailand, women serve as cheap labor in households, agriculture, factories, and in the sexual services industry. In export-oriented industries, women occupy up to

80% of the workforce. On average, women workers are given two-thirds of the wages of men. Their subordinate status makes them not only cheap labor, but also a compliant source of labor. In tandem with urbanization and capitalist organization of agricultural production, many women migrate from rural areas to urban areas searching for survival means. Often times, they enter commercial sex work or low-paid factory and domestic work (Lewis 1997: 7).

Due to the fact that women are denied equal rights and men control women in many social arenas, gender inequality fuels a booming illicit sex trade. In the region where women and girls lack social, educational, and economic power, many women find it difficult to obtain employment. Poverty and lack of opportunity drive many into sex work, where they cannot negotiate condom use.

In the absence of social welfare programs, urban-based sex workers cope with poverty and unemployment by remitting funds to their rural families. In Thailand for instance, urban sex workers sent $300 million annually to their rural families. As in many other Asian countries, it is the sex workers' remittance that compensates for the government lack of concern for rural welfare and allows the poor to survive.

Women and girls who are trafficked for sex work also face a high risk of HIV infection. Research has revealed a 38% HIV prevalence among trafficked women and girls who have been repatriated to Nepal, and 50% HIV prevalence among those trafficked to Mumbai and India (UNAIDS 2008). In India, a 16% HIV prevalence has been found among home-based sex workers, 26% among street-based sex workers, and 47% among brothel-based sex workers (UNAIDS 2008).

If women and girls were found to be HIV positive, it was reported that they were not only often beaten, abandoned, or killed by their husbands and families, but also suffered discrimination in housing, employment, and inheritance (Hunter 2005).

In certain areas such as China, because the favor of sons to carry on lineage is so prevalent, sex ratios of 120 men to 100 women have been noted.

In countries such as India, Afghanistan, and Pakistan, women are not allowed to own or inherit property. In Nepal, an amendment of the 2002 civil code allowed daughters to share equal status with sons to inherit property. The amendment law also required parents to provide the same kind of care and protection for their daughters as their sons. According to the 2004 report however, less than 1% of the women legally owned their land, homes, livestock, or other assets. Only 16% had certain kinds of regular income; most women worked in the fields or attended to housework chores (Hunter 2005).

In Laos, truck drivers seek clean girls who do not ask for condom use. Many truck drivers have more than one extramarital wife. Infections have been reported in farmers, businessmen, hotel and service sector workers, and the unemployed (Hunter 2005). In Vietnam, half of the HIV/AIDS cases are found among 20- to 29-year-olds, three-fourth of whom are heterosexuals (Hunter 2005).

Health Care System

According to Susan Hunter, the inadequate health care system has left a great number of HIV-positive people unaware of their status, and 40–50% of AIDS sufferers without medical attention of any kind (Hunter 2005).

The Government and Prevention

Due to the lack of prevention messages and many Asian governments' conservative approach to sexuality, many many people have been left ill-informed about how to protect themselves. On top of that, the U.S.-funded abstinence program has also pressured many Asian governments to participate. This program has been the mainstay of the Bush administration's foreign policy on HIV/AIDS. For years, the Bush administration has been supporting a foreign policy that interferes with condom use and promotes abstinence only for the prevention strategy. In 2003, Catholic cardinals preached that condoms were so unreliable that their use "is like betting on your own death" (Hunter 2005). They offered the advice of "natural family planning" to discourage condom use, and argued for total abstinence from sex. In some Asian countries, the Vatican's anti-condom stance was adopted and the police can arrest a prostitute for possession of condoms (Hunter 2005).

In the Philippines, the government has recently been in the process of adopting the prevention strategy of condom promotion and putting in place a solid national AIDS prevention program. However, impacted by the U.S.-advocated abstinence-only policy, President Arroyo started making false statements about condom effectiveness and prohibiting condom distribution in public health facilities. The president blocked availability of free condoms, terminated programs of condom promotion, and ceased supplying condoms to local clinics (Hunter 2005). Along with the anti-condom stance of the president, 85% of the Catholics utilize moral arguments to oppose condom use and claim that condoms contain microscopic pores that are permeable by HIV pathogens (Hunter 2005).

Because HIV was first discovered in a Filipino national who returned from overseas on contract labor in 1984, and subsequently in prostitutes, the government and media agencies in the Philippines have portrayed the spread of HIV in the Philippines as a problem of foreigners, and prostitutes became the target of social hostility (Law 2000: 83). The Catholic Church (and its related groups) generates a "medico-moral" discourse that seeks to control sexuality by condemning "three P's"—Premarital sex, Promiscuity, and Prostitution—and opposes condom use as it promotes promiscuity, and legitimizes prostitution (Law 2000: 83).

Working within such a conservative environment, local health workers in the Philippines united together to pool their own funds, purchase condoms in bulk, and sell them at discount prices to the poor (Hunter 2005).

In other countries such as Laos, the government has no money for prevention campaigns or HIV testing. Due to the lack of government-initiated prevention programs, condom use is very low in the region. For instance, in Indonesia, each year only 10% of 10 million men who visit sex workers use condoms (Hunter 2005).

Government Inertia

With the exception of Cambodia and Thailand, many Asian governments such as India and China have exhibited a reluctance in acknowledging the extent of the HIV epidemic, and have shown an inertia in establishing effective measures to curb the spread of the disease and combat the stigmatization against the HIV infected.

In some Asian countries, the governments were responsible for the tainted blood supply that caused many casualties and HIV infection. For instance, in 2001, the Japanese court convicted a Ministry of Health bureaucrat for being responsible for the death of 500 people due to the tainted blood supply. In 1998, WHO (World Health Organization) estimated that one-fifth of India's HIV infections were from improperly screened blood and blood products. Blood supply became a national scandal in the early 1990s. Studies in 1996 estimated that 95% of India's blood supply was unsafe. In India, blood supply also became a national scandal in the early 1990s. In China, as I will illustrate below, local governments were involved in an illegal yet highly profitable blood trade where unsterilized needles were used and reused; 1.5 million people in central China were infected with HIV through the blood trade, yet for years the central government had been instrumental in concealing the HIV epidemic as a national secret.

Drug Users and Sex Workers

"In countries without laws to protect sex workers, drug users, and men who have sex with men, only a fraction of the population has access to prevention. Conversely, in countries with legal protection and the protection of human rights for these people, many more have access to services. As a result, there are fewer infections, less demand for antiretroviral treatment, and fewer deaths. Not only is it unethical not to protect these groups: it makes no sense from a health perspective." Secretary-General Ban Ki-moon's speech at the International AIDS Conference, cited from UN News Centre. 2008. "Address to the International AIDS Conference."

Growing poverty and economic disparity have impacted those who have not benefited from Asia's participation in the global economy. The disappointment and frustration have caused increased injection drug use and sex work, and the region has seen a serious overlap of injection drug use and sex work. Few countries have been able to develop effective programs such as peer education or syringe exchange programs to help with the drug users and sex workers, because most governments hold antagonistic and hostile attitudes toward them. Their major measures in dealing with the drug users and sex workers have been crackdown and punishment.

Many Asian countries such as Vietnam and China perceive drug use and commercial sex as social evils. Upon discovery, drug users and sex workers are imprisoned in rehabilitation centers. Yet at the same time, local governments profit from the sex industry through bribes from the sex business.

WHO, UNODC (United Nations Office on Drugs and Crime) and UNAIDS recommend a compressive harm reduction interventions that comprise multiple strategies, the mainstay of which include needle and syringe programs (NSPs), outreach and peer education (safe sex and condom distribution), primary health care (STI treatment) and Opium Substitution therapy (OST) and other substitution therapies. Harm reduction has been acknowledged as the most effective approach to curb HIV transmission (UNAIDS 2010).

WHO, UNODC (United Nations Office on Drugs and Crime) and UNAIDS argue that if these strategies are implemented together, they can greatly reduce IDUs' risk of contracting HIV and radically diminish the spread of HIV as well as Hepatitis B and C (UNAIDS 2010).

Needle and syringe exchange programs are critical in providing clean and safe injection equipment for drug users. Substitution therapy wherein synthetic substitutes such as methadone and buprenorphine are provided and taken orally can diminish injection frequencies and reduce cravings (UNAIDS 2010). We will discuss the needle and syringe exchange program further in Chapter 8.

Several countries in Asia have started implementing the harm reduction programs. For instance, Indonesia revised its national AIDS strategy in 2007 to include harm reduction and a court ruling called for the prioritization of drug rehabilitation over imprisonment for drug users. China and Malaysia have greatly increased the number of Opium Substitution Therapy sites. China, Indonesia and Malaysia have implemented the most increases in the number of Needle and Syringe Exchange Program sites (UNAIDS 2010).

A study of 103 cities showed that HIV incidence declined in 36 cities with NSPs by an annual rate of 18.6%, whereas HIV incidence increased in 67 cities without NSPs by an annual rate of 8.1%. Another study in Manipur, India, has shown that following the implementation of NSPs, needle sharing among IDUs has sharply decreased over the period of six years, yielding a decrease in HIV prevalence among that group (UNAIDS 2010).

Methadone treatment in China has also demonstrated a lower HIV incidence (0%) and reduced needle sharing (2 injections per month) among those who accessed the treatment, juxtaposed by the 3–9% HIV incidence among non-treatment groups (90 injections per month).

Despite these exemplary cases, in general, Asia has extremely low coverage of these harm reduction programs, with only one in 50 IDUs being reached. In 2007, only 3% of IDUs had access to harm reduction programs and only 8% had access in East Asia, most of whom were in China). In 2007, in East, South and South-East Asia, the median number of syringes distributed by NSPs per IDU per year was about 27, far below the internationally recommended target of 200 syringes provided per IDU per year (UNAIDS 2010).

Since drug use is often illegal, drug users tend to be 'hidden' and clandestine. Therefore, harm reduction programs are hard to implement without a supportive government policy, cooperation from local police and authorities, and outreach and peer education which can help bring IDUs to NSP or substitution clinics.

Because sex work is illegal in most parts of Asia, the sex industry is run, managed, and controlled by male thugs, and usurped and exploited by local officials (Zheng 2009b). In Zheng's research on the sex industry in urban China, for instance, the state policy against sex work was distorted and even derailed by the interest-seeking behavior of local officials. Officials extracted economic benefits from clandestine brothels and arrested sex workers through a combination of bribes and fines. In this sense, the state policy was high-jacked by the service of officials' personal economic interests (Zheng 2009b).

Drug use flourishes in many countries in Southeast Asia and in Yunnan province of China. In 1999, surveys in 19 cities of Nepal revealed that 40% of injecting drug users were infected. By 2001, in Jakarta, Indonesia, the infection rate in this group was also 40% (Brown 2003).

Central Asia is another region where drug use is prevalent in the environment of poverty and organized crime. In Central Asia, injection drug use is responsible for 30 to 90% of HIV infection. Moscow alone has more than 1 million drug users, including 150,000 needle-using cocaine and heroin addicts (Hunter 2005).

The drug use in Central Asia is increasingly associated with the youth culture. Drastic social transformations such as economic liberalization and globalization have spawned massive unemployment and a bleak view of the future. Feeling lost and frustrated, young people resort to sex and drugs for release or rebellion.

Drug Trafficking

Drug trafficking is intersected with trafficking in women and other laborers, led by gangster bands that operate across the heart of the region (Hunter 2005). India not only produces opium, heroin, and marijuana, but also serves as an international node for drug trafficking. Heroin is trafficked from Myanmar and Laos to India, and India is a major center where the drug money goes through laundering. As the drug trade and human trafficking flourish in this area, the Indian government cracked down on drugs in 2003, resulting in 2,000 deaths (Hunter 2005).

Migration

Migration has been identified as one of the most important risk factors for HIV transmission around the world. Due to the economic upheaval and economic disparity, to maintain survival and combat poverty, both men and women circulate within and between China, Japan, India, Singapore, and other countries in Asia to work in mining, construction, seafaring, fishing, and the sex industry, as demanded by the market. Male migrants can pick up HIV virus from visiting sex workers during their lonely years of migration labor in a distant city or country. Upon returning home, they can transmit the virus to their wives. Female migrants can participate in lucrative sex work for its fast profit, thereby subjecting themselves to possible HIV infection.

Ethnic Inequality

Many Asian countries operate a prejudiced and stigmatizing view of ethnic minorities, leading to their poverty and vulnerability to HIV infection. In many countries, ethnic minorities hold a low social status and poverty drives them into the drug industry and sex work. For instance, in India, the Hindu caste system classifies the society into a hierarchical social status, from Brahmins or priestly teachers to soldier-nobles, and from merchants to Dalits, and finally to the lowest Chandals. Ethnic minorities are despised as the lower-caste Indians and have less access to health care (Hunter 2005).

In Thailand, the majority group enjoys high levels of school attendance and literacy. However, for ethnic minorities, access to social benefits and services is restricted (Hunter 2005). In Bangladesh, ethnic women are often raped to maintain discipline as militarization is the government's major vehicle for subjugation (Hunter 2005). In China, the Han Chinese deem ethnic minorities to be morally loose, economically primitive, and sexually promiscuous. Similarly, rural migrant workers are also stigmatized and despised for the same stereotypes.

During the early days of the Chinese HIV epidemic, China mapped HIV/AIDS onto minority prefectures in Yunnan because of these prejudiced perceptions about ethnic minorities. As Sandra Hyde has shown in her book, although the Chinese public health services and social scientists responded to the epidemic by linking HIV/AIDS to ethnic cultures and their cultural behaviors, in reality, it was poverty and drug trafficking that drove the epidemic in this area (Hyde 2007).

Hyde contends that the Chinese government was unwilling to acknowledge the problem of poverty and blamed it on the minority borderlands, reflecting the Han stereotype of ethnic minority groups as loose and sexually uninhibited. She argues that the underlying goal was to control China's borders through controlling borderland bodies. Through examining surveys and collections of statistics about minority populations in Yunnan, Hyde argues that the purpose of this process is control and surveillance. She asserts that it is through this process that the Chinese state maintains control over the border regions (Hyde 2007).

Nationalism

In many parts of Asia, in the early days of the AIDS epidemic, AIDS was considered as an imported product from the West. Nationalism and anti-foreign sentiments abound in the region's responses to AIDS. As HIV/AIDS was represented as a product of sexual promiscuity and bad morals, those infected were said to "lead a western lifestyle" and exhibit weak will, poor self-discipline, poor morality, and a heavy reliance on drugs. Since foreigners were identified as harboring these "bad" and "abnormal" sexual values, AIDS was construed as mainly the problem of foreign countries and as evidence of capitalist corruption and decadent lifestyles.

In the late 1980s, HIV/AIDS was perceived as a foreign import in Thailand. In 1989, the oldest university in Bangkok set up a regulation to screen foreign staff for HIV status. In India, facing the onslaught of HIV infections at the end of the 1980s, the director general of the Indian government's Council for Medical Research declared, "This is a totally foreign disease, and the only way to stop its spread is to stop sexual contact between Indians and foreigners" (Sontag 1989: 80).

In Hong Kong, a survey in 1993 revealed that 70% of respondents attributed the low HIV rate in the region to the small number of homosexuals in Asia, and Asian people's nature to be sexually conservative, unlike the promiscuous West (Lewis 1997). In Indonesia, the initial response was to blame the foreigners for the disease and prevent foreigners from entering prostitution establishments (Lewis 1997).

In China, when the first AIDS case was reported in an American patient who died in Beijing in 1985, he was reviled as a foreigner who was alleged to have engaged in "abnormal" (homosexual) behaviors. After he died, his room was disinfected for 24 hours and all his clothes, the nurses' clothes, and medical equipment were burned. He was hated and detested, for he had brought terror and fear to everyone in the hospital. Thereafter it was reported that foreign males had infected Chinese nationals in China and Chinese immigrants were infected abroad. This official discourse evinced a law on the mandatory testing of all foreign residents. Since 1992, national sentinel surveillance sites have been set up in a number of cities to screen the blood of foreigners, returnees from abroad, international marriage spouses, and other "high-risk groups" (Li 2000; Lin 2000).

In 1987, the head of the Hygiene Ministry declared that AIDS could be controlled in China because the two means of transmission, gay relationships and promiscuity, were prohibited in China. After several years, the mayor of Kunming, Yunnan, reiterated the message in conferences that AIDS was the problem of foreigners. Hence it was necessary to proceed with the most severe checks of foreigners at the airport.

Surveillance stations were established at various airports to mandate AIDS virus tests for foreigners and returned workers from abroad.

Media in South Korea also invoked the menace of AIDS from the outside and the fear of foreign sexual contamination (Cheng 2005a). In 1985, the first case of HIV was identified in a man who reportedly got infected abroad. This first case confirmed that the virus belonged to the outside world (Cheng 2005a). In 1987, the AIDS Prevention Act introduced measures to screen the HIV status of migrant workers and foreigners who intended to stay long-term in South Korea. Any HIV-positive non-Korean, upon discovery, was deported. By 2002, 260 foreigners had been deported due to their HIV-positive status (Cheng 2005a).

Their neighbor nation, Japan, has also construed AIDS as a foreign disease. The fact that the infected blood in Japan came primarily from the United States contributes to the constructed foreignness of the disease. Hence the Japanese government blamed foreigners, especially migrant sex workers, for sexual transmission of HIV (Buckley 1997). The Japanese official figures always separate foreigners from the Japanese, resulting in the stigmatization of the illegal immigrant women in the entertainment and sex industry. Japan also emphasizes the lifestyle of avoiding gay sex and sex work, and perceive homosexuals, foreigners, and drug users as threats to the happy, risk-free, heterosexual family (Cheng 2005a).

Other countries such as Taiwan, Thailand, Nepal, and the Philippines also echoed this pattern (Hsu 2004; Pigg 2001; Smyth 1998).

Exemplary Countries

At the advent of HIV/AIDS epidemic in Asia, the governments' responses were generally weak, either in denial or in silence. Among the Asian countries, Thailand and Cambodia have launched comprehensive control programs that have been considered successful. Both Thailand and Cambodia have shown that strong government commitment, early and active response with substantial funding, and targeted intervention can have a successful effect on the STD and HIV epidemic.

Cambodia and Thailand are the two exemplary countries in Asia that have effectively curbed the spread of HIV and reduced the growth of HIV infection rate. Both countries have employed a solid legal system to provide protection for sex workers. However, none of the other countries have been able to follow suit or take such a strong preventive stance. In other Asian countries, women in the sex trade are harassed, abused, and arrested. In Thailand, the government has been active in setting up well-rounded strategies including the health and social dimensions in response to HIV/AIDS-related issues. During 1984 and 1990, the government established the reporting system of HIV/AIDS cases and implemented strong health education programs (Chitwarakorn 2004). In 1990, Thai Prime Minister Chatichai promulgated a national policy to control and curb HIV transmission.

During 1990 and 1996, the government drastically increased the national budget allocations for HIV/AIDS, and this is a period that witnessed extensive national activities due to the government commitment to keeping the AIDS issues on the top of the government agenda. In 1991, the government set up the National AIDS Prevention and Control Committee, chaired by the prime minister. The Committee established a multi-sector collaboration with nearly 300 nongovernmental organizations, involved in prevention, care, and support of AIDS-related issues (Chitwarakorn 2004).

During this period, mass media, advertising, and the marketing industry played a vital role in creating popular awareness of HIV/AIDS. For instance, HIV/AIDS education was aired on television and radio stations hourly. In 1991, when 1 million people were infected with HIV, the government initiated a 100% condom use program and made it a national policy to reduce the HIV risk in commercial sex.

The 100% condom campaign started in licensed brothels. Along with this campaign, the government also instituted voluntary counseling and testing, public education, and prevention of mother-to-child transmission. STD treatment programs were strengthened nationwide, and NGOs promulgated HIV education and prevention programs to the young people outside of schools. Many private firms disseminated AIDS education in the workplace and the Thai Business Coalition on AIDS was established to promote workplace policies and prevention efforts (Chitwarakorn 2004). The Thai Red Cross Society set up the first anonymous HIV counseling and testing center. Later the Ministry of Public Health implemented such a center nationwide. Thailand is also renowned for implementing anti-retroviral treatment nationwide and manufacturing its own generic anti-AIDS drugs.

Thailand has enjoyed great success in implementing 100% condom use in brothels, with support from the owners and local governments. The Thai government mandates that brothel owners enforce condom use in every paid sex act. Uncooperative owners are identified through STD surveillance among sex workers and clients and receive sanctions. Since health officials worked with brothel owners on instituting 100% condom use in all brothels, condom use has reached more than 90% in commercial sexual encounters and the proportion of men visiting sex workers has fallen by half. The government did not directly discourage commercial sex, but mandatory condom use and the awareness of risk caused many men to give up paying for sex. Thai men also reduced the number of their unpaid casual partners. Rates of STDs fell rapidly and HIV incidence and prevalence are declining.

Thailand's experience has also shown that with an intense 100% condom use promotion program, condom use in brothels has risen from about 14 to more than 90% (Rojanapithayakorn 1996), and 89% of indirect sex workers have used condoms with paying clients, as compared to 19% with nonpaying clients (Mills 1997).

Starting in 1997, the government emphasized the participation of all sectors of private, public, and communities, in solving AIDS problems (Chitwarakorn 2004: 148). The holistic approach of management required the collaboration between private and public enterprises. The goal was to reduce the HIV prevalence to less than 1% and make sure that 80% of HIV/AIDS patients have access to quality health and education support from the community. The government also ensured that local administrations and community organizations across the country efficiently continue the endeavor of HIV/AIDS prevention and alleviation (Chitwarakorn 2004: 148).

The Cambodian government was also committed to the endeavor of HIV/AIDS prevention. Cambodia, the country that originally had the highest HIV rate in Asia, with a high proportion of transmission occurring through commercial sex (Chanpong 2001), also instituted a 100% condom program in the mid-1990s, after learning that three-fourths of the police and military and two-fifths of male students reported using sex workers. After the implementation of the program, STD rates among sex workers fell substantially, and so has HIV prevalence (Hearst 2004).

Experiences in Thailand and Cambodia have shown that aggressive prevention programs can lower HIV transmission rate by promoting condom use and improving STD care.

HIV/AIDS in China

Below I will discuss the cultural, social, and political factors that are involved in China's attempts to manage its growing HIV epidemic.

HIV infection was first reported in China in 1984. An American man was identified as HIV positive and was quickly deported. Since then there have been three phases to the AIDS epidemic.

The first phase began in 1985 and ended in 1988. During this phase, a small number of AIDS cases were found in coastal cities and those infected were mainly foreigners or overseas Chinese. In 1985 four Chinese people with hemophilia were found infected by factor VIII sera produced in the United States. In July 1988, sexual transmission was discovered in a Chinese male who was tested HIV positive. He confessed that during the previous September he had homosexual contacts with foreigners.

FIGURE 4.2 HIV Prevalence among Injecting Drug Users, 2002–2006

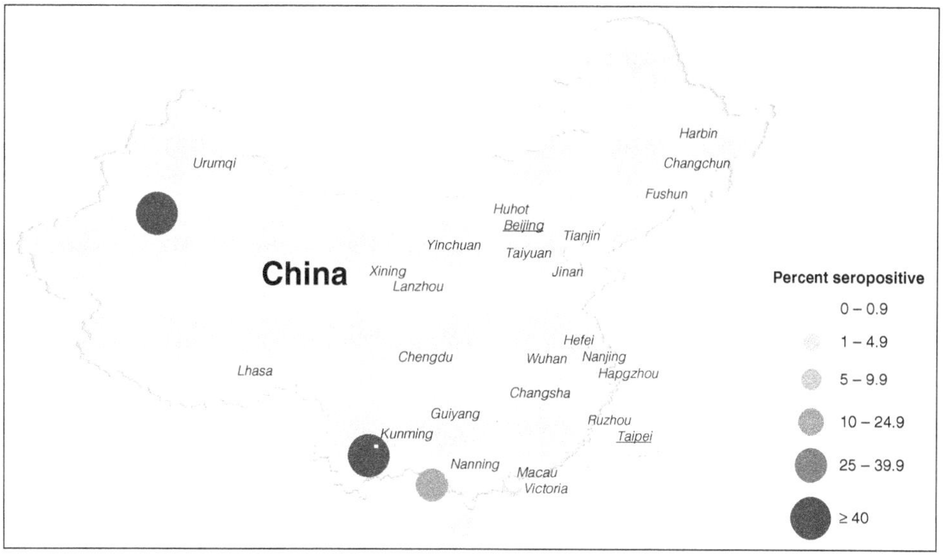

The second phase started from 1989 and ended in 1993. This period was marked with a limited epidemic. Since 1988, an HIV epidemic has been found in Yunnan province. Located in southwest China, Yunnan province is a predominantly agricultural region along the border of Myanmar, Laos, and Vietnam. The majority of the reported HIV-positive population was among drug users in Yunnan.

For centuries, there has been a tradition of smoking opium in this region. The recent trend has turned toward intravenous use of drugs, particularly heroin. Since the 1980s, drug use has greatly increased in Yunnan province and the adjoining provinces. According to official reports, the number of the intravenous drug users was over 100,000. Due to a shortage of drug-injecting equipment such as syringes, communal use of syringes put the drug users at high risk. By 1990, the number of HIV-infected people in Yunnan accounted for 87.2% of China's total HIV prevalence. While the country of China is dominated by the Han Chinese, this region is populated by the minority people, referred to as non-Han such as the Jingpo and the Dai people, who are originally related to Thai farmers across the border. In 1990, the Dai people accounted for 68.6% of those infected locally. As reported by *China Daily*, the Dai people demonstrated the strongest pattern of infection, especially in drug use. Another ethnic minority, the Jingpo people, accounted for 17.7% of those infected in 1990. As shown, in 1990, the overwhelming majority of HIV-positive cases was among ethnic minorities, especially young males ages 20 to 39, who were tied to land and engaged in drug use. Meanwhile, in Special Economic Zone areas, the number of expatriate Chinese who were found HIV positive was also very high.

The third phase began in late 1994 when HIV transmission spread beyond the Yunan province. The HIV epidemic was reported not only among drug users, but also among commercial plasma donors and others who were infected via sexual contact. The Chinese Ministry of Health announced that China has entered a rapid expansion of HIV epidemic ever since 1998. In December 2001, the Chinese government estimated the number of HIV-infected people at 600,000. In April 2002, the official estimate was revised to 850,000. During the first half of 2002, the HIV infection rate had increased by 70% (Micollier 2003). Although the Chinese government publicized this estimate, most national and international experts surmise that over 1 million—up to 1.5 million—people were probably infected. By 2010, the Chinese Ministry of Health predicts that up to 10 million people will be infected, whereas other experts expect 20 million HIV-positive people in China (Micollier 2003).

Modes of Transmission

There are three main modes of HIV transmission in China: sharing infected needles among drug users, reusing infected needles in blood trade, and unprotected sexual practices.

As mentioned above, Southwest China is the main region for producing opium and heroin. The region is known as the golden triangle, near the borders of Laos, Myanmar, and Thailand. Injected drug use and needle sharing has led to a very high level of HIV infection in this region. It is difficult to eliminate and control drug use effectively, due to the large market for drugs and the geographic environment. Another mode of transmission is through blood trade. Blood selling is a very lucrative business, and poor peasants in central China sought for survival by selling their blood. Henan province, the second most populous in China, has been hit the hardest. In Henan alone, some estimated that 1.2 million people were HIV positive. In some "AIDS villages," 80% of the inhabitants have contracted the virus and more than 60% have already suffered from AIDS.

In 1988, the Chinese government prohibited imported blood and blood products in order to prevent the transmission of HIV by blood products. In China, it is the Communist Party members who are required to donate blood without payment. Beyond the Communist Party members, the majority of the Chinese population would refuse to give blood because of their Confucian and Taoist belief that perceives blood as a body fluid that is transformed from sperm (jing) and life force (qi), and it is crucial to respect the integrity of the body. Because of the limited supply of blood products, to generate enough blood products in hospitals, blood products mostly come from blood donors who receive payments.

In central China, some blood banks run by local governments started collecting and buying blood from local peasants. The plasma was removed from the pooled blood and the remaining blood, the mixed blood of all donors, potentially contaminated with HIV, was injected back into the donors. Between this procedure and the reuse of unsterilized needles, the local population was ravaged by the HIV epidemic.

During the process, more women sold blood than men either because men's blood is considered to be more precious, or because women were believed to lose blood anyway during the time of menstruation (Micollier 2003). After all, men believed that it was necessary for them to preserve their blood because they were the heads of their families and they were responsible for most heavy labor outside the house. Poverty drove villagers into a frenzy of selling blood, and many had even built their houses by selling their blood. Some even bribed the blood heads to allow them to sell more than once a day. Doctor Gao Yaojie related that she saw hundreds of people queued at the entrance of their village. At the beginning she thought it might be a vegetable market or a movie, but it turned out to be blood selling. Without any sterilized equipment, villagers waited for their turn to tell the blood heads their blood type, and then they lay down on the ground to offer blood.

At the end of 1994, there was a severe outbreak of HIV among paid blood donors in central China.

Government Inertia

The governments of India and China, for a while, refused to acknowledge the extent of the disease and failed to establish responsible and reliable strategies to control the epidemic.

In the case of China, it was not until August 2001 that the Chinese government finally admitted that China was facing a serious AIDS crisis. Prior to 2001, denial, suppression, and institutional inertia characterized the government's response to the HIV/AIDS epidemic.

The Chinese government's first reaction to AIDS was to isolate and purge infected individuals, which led to stigmatization and marginalization of this group. In 1988, the Chinese Ministry of Public Health promulgated regulations concerning monitoring and control of HIV/AIDS. In 1989, People's Congress endorsed the Law of Preventing Infectious Diseases. This law singles out the non-Chinese foreigners and Chinese expatriates returning to China as a potentially infected group. The regulation requires those who intend to stay in China more than one year to demonstrate proof of their HIV-negative status. If identified, any HIV-positive person could be criminally prosecuted if s/he knowingly transmits the virus to another person.

According to the regulation, provinces have the right to restrict the movement of seropositive individuals to ensure local quarantine measures and the provision of medical care to the HIV infected. In the province of Yunnan, authorities issued registration cards to HIV-positive individuals to trace their movements. Those infected were not allowed to travel unless they could provide appropriate notification or release paperwork from the local epidemiology station.

The rationale for limiting movement of seropositive individuals is that the infected few can sacrifice themselves for the common good. Restriction on movement was not new in China. The 1958 law barred rural people from entering the city on the premise of allocation of resources, leading to a rural-urban apartheid.

The 1988 law stipulates that drug dealers, drug users, and traffickers, upon discovery, should be immediately prosecuted, as the activities they engage in are categorized as illegal by law. The government strongly cracks down on prostitution and drug abuse, and operates rehabilitation centers to incarcerate arrested prostitutes, drug users, and drug dealers. The government has intensified surveillance and anti-vice campaigns to combat the "vicious" and "evil" cultural phenomenon.

Illegal Blood Trade and Government Suppression in China

The mid-1990s witnessed the grand opening of several hundred illegal blood banks in Henan province. A frenzy of illegal blood trade arose as a result of their purchase of peasants' blood. During the process, unsanitary and unsterilized needles were used and reused. Each peasant seller was drawn around 800cc of blood. The blood head mixed six to eight sellers' blood all together and centrifuged them to separate plasma. The remaining red blood cells were reinjected into the sellers. Each time the seller was paid 40 yuan, which was a handsome amount for the peasants. Many peasants sold their blood multiple times.

The illegal blood trade and the continuous use of unsterilized needles led to a virulent HIV epidemic in Henan. Between 500,000 and 700,000 blood sellers were infected by HIV. In Houyang village, Shangcai county in Henan, 90% of farmers ages 16 to 55 had sold their blood in those years. Among them 90% are HIV positive; over 400 people manifest full-blown AIDS. In the year 2001 over 150 youths died of AIDS. All the villagers had sold their belongings to seek a cure, even the trees in front of and behind their houses. In that year, not one family was debt-free, not one family could afford the expensive medicines, not even those for fever or diarrhea.

In 1994, Wan Yanhai reported to the Beijing government that he discovered some contaminated blood with HIV virus in Henan. Both the central and local governments were offended by his report and condemned him as a disobedient troublemaker. Wan was removed from his office in 1997, as the central and local governments were afraid that he would blemish their reputation with the incident. After losing his job, he did not have any means of living for two years, exclusively relying upon his friends' financial aid. He set up an NGO in China, publishing fliers and newspapers, establishing hot lines, and organizing the gay community to fight against the AIDS epidemic.

In 2000, Wan Yanhai publicized the news on his AIDS e-mail list about the HIV contaminated blood in Henan and the associated illegal blood trade run by local blood heads. Charged with disclosing national secrets and sympathizing with gay and sex workers, Wan was imprisoned for two months. The government not only prohibited discussion of the illegal blood trade and HIV outbreak in Henan by news media and health workers, but also barred outside researchers from learning about it or entering Henan to study it. It was taboo to even mention this outbreak. This tenuous situation continued until 2001 when the government finally admitted the devastating HIV epidemic in Henan due to illegal blood trade.

Since some local government officials were involved in the illegal blood trade, local authorities attempted to cover up the situation and conceal their participation in these practices. Because local officials have blocked and thwarted government scientists' efforts to survey these areas, the magnitude of the problem is left unknown. The hidden HIV epidemic in Henan undoubtedly stripped local citizens of their timely attention to the epidemic and concomitant precautions. Consequently, it fostered the continued spread of the disease.

In 2001, when village protestors traveled to Beijing, they were barred from entrance to the first national AIDS conference. By 2003, when protests intensified, village protestors were arrested and beaten, and journalists were harassed and expelled.

The Government and Six Risky Groups

In the early stage of HIV/AIDS, the government identified six risky groups of HIV/AIDS: street prostitutes, aspiring industrialists/businessmen, young women longing to study abroad, teenage women who have been raped and thus are indifferent to sex, young women with vengeance toward men, and people in general who are indifferent to risks of STDs.

It is evident that these six risky groups are predominantly female (four of the six groups). In fact, it is the foreign businessmen with decadent capitalist lifestyles and Chinese women with immoral values that are deemed to be the mediums of transmission. The intersection between foreign men and Chinese women is a highly contentious issue in China. The Chinese state has striven to police Chinese women's bodies to protect national integrity. For instance, the 1984 criminal law defined women who "seduce foreigners and have intercourse with foreigners" as "female hooligans." In one popular movie, female "hooligans" who seduced and slept with foreign men were tracked down by government agents.

This first film on AIDS was titled "AIDS patient" and was released in 1988. In this mystery, Tony, a foreign teacher at a university on the east coast, died of AIDS. The police organized an investigation unit to collect Tony's relics and track down the three Chinese females who had had sexual relationships with him. This investigating unit also included the female secretary from the foreign affairs department, Xiaoyu Wang. The unit screened the blood samples of all the teachers, staff, and students under the pretext of physical examinations. The result showed that two women were infected. The first infected female student was found immediately. The unexpected blow made her desperate to commit suicide, but she was stopped by the police. She told the unit that Tony used to know a woman at a restaurant, but it was impossible for the unit to locate this woman. The second woman infected had used a fake name on the name list, so the investigation was stranded. At this time, more relics of Tony's were shipped from abroad, including a picture and a shopping receipt from a Friendship store. From the picture, the unit located the woman, who had married a rich Japanese businessman and had gone to Japan. The second piece, the shopping receipt, showed that Tony had bought a record of Madame Butterfly. It so happened that Xiaoyu Wang, the female secretary in the foreign affairs department, also had the same record. Was it a coincidence? After a thorough investigation, the truth was revealed: Xiaoyu was the infected female they had been looking for. Xiaoyu went to a room at the seaside where she had had intercourse with Tony and committed suicide by setting herself on fire.

The film targets women who might have had sexual relationships with foreigners and portray how they are doomed as a result of their "immoral" behaviors. This cautionary tale is intended to warn women against getting too close to foreigners, because the foreigners will corrupt them and infect them. While the mass media stress that foreigners are the vectors of disease, they also shows the catastrophic consequences of women's immoral behavior.

Women with corrupted morals were depicted as the major source of HIV/AIDS transmission. Categorized as "female sex criminals" (xingzuicuo funu) or "clandestine prostitutes," they were reported as "the most dangerous group" that spread the disease to the general population. A proliferation of journal articles illustrated how the infected prostitutes endangered the society by deliberately transmitting their disease to the general public, although the results of the national sentinel surveillance surveys continued to show that HIV-infection prevalence was very low in these selected populations.

The Government and Prevention

The government believes that HIV/AIDS can be prevented in China by practicing the traditional Confucian ideology of sex, that is, sex is only permitted within the bounds of marriage. Premarital and extramarital sex are prohibited, therefore condom dissemination is restricted to married couples.

Prior to the market economy, condoms were only available for married couples in the state-run pharmaceutical stores and health clinics. After the initiation of the market economy in the 1980s, anybody could purchase condoms in the street drug stores, supermarkets, adult health shops, and convenience stores, away from the regulations of the state. As Hyde argues, despite the state birth control ethos that emphasized the IUD (intrauterine device) and sterilization, the market provides condoms, which creates potential weapons against sexually transmitted infections and HIV/AIDS and helps circumvent state regulations. In a nutshell, the market provides a space where people can procure condoms to prevent possible transmission of HIV/AIDS (Hyde 2007).

However, sexuality is still moralized by the government and condom advertisements still remain taboo. The taboo against condom advertisements originated from the 1989 regulation titled "About Prohibition of Advertisements of Sex-Life Related Products." This law stipulated that any medical equipment designed to cure sexual malfunction or aid sexual life, although they are allowed to be produced, may not legally be advertised. This law and the series of setbacks to condom advertising ushered in a proliferation of debates by medical experts, scholars, government officials, and the general public on whether "family planning products can be advertised."

What was the ground for this regulation? It was argued that during the late 1980s, the government was concerned that the society was not ready for condom advertisements due to the so-called "social ethics." This ethics considers condoms a product related to sex and determines that condom advertisements will encourage prostitution and exert a deleterious effect upon children and society. According to a government official in Wuhan in 2002, "If we advertise condoms among the youth, it is equivalent to issuing sexual licenses and giving up on sexual morality. Abstinence is the best method to prevent AIDS. The best place to sell condoms was the check-out counter so that many people could furtively add a condom when paying for everything else." According to the officials in the Industrial and Commercial Department in Guangzhou, condom advertisement is adverse to the construction of spiritual civilization. Officials in Shenzhen Industrial and Commercial Bureau also commented that condom advertisements are not appropriate in China because the influence of media is too much for the youth, whose sexual knowledge is far less than their counterparts in foreign countries. According to the current level of sexual education, "it is not good to advertise condoms on a large-scale." In a nutshell, the advertising regulations reflect a government's discomfort with a sexual discourse.

Some experts exerted themselves to change this law and publicize condom use in the media. For instance, Li Jihong, the Deputy Secretary in the Sexology Committee, argued that we should allow condom brands to appear in public interest advertisements to encourage condom companies to support the dissemination of information on HIV/HIDS prevention.

In March 2002, Li Honggui, the Vice President of the Chinese Population Association, forwarded a plea to the National Congress for a lift of the ban on public interest condom advertisements as long as the ads were under supervision. The plea was signed and supported by more than 100 representatives of medical and other professions. Li contended that defining condoms as sex equipment and banning their advertisements prevent the consumers from obtaining information from normal channels, stymie the enhancement of condom quality, and hinder the establishment of superior condom brands. In June, the Industrial and Commercial Bureau replied to the plea, agreeing to lift the ban and allowing condom advertisements "under special conditions and with limitations."

After long appeals for condom advertisements by the family planning committee, experts from the CDC, and so on, June 2003 witnessed a change in regulations whereby *limited* advertising of condom use was allowed. In July 2004, six departments of the government, including the Hygiene Department, Family Planning Committee, Food and Medicine Supervision Bureau, Industrial and Commercial Bureau, Broadcast Bureau, and Quality Supervision Bureau, promulgated a regulation titled "About Condom Use for HIV/AIDS prevention" to encourage public interest advertisements on use of condoms for prevention of diseases.

Although the government had lifted the ban on condom advertising since 2002, in 2007, when I conducted my fieldwork, workers in the Dalian TV station told me that they still rejected condom advertisements. When I asked why, the answer I received was, "We have government documents that forbid condom advertisements. After 11pm, products that cure impotence and so on are allowed to advertise, but not condoms."

Post-2003 Government

Until 2002, the government's overall response to AIDS was silence and denial (Gill 2002). This response shifted to commitment by the end of 2003, signaled by the China CARES program implemented by the State Council in March 2003, designed to provide care and treatment to those most affected by AIDS (Kaufman 2006b). In February 2004, the State Council formed a multi-sector State Council AIDS Working Committee chaired by Vice Premier Wu Yi, soliciting participation of senior officials from all provinces to address the AIDS issue. This new committee implemented a policy of "Four Frees and One Care"—free anti-retroviral treatment, free counseling and testing services, free treatment for pregnant women and testing for their babies, free school fees for orphans, and financial support for affected families (Kaufman 2006b: 4). Since then, AIDS has become a priority of the State Council (Yip 2006: 179–180).

In the society, over 200 NGOs, both local and international, are at work, dealing with HIV/AIDS in China. These organizations include Action Project against AIDS, launched by Wan Yanhai, the most prominent AIDS activist; GONGO, Government-Organized Non-Government Organizations (puppet NGOs actually run by government officials); and research centers, networks and forums, and clubs and salons with restricted memberships (Micollier 2005).

Despite government efforts to disseminate information and reduce the stigma associated with AIDS through the policy of "Four Frees and One Care," China faces pressing challenges in implementing the policy, raising HIV awareness, and reaching and treating sex workers and their clients, as well as drug users (UNAIDS 2006). Research has demonstrated deficiencies in the surveillance and care reporting system, paucity of social science evidence, lack of coordination between CDC and hospital systems, poor health-worker attitudes, overcharge of drugs and services by health providers, deteriorating health education and preventive health care, lack of health insurance coverage for most rural citizens, and other limitations that have thwarted the government's endeavors (Kaufman 2006a).

Despite the announced policy of "Four Frees and One Care," it is also worth noting that there are few care facilities or programs for HIV-positive patients in China (Micollier 2003). The majority of the HIV-infected patients receive treatment from the medical staff of the Epidemic Prevention Stations and those assigned by the national health authorities. However, as Micollier points out, psychosocial care is neglected given the few networks for HIV-positive people and no home health care facilities (Micollier 2003: 39).

Currently, two support structures for the HIV-infected patients are in place in Beijing. Established in 1998, the first support structure is the Home of the Red Ribbon in Ditan Hospital. Ditan Hospital was designated as the referral hospital in China for HIV/AIDS treatment and research. It is here that researchers conduct studies on how to utilize both the biomedical anti-retroviral drugs and traditional Chinese medicine to produce the most effective medicine for the HIV positive patients. Their research is under the auspice of the Ministry of Health Center for AIDS Prevention and Control (Micollier 2003).

The second supportive structure is the Home of Loving Care within You'an Hospital. HIV positive patients, either hospitalized or not, can receive medical care and support in this Home. The Home absorbs quite a number of volunteers from surrounding universities in Beijing, who help with the medical care and fight for HIV-related discrimination.

Health Care System

The UNAIDS report in 2002 identified the unequal public health system in China as one of the key factors that have fueled the spread of HIV/AIDS. In China, the public health system excludes many people from the health care and prevention system and severely stigmatized AIDS patients. Despite the fact that the Chinese Ministry of Health took the rehabilitation measures at the end of the 1980s, the rural health system has relentlessly deteriorated (Micollier 2003).

Tony Saich, in his article "Social Policy Development in the Era of Economic Reform," has reviewed the 20-year trend in underinvestment in health in rural China and outlined its impact on numbers and quality of health personnel and facilities (Saich 2006). He points out that rural spending for health care was two-thirds of the national average, whereas urban spending for health care was almost twice the national average (Saich 2006: 20). His research concludes that there is a social stratification in access to health care between urban and rural population. In addition, there is also a discrepancy between the central and the local governments (Saich 2006).

Saich points out that unequal access to heath care is combined with the rising income inequality and the unequal distribution of resources that account for the huge variation in the provision of public goods and services between the rural and urban regions. Indeed, there is a conspicuous policy discrimination against the poor, particularly against the rural population, leading to poor-quality or non-public medical care in many rural areas (Saich 2006).

Despite the fact that the central government aims at restoring equal access to quality health care, local authorities ignore the policy and even underreport HIV prevalence in the region for fear of the effect of being open about HIV. To this date, we have yet to hear of any local leaders who have followed the previous President Jiang Zemin's lead to visit HIV/AIDS patients or publicly embrace any HIV/AIDS patients. Because local regions are self-financed and do not have sufficient funds to implement high-cost health care services, local systems can either neglect or undermine national policy (Saich 2006).

Migration and Prostitution

Since the 1980s, there has been a resurgence of prostitution in China, originating in coastal cities and large metropolitan areas, and gradually extending inland to smaller townships. Prostitution in China is closely intertwined with rural-to-urban migration and the entertainment industry. During the communist era, the 1958 household registration policy outlawed rural migration through the management of resource distribution and thereby established a two-tier urban-rural caste system in the society.

After the state initiated the market reform and open policy in 1978, the loosening state policy led to a flood of rural-to-urban migration. Institutional (that is, household registration policy) and social discrimination have forced the vast majority of these migrants onto the lowest rung of the labor market. Without the benefit of housing subsidies, health care, or education, many rural migrants remain undocumented and unregistered, living a semi-clandestine life beyond the reach of the authorities. Willing to take on low-paying or illicit employment disdained by city-dwellers, rural migrants commonly work as construction workers, garbage collectors, restaurant waitresses, domestic maids, factory workers, and bar hostesses. A substantial number of female migrants find employment in the booming sex industry.

The new consumption spaces concomitant with the Chinese market economy include nightclubs, beauty parlors, massage parlors, sauna bars, and karaoke bars. These places provide sexual services offered by female hostesses. For the rising entrepreneur class, it is a status symbol to visit these high-level consumption places and consume the services of the hostesses. In addition, keeping a second wife or mistress also denotes the prowess, wealth, and prestige of the male patrons. More often it is the clients who have the power to decide whether or not to use condoms during sexual intercourse.

Homosexuality

In China, although homosexual activities are not illegal, they are not socially acceptable in the society. Social stigma and marginalization force most homosexual people to conceal their sexual orientation and get married. World-renowned activist Wan Yanhai has been successful in organizing many homosexual people into his active AIZHI (AIDS) Action Project, a nongovernment organization he founded in 1994. During my fieldwork in one of his subsidiary organizations in a northeastern city of China in 2007, 99 % of the health educators working in that organization were homosexual men. They managed an AIDS education hotline, HIV voluntary testing and counseling, and distribution of AIDS information flyers and free condoms to the gay population, the dancing hostesses, and migrants in the city.

Fear and Discrimination

Fear and discrimination against the HIV infected constitutes a major obstacle to the implementation of prevention polices. As scholars have pointed out through their research, there has been a considerate gap between official policies and actual practices (Micollier 2003). The Chinese government has promulgated laws against AIDS discrimination, yet neither authorities, the health personnel, nor the general public accept the nondiscrimination law.

As Micollier points out, each national law prohibiting discrimination encounters a local regulation that contradicts it (Micollier 2003). For instance, local regulations such as provincial laws prevent HIV-infected people from getting married, continuing to work, or using public swimming pools (Micollier 2003). The police can issue warnings to companies run by HIV-positive people and even seize their merchandise. Due to the lack of confidentiality, doctors could potentially disclose their patients' HIV status to their employers. As Micollier notes, "of the 10 principles on which there is consensus in China and which sum up the content of current medical ethics, not a single one concerns patient confidentiality or anonymity" (Micollier 2003: 37). She points out that even medical staff refuse to provide care for HIV-positive patients for fear of transmission of the virus.

This finding is not surprising. Indeed, research has shown that Chinese health care workers not only exhibited a lack of knowledge of HIV, but also manifested overwhelming fear of transmission by HIV patients. In 2003, Allen Anderson of Indiana University and his Chinese research colleagues reported this finding. In the study, a questionnaire was circulated among the health care workers in three different hospitals in South China. The questionnaire consisted of questions on the knowledge of HIV transmission, HIV/AIDS control policies in their facility, and their personal attitude to the HIV infected. Despite the fact that it was common knowledge that blood, semen, and vaginal fluids were potential transmission vehicles for HIV, the result was alarming: 92% were concerned about becoming infected in their health care position; 27% did not believe that accidental needle sticks could transmit HIV; 34% considered saliva as a source of transmission; 4% believed transmission occurred by breathing air in the patient's room; 22% believed in transmission via toilet seats; 33% believed in transmission via mosquito bites (Stine 2007: 236).

If health care workers in hospitals are so deplorably ignorant about HIV and so apprehensive about casual contact with HIV patients, it is not at all surprising to find that lay people hold an immense amount of prejudice, animosity, and fear against HIV patients. Micollier relates the story of a group of HIV-infected patients searching for living accommodations. They were evicted from a legally rented apartment, rejected by landlords in their search for lodging, and forced to leave the district where they lived (Micollier 2003).

A 2005 survey found that 63% of respondents thought that it would be unsafe to work in the same office as a person infected with HIV, and 74% thought that those living with the virus should be banned from public places such as public swimming pools (Cheng 2005b). Negative perceptions of people with HIV/AIDS were also recorded: 44% of respondents thought that most people with HIV are promiscuous and 21% felt that they are merely receiving the punishment that they deserve (Lau 2005).

Jing Jun (Jing 2006), in his article "The Social Origin of AIDS Panics in China," reports the fact that the Chinese news media criminalize people with AIDS. Media are replete with scary stories of how HIV-infected patients carry a needle with them and attempt to inject their infected blood into healthy people's bodies indiscriminately. Jing argues that the very words "AIDS criminals" in the Chinese news media are based on an extremely thin layer of evidence. Yet the stories of AIDS criminals get amplified, sensationalized, and distorted to serve the purpose of criminalizing marginalized sufferers of AIDS.

Jing points out that when the Chinese government claims to have done a great deal to combat the AIDS-related stigma, no officials have tried to examine or critique the news media's role in creating an environment of public opinion hostile to AIDS patients. Jing concludes, "China encountered a multiplication of such rumors in many cities by the end of 2005. The progression of these rumors and associated panics indicates that China has a long way to go in combating social discrimination against AIDS patients" (Jing 2006: 168).

NGOs and GONGOS

In countries such as Thailand that have adopted effective strategies to fight the spread of HIV, the government has fostered strong collaboration with nongovernment organizations(NGOs). It has proven that the government's partnerships with NGOs are effective in mobilizing the resources of civil society and community-based organizations.

In China, despite the increasing number of NGOs that engage in AIDS-related activities, the government remains ambivalent and distrustful of the development in this sector. In China, over 200 NGOs, both local and international, are at work, dealing with HIV/AIDS in China. These organizations include Action Project against AIDS, launched by Wan Yanhai—the most prominent AIDS activist, GONGO – Government-Organized Non-Government Organizations (puppet NGOs actually run by government officials), research centers, networks and forums, and clubs and salons with restricted memberships (Micollier 2005).

The government's suspicion of NGOs has led to its strong control and surveillance over the sector. As a result, the NGO sector is still dominated by the government, especially those organizations where the government plays a significant role. However, at the same time, the government recognizes the fact that its obligations on AIDS-related issues are too many for it to handle single-handedly. Therefore, the state has allowed for expansion of community-based organizations to provide a wide array of social services. Indeed, in 2004, Premier Wen Jiabao announced that the government would defer certain responsibilities to enterprises, NGOs, and intermediary organizations (Saich 2006).

In China, domestic, international, and government-led NGOs are playing an important role in HIV/AIDS prevention and HIV-related work. International NGOs such as Save the Children UK have been actively working with AIDS orphans in Yunnan and other provinces such as Henan and Anhui (Saich 2006). Meanwhile, HIV-positive patients have also set up quite a few self-support groups in Xinjiang, Shaanxi, Shanxi, Guizhou, Shanghai, Beijing, Guangdong, and Sichuan (Saich 2006: 38).

The government has set up many large organizations called GONGO—Government-Organized Non-Government Organizations. GONGOs operate at three administrative levels: local, regional, and national, linked to a government body organization. GONGO staff are paid by the government and the government administration has the files on the staff (Micollier 2004b). They even attend the same political meetings as their civil service counterparts.

These are quasi-official organizations and the preference for them instead of NGOs is apparent. Regulations on social organizations require that "similar" organizations should not coexist at the various administrative levels. This requirement has been used to deny registration for some groups. In so doing, the GONGOs such as the All China Women's Federation and the All China Federation of Trade Unions can enjoy monopoly representation of the interests of women and workers. Establishment of any smaller local organizations of similar nature is prohibited. As a result, certain social needs of women and workers are silenced due to the monopoly of the GONGOs (Saich 2006: 38).

Academic NGOs, referred to as "secondary organizations," play an active role in combating AIDS. Examples of NGOs are: the China AIDS Network, the Beijing Preventive Medical Association, and the Institute for Research on Sexuality and Gender at Beijing People's University. The Beijing Aizhixing Institute is the foremost AIDS NGO in China. The Institute works on HIV/AIDS and public health–related policy, legal aid and human rights, and community outreach among the most vulnerable populations. The Institute has also organized several challenging campaigns in China, including a national compensation campaign for the victims of HIV infection caused by blood transfusion; a national working group for the educational rights of those with HIV, hepatitis, or other health problems; and a China HIV/AIDS NGO Network. The organizer of the Beijing Aizhixing Institute, Wan Yanhai, holds the belief that the widespread social prejudice against gays, lesbians, bisexuals, and intravenous drug users undermines efforts to combat the spread of disease. His approach to conveying this message has challenged the government official perceptions and policies on health and human rights.

Given the severity of the HIV epidemic in China, it is crucial that the international and local NGOs and GONGOs should collaborate in a partnership, working to improve the environment and reduce the HIV infection rate by fighting against stigma and prejudices, disseminating HIV prevention knowledge, and providing care for the HIV infected. It is our hope that the successful examples led by Thailand and Cambodia can be followed by more and more countries in Asia, including China, in effectively curbing the spread of HIV.

Summary

This chapter discusses the geographic case study of Asia in general, and China in particular, and pinpoints the cultural, political, and economic factors that have fueled the AIDS pandemic in this region. More specifically, these factors include authoritarian government, a colonial history, gender imbalance, intergenerational imbalances of power, migration of labor, economic disparity, and social stratification. In Asia, as a result of the global capitalist economy, unequal distribution of global income, unequal allocation of resources, and unequal access to health care have left those at the bottom of the society vulnerable to infections. Due to the drastic inequity among sexes, classes, and generations, most of the infected are marginal to their own societies and the global economy. Moreover, due to the European colonial exploitation in Asia, wealth, resources, and treasure had been plundered away from Asia. The colonial history in Asia has a profound impact on the spread and prevalence of STDs.

Name: ______________________ **Date:** ______________

Chapter 4 HIV/AIDS in Asia

Exercises

<u>Exercise 1</u> Discuss with your partner your cultural knowledge of Asia. Tell a story about your first encounter with Asia, including people you met, TV programs you have seen, etc. What is your impression about Asia? What are the routes through which you acquire knowledge about Asia?

<u>Exercise 2</u> Reading Comprehension:

1. Why did the epidemic surge without any warning in Asia?

2. What are the factors that have fueled the AIDS epidemic in Asia?

3. How did the colonial history contribute to the spread of STDs in Asia?

4. Please discuss the correlation between gender dynamics and the spread of HIV in Asia.

5. Why are women in general less informed about sex than men in Asia?

6. How were Asian governments affected by foreign policies in their approaches to sexuality?

7. How was the prevention program hampered by government politics?

8. Which two countries are the exemplary countries in Asia, and why?

9. What are the three phases of HIV epidemic in China?

   1st phase:

   2nd phase:

   3rd phase:

10. What are the cultural, political, and economic factors that affect the spread of HIV in China?

    Cultural:

    Political:

    Economic:

11. Please discuss the progress and status of NGOs in China, and the government's attitude toward NGOs in China.

    Progress:

    Government's attitude:

Exercise 3 Discussion Questions:

1. If you were the president of China, how would you cope with the issue of illegal blood trade, and why?

2. If you were the president of China, India, or Nepal, what measures would you enforce to curb the spread of HIV?

   China:

   India:

   Nepal:

3. The Chinese government has listed six risky groups of HIV/AIDS. What do you think of this phenomenon? Should these vulnerable groups be blamed for spreading the disease and should this deepen their social stigma? If we fail to recognize the link between AIDS and high-risk groups, will it be difficult for us to know where to concentrate our energies as public health activists? If you were the policy makers in China, how would you deal with this dilemma and balance these two issues so that we avoid blame and enforce effective interventions?

4. Given the entrenched gender hierarchy in many parts of Asia, what, in your opinion, are the measures to be taken in order to bestow more power upon women?

5. Do you think the 100% condom campaign can be carried out in countries other than Thailand and Cambodia? What kind of predicament do you think it will encounter in other Asian countries such as China, India, and Nepal?

Exercise 4 Test Your Knowledge:

1. Asian countries experienced a major AIDS epidemic prior to the late 1980s.
   a. True
   b. False
2. Asian governments are very open about their HIV statistics.
   a. True
   b. False
3. In Asia, there is no correlation between migration of labor and the HIV epidemic.
   a. True
   b. False

4. The European colonial exploitation has created poverty, illiteracy, violence, and polarized social stratifications in many Asian countries.
   a. True
   b. False
5. Colonization has led to a more rigid regulation of STDs.
   a. True
   b. False
6. Many Asian governments reacted very quickly to establish effective measures to curb the spread of the disease.
   a. True
   b. False
7. There is no correlation between increased injection drug use and growing poverty.
   a. True
   b. False

Chapter five | AIDS in Africa

Africa, as we saw in chapter one, is where the AIDS epidemic began. It was probably in west Africa where the disease moved from being a relatively benign malady in chimpanzees and monkeys to a deadly disease in humans. West Africa was the origin of both the virulent HIV-1 virus and the less virulent but still deadly HIV-2 virus. What is curious and not entirely understood is that it was not in west Africa that HIV-1 became the deadly epidemic that spread around the world and killed millions. It was in Kinshasa in the eastern region of the Democratic Republic of the Congo that AIDS first reached epidemic proportions. From here it spread into eastern and southern Africa and eventually around the world. There are river connections between western Africa and Kinshasa; presumably an infected person carried the virus from western Africa to the Kinshasa region, where the political turmoil and urban environment allowed the epidemic to get started. Ironically, the relatively small epidemic in western Africa seems not to have sprung from indigenous sources, but to have spread from the epidemic in southern and Eastern Africa. Thus the disease has come full circle. Along the way it infected Europeans working in former colonies and Haitian workers who carried the disease back to their corner of the globe. The disease was probably transferred to the United States by sex tourists in Haiti. Interestingly, the disease first was identified as an epidemic in the United States where it was thought to be a disease peculiar to gay men. By the late eighties the disease had become an epidemic among drug users and heterosexuals. By the nineties, as the epidemic waned among middle class gay men, it exploded in the African-American underclass.

We earlier quoted Merrill Singer, who defined AIDS as an epidemic of the poor. At first glance this seems to apply to sub-Saharan Africa, the world's poorest region. However, as we will see as we examine the contours of AIDS in Africa, there are few easy generalizations we can make about this epidemic as it turns into a worldwide pandemic. As we will see, this is especially true of AIDS in Africa, where the disease has made a unique pattern and has reached numbers greater than the rest of the world combined. It is true that poverty has played a big role in making the disease so devastating in Africa, but within the society it is not just a disease of the poor. In some regions it is the more affluent and better educated who have become infected.

In 2007 about 1.5 million Africans died of AIDS and an estimated 22 million more were living with the disease. There were an additional 1.9 million new infections in that year, meaning the disease was growing even faster than it was killing people.

In southern Africa seven countries had infection rates of over 15%: this included Botswana, Lesotho, Namibia, Swaziland, Zambia, Zimbabwe, and South Africa. Swaziland, with 26% of the population infected, had the highest infection rate in the world, while South Africa, with 5.7 million

FIGURE 5.1 African HIV1 Seroprevalence for High-Risk Urban Populations

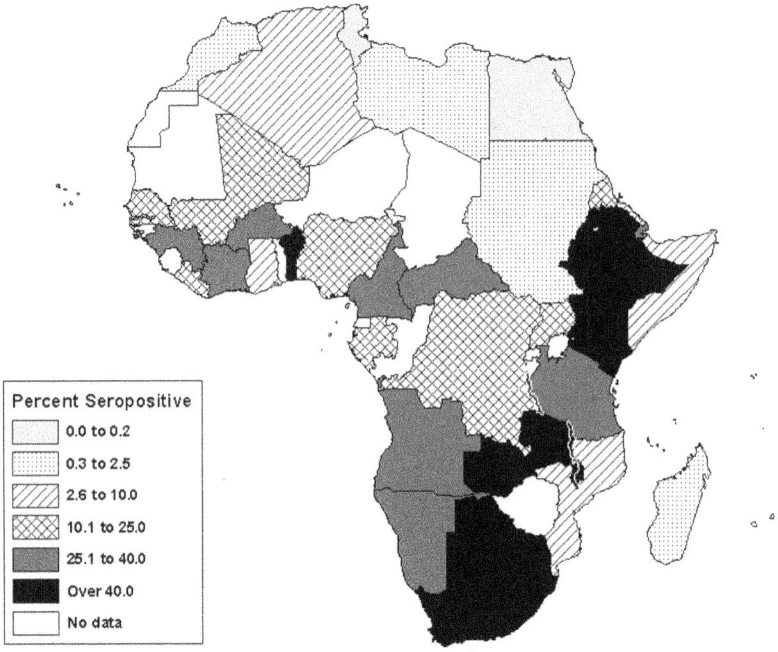

Source: U.S. Census Bureau, Population Division, International Programs Center, HIV/AIDS Surveillance Data Base, December 2006.

infections (18.1%), had the highest number of infections in the world. Tragically, there were over 11 million orphans left behind as of 2007.

Both the pattern and the numbers are unique in sub-Saharan Africa, which raises many important questions. The most obvious question is: Why is HIV/AIDS so much worse in sub-Saharan Africa than anywhere else? An easy answer would be that it started in Africa and has had more time to develop there than anywhere else. However, at one point, in the early 1980s, it was apparently worse in the United States, but has now declined relative to the African epidemic. At one point it was feared that rates in China, Southeast Asia, Russia, and India would follow the African model, but that has not happened, at least not yet. What is driving the numbers in sub-Saharan Africa? As mentioned earlier, American anthropologist Merrill Singer believes AIDS is a disease of poverty and Africa is a poor continent, especially south of the Sahara; but some of the poorest countries have not been as heavily affected and some of the richest countries, South Africa for instance, have been hardest hit. Even within countries, unlike the United States, the most afflicted are not necessarily the poor. In some areas, the heaviest infection rates are among the most affluent. As we will see, there are many variables influencing this unique disaster in Africa.

To begin, let's trace the spread of the disease through the continent south of the Sahara, beginning in the eastern region of the Republic of Congo. In the mid-1980s, after testing procedures for HIV became available, 672 frozen blood specimens taken from various parts of sub-Saharan Africa revealed a single case of HIV/AIDS taken from a specimen collected in Kinshasa in the Eastern Republic of Congo in 1959. HIV/AIDS only became an epidemic in the Kinshasa area during the 1970s. Why did it take so long to reach epidemic stage? One answer is the relatively long gestation period during which the HIV infection may not immediately turn into full-blown AIDS; however, probably more significant is the relative isolation of the region infected. This was changed when the disease began expanding rapidly into the city of Kinshasa. The key was a network of sexual relations through which the virus spread rapidly and silently. Here the long gestation period did play a role. It is during the early stages of this gestation period when there are no symptoms to alert people that the viral load is most deadly, and infection is most likely. Because there were no symptoms and because the disease was still believed to be primarily a disease of homosexuals, there was no reason to be suspicious until the disease had established a strong foothold. From Kinshasa, a major urban center with traffic to and from other parts of Africa, the epidemic spread first into East Africa and then into southern Africa and later, finally, into West Africa.

Why did a disease that had, through the mid-eighties, been a disease of homosexuals become, in Africa, a disease of heterosexuals? Why, as the disease spread, did it cause epidemics in some parts of Africa and barely affect other areas? The answers to these questions are inseparable from the specific local conditions of the areas into which the disease spread. In some areas prevalence was less, partially because of traditions of circumcision. As it turns out, circumcised males are significantly less likely to become infected, and therefore less likely to spread the disease. The presence of sexually transmitted diseases (STDs) was also a major contributing factor. Because HIV is passed through bodily fluids, most commonly blood, STDs that created lesions on the genitals became a major factor in making HIV/AIDS a heterosexual disease in Africa. Related to this was the often poor and inaccessible medical facilities in Africa. In the United States, STDs can be easily treated; in Africa they are more likely to be out of control.

Most significant of all, and perhaps the key factor in the African epidemic, are cultural habits that are common throughout equatorial Africa, but for economic and political reasons are more pronounced in some areas, the areas that experienced, and in most cases continue to experience, the worst of the epidemic. AIDS researcher Helen Epstein refers to these practices as concurrency, that is, long-term multiple sexual relationships. It should be emphasized that these relationships should not be construed as an example of the stereotype of African hypersexuality. Surveys suggest that the number of sexual partners in African society are similar to averages in the United States or Europe. What is unique is the factor of concurrence. A man may have a long-term relationship with three, four, or even five women. These women, or some of them, may also have long-term relationships with other men. What is different is that in the United States or Europe it is more likely that a similar number of relationships will be in succession rather than concurrent.

Why should this make a difference in infection rates, and how does this contribute to a heterosexual epidemic? It is important to remember that HIV is not easily transmitted through vaginal sex. It is much easier to transmit through anal sex, because the anus has thinner, more vulnerable walls, making blood contact much more likely. This is the major reason that AIDS was originally identified as a disease of homosexuals. HIV spread through the homosexual community so easily because of the prevalence of anal intercourse. It is estimated that transmission through vaginal sex happens on the average only in about one out of every one hundred incidents. Of course, as noted above, STDs can change the odds by creating open sores in the vagina or on the penis. It is also an important factor that the viral load an infected person carries is much greater during the early period of infection. What this means is that if one is infected by a person in his/her network, that person has a heavy viral load with which to infect others in that network with whom he/she is having concurrent sex. In this way the disease can spread like wildfire through an extended network, where everyone is at maximum viral potency.

It is important to remember the old maxim that when it comes to disease, you are having sex with everyone with whom your partner has had sex. In the case of AIDS this is especially true if you are having concurrent sexual relations with people in a network as opposed to having serial relations with a series of people one at a time. Serial relations, as are more common in the United States or Europe, mean that by the time you move on to a new partner, chances are that the disease will have lost its potency, and even if you do pass it on, it will be to one person, not an entire network. (This should not be interpreted to mean that sex with a person long infected is safe. One single encounter with an infected person can pass on the disease. At best, assuming other variables such as STDS are not present, it simply gives you better odds.) Because HIV can be latent for many years, it is easy to see how whole areas can become silently infected with no warning.

HIV/AIDS Spreads into East Africa

By the late 1970s, AIDS had moved out of the Democratic Republic of Congo into Rwanda and Burundi. By the early 1980s, HIV/AIDS had reached epidemic proportions in Rwanda. In 1982 about 12% of blood donors in Kigali, the capital and a major city, tested positive. In Burundi as early as 1980–1981, blood supplies from patients suffering from hemorrhagic fever tested 4.4% positive. By 1986, 16.3% of women tested in antenatal clinics in Bujumbura, the capital of Burundi, tested positive for HIV. The disease continued to expand, but in these two countries, in contrast to other areas, the disease was concentrated in the cities.

The regional uniqueness of the disease is nicely illustrated by these two countries. The region is heavily Christian, largely Roman Catholic, and sexual behavior is restrained. According to historian John Iliffe, "In a survey conducted during the late 1980s, only 10% of men and 3% of women aged 15–19 reported sexual intercourse during the past twelve months, compared with 51% and 30% respectively in the central African Republic."

Given this relative inactivity, why did the disease spread so rapidly? The key is commercial sex, rather than concurrent sexual partners. There are several contributing factors: first, the already noted celibacy of a high percentage of the population; second, the relatively late marriage age (24 for men). Other reasons include the disproportion of men and women, with many more men than women; and finally, the rejection of condom use, and the lack of circumcision. HIV established itself among sex workers and their clients before moving into the general population. Eventually, the disease spread into the countryside, apparently carried by male visitors to the cities; however, because of the strict moral code, it never became as serious a problem in the countryside as elsewhere.

In Uganda and Tanzania the disease was probably present as HIV by the mid-1970s and erupted into AIDS by the late 1970s. The plague became especially serious in Uganda, where it was initially spread by soldiers and long-distance truck drivers. General Amin's troops had been stationed on the border with Rwanda where the infection was already high. When they retreated into the interior they carried the disease with them. That the trans-Africa highway also ran through Uganda was another contributing factor. Long-distance truck drivers contracted HIV from bar girls and spread it along the highway to other bar girls and ultimately to their families. When Amin's troops moved into northern Uganda to suppress rebellion, they carried the disease with them and from there it later spread into northern Kenya and Ethiopia. Uganda was probably also infected by migrant workers who carried the virus back to their rural homes, a pattern we will see even more pronounced in southern Africa. By 1987 the infection rate among pregnant women in Kampala, the capital of Uganda, was 24%, which, along with Kigali, was the highest rate in the world at that time.

In Kampala, HIV infection was not primarily a disease of prostitutes and their clients, as in Rwanda and Burundi. In Uganda, as in Kinshasa, there were more women than men. They began sex early, typically at the age of 14 and married relatively late. Because of the economic dislocation caused by Idi Amin's rule, many of these young women were part of an economy that made them dependent upon gifts from relatively wealthier men. As we will see later, this is a situation common in southern Africa as well, and deprived young women of control over their sexuality. It created the conditions that led to concurrency, that is, having multiple partners during the same time period. This was not a choice these young women freely made; it was dictated by their powerlessness and poverty and their need to survive. Presents of cash or food were often the difference between survival or not. The result was a perfect environment for an AIDS epidemic. By the peak of the Ugandan epidemic in 1991 about 1.2 million people were believed to be infected.

In Kenya, as in many other African countries, the authorities were reluctant to admit that there was an epidemic in their country. This was among many negative consequences of colonialism. The spread of AIDS fit too easily the European stereotype of Africans. Nations recently escaped from colonial rule were dominated by the pride of intense nationalism. To admit to a disease associated with immoral behavior was more than some could swallow. Unfortunately, the failure to face the disease early only added to the tragedy. By 1985 the disease was so well established that authorities were forced to face up to the crisis. It was also true that authorities faced with other devastating diseases, such as malaria, and limited health facilities and budgets, were inclined to look away from what seemed an impossible task.

In Nairobi, the capital of Kenya, the disease began among sex workers and was passed to their clients and then into the general population. This was a frequent pattern, as we have seen in Rwanda and Burundi, but not the exclusive pattern. As in Rwanda and Burundi, this was a common pattern when there was a large gender imbalance, encouraging the use of sex workers. Nairobi, with 138 boys for every 100 girls, encouraged and supported prostitution.

Within Kenya, the Luo people represented an instructive subset. Unlike most Kenyans, most Luo men were not circumcised, which greatly increased the chances of infection, perhaps doubling transmission chances. Even more relevant was the prevalence of concurrent sex. Luo society had been in economic decline for a long time and as a consequence was experiencing social disintegration, ideal conditions for the practice of concurrent sexual patterns. As we saw in Uganda, young girls without means depended upon the help of a network of men who provided them with resources and passed on the disease. The Luo also practiced a system of bride inheritance, where a brother would inherit his brother's widow. This was a practice designed to provide a kind of insurance for widows and care for children, which in normal times it did. But because so many men were dying of AIDS, this became an efficient way to pass the virus to the surviving brother.

There is a puzzle about the epidemic in Ethiopia. HIV-1 mutated into four subgroups. The dominant subgroups in East Africa were types A and D, but in Ethiopia the dominant subgroup of the virus was type C, which was also dominant in South Africa. Looking at the map one can see what would seem to be a natural progression of the disease from Uganda through northern Kenya into Ethiopia. Southern Africa is separated from Ethiopia by about 1,000 miles.

What is clear is that in Ethiopia the disease radiated out from the capital, Addis Ababa, and other major cities. At its peak in the early twenty-first century about 1.5 million Ethiopians were infected. Given the size of Ethiopia, about 80 million people, this is a relatively small number, probably because the disease arrived late in this relatively isolated country.

Once again we can see that Ethiopia fit the common, if not universal, pattern we have seen in East Africa in which women in particular are impoverished and dependent. As in Kigali, commercial sex had a major role, because of the emphasis upon premarital virginity in this ancient Christian country. The predictable result was a thriving sex industry that formed the core of the disease.

Also contributing to the epidemic was the large population of women in Addis Ababa who were without a conventional means of support. The low status of women and the ease with which they could be divorced was the key contributing factor. Women of this status, deprived of land or other capital, could not survive in the countryside and flocked into the cities. Prostitution was their main option, and prostitution in which their ability to demand condom use was weak. The critical period of infection was in the late 1980s. By 1990, 54.2% of sex workers were infected.

Fortunately, what did not happen in Ethiopia was a significant spread of the epidemic to the countryside. Ethiopia was undeveloped commercially and the countryside was relatively isolated. In other countries, rural men visiting the city became infected and brought the epidemic home to the countryside. In Ethiopia, the large numbers of women from the countryside stayed to die in the cities.

AIDS in Southern Africa

Southern Africa would eventually become the most afflicted region in all of Africa, containing over half of all HIV-infected victims in the world. In the nation of South Africa over 5 million people would become infected by 2003. In Swaziland, 26% of the population became infected with AIDS, the highest rate in the world. AIDS came late to southern Africa, but the failure of government to respond adequately allowed the disease to expand rapidly, a problem that has still not been resolved, particularly in the Union of South Africa.

The first indications of the disease were in northern Malawi that bordered the infected East African nations of Tanzania and Zambia. Blood samples taken in 1981 showed no indication of HIV, but by 1984, 11 cases had been established, still a minor number. Four of these cases were from outside Malawi. Because the dominant strain of HIV in Malawi and in southern Africa generally was subtype C, it is assumed that the infections originated in the Democratic Republic of Congo and reached southern Africa through Zambia, rather than traveling through East Africa.

As elsewhere in Africa, the long incubation period was critical in allowing the disease to get a foothold before public officials could respond. It is also the case that, as was frequent in Africa, that nationalistic pride made officials reluctant to acknowledge the disease even after it was obviously established. This was and is especially true in South Africa where President Umbeke is still in a state of denial, much to the detriment of his country.

In South Africa as in the United States, the first serious outbreak was among white homosexuals. In 1982, the first case was an airline steward who had probably contracted the disease on a layover in New York. In spite of a South African law declaring homosexuality illegal, the response was vigorous, including blood screening and hospital wings created just for AIDS patients. By 1990 the gay epidemic was under control. It was clear that gays had not infected the heterosexual community since the subtype B characteristic of American and South African homosexuals was not the strain in the heterosexual community. By the early 2000s, AIDS had become a largely black heterosexual disease in South Africa. As early as 1987 blood testing showed a black rate of infection eight times higher than whites, and doubling every six months.

In South Africa there was no core group such as sex workers who were causing the infections. Rather it was the strength of the South African economy that was attracting immigrants from infected areas such as Malawi. The possibility of jobs in the mines was a particularly strong motive and attracted many people from surrounding countries.

Because of apartheid, the black population was especially vulnerable. Poverty and poor health care meant malnutrition and preexisting untreated STDs that made already weakened immune systems more vulnerable and allowed contamination through open genital sores. Poverty, an inevitable consequence of apartheid, led to more risky behavior, particularly by women without resources. As we have seen elsewhere in Africa, there existed a network of sexual relations in which young women depended upon men for money and gifts to survive. Concurrency played into the requirements of the virus. By tapping into a wide network of sexual partners it increased the odds of someone getting infected. Because the viral load was heaviest in the newly infected, it created the best chances for passing it on to the maximum number of people. The result was an exploding epidemic, the worst in the world.

The complexities of the ways in which the disease spread is illustrated by the strange places that suffered the most. One would expect the highest rates of infection to be in cities like Johannesburg, but the highest rate was in a rural tribal area, KwaZulu-Natal. KwaZulu-Natal was close to the major city of Durban and the easy communication between the city and the densely populated countryside was clearly a factor. The Zulus had also given up circumcision two centuries earlier, making them twice as vulnerable as the circumcised. There were also very high rates of STDs that greatly increased the odds of infection. Finally, the area was crisscrossed by truck routes, providing connections to the outside world, and these routes attracted migrant women hoping to benefit from the truckers.

Within South Africa are two independent tribal homelands, Lesotho and Swaziland, that are more or less independent countries, but economically dependent upon South Africa. Lesotho, in particular, sent large numbers of laborers to the mines. This practice also led to dangerous behavior. Large numbers of men away from home, doing dangerous work but making relatively good wages, was a situation that encouraged risky behavior. By 2000 it was estimated that 48% of the workers returning to Lesotho were infected. This then spread into their families. As we have seen, the practice of concurrency helped it spread rapidly through the population once it was introduced. The condition where absent husbands frequently did not send adequate money home to their families further encouraged the practice of concurrency, since the women left behind had few resources.

The situation of women in South Africa was generally one of powerlessness. Their lack of independent means of support made them economically dependent upon men. Even when they were not dependent, they faced the danger of rape that was common. There existed an attitude of entitlement among men. A kiss could mean a green light to go ahead. The slightest unintended gesture could be seen as an invitation. Rape was not easily or often prosecuted. Also, economic dependency led to emotional dependency. Young women needed to attach themselves to men and wanted to feel cared for. The result was skyrocketing infection rates among women.

Another aspect of gender relations was a past tradition of polygamy. This tradition contributed to the attitude of entitlement, and reinforced the practice of concurrency. Perhaps even more relevant was the male romantic ideal of the Isoka that was popular among poor township boys with few real prospects. According to historian John Iliffee, the Isoka was "the handsome, popular and irresponsible hero who displayed his masculinity, in one of the few ways available in a township, by having penetrative sex with girlfriends whom he could not afford to marry." This narrative is reminiscent of American inner-city patterns of behavior where a kind of bravado grows out of grinding poverty and a sense of hopelessness about the future. Young men find compensation in constructing what they consider a romantic and heroic narrative about themselves as Don Juans. One can see how the concept of conquest in this narrative can easily cross the line into rape. This narrative includes a cavalier attitude toward danger and eschews the use of condoms, which limit the free reign of pleasure and do not fit the devil-may-care narrative to which the young men are subscribing. In fact, perhaps less bravery than ignorance seems to be involved in these behaviors. Studies indicated that as late as 2003, 62% of HIV-positive respondents believed they were not engaged in a dangerous activity. Tragically, unbeknownst to them, their fate was already sealed.

Perhaps more tragically, young girls were not free to create a romantic narrative to make sense of their dilemma. A 1999 interview at Carletonville revealed that 16% of girls between the ages of 14 and 24 had been raped. Indicators are that rape was only one form of coercion. Most common was constant pressure on girl friends with the threat of abandonment.

Underlying all of this was a breakdown in traditional village values regarding premarital sex and violence. Rural South Africa was undergoing dramatic change. Men were forced to leave the community for work. Traditional agriculture was less viable as a means of sustenance. Traditional marriage was giving way to informal relationships, and even marriage when it occurred did not provide security from disease for women, who were frequently infected by their husbands. The breakdown in traditional values under the impact of colonialism, urbanization, and modernization was a recurring theme throughout Africa and throughout the developing world, although nowhere else with the tragic results characteristic of sub-Saharan Africa.

Epidemics in Malawi, Zambia, Zimbabwe, and Botswana began to level off in the late 1990s, but only after reaching very high levels of infection. Botswana provides another example of variations on a theme so common in sub-Saharan Africa. Botswana is described by its own citizens as a rich nation of poor people. Newly discovered diamond wealth caused a huge expansion in economic growth, making Botswana a rich nation by African standards. However, as is usually the case when wealth comes in the form of precious natural resources (oil being a good example of this), it is not distributed equally across the population. The new economic growth enriched some and left the majority behind. As we witnessed elsewhere in Africa, this discrepancy in wealth combined with the weak social and economic position of women led to risky behavior by both rich men and poor women. Here also the discontinuation of the practice of circumcision sped up the contagion. Men were able to use their wealth to support sexual relations with a large network of women, many of whom were part of other networks. Poor women used their sexuality to access the networks of rich men or at least to try to gain enough of it to survive. The result was an HIV infection rate of slightly over 17% by 1997.

A variation on this theme was also taking place in Namibia, where relatively rich men and poor powerless women gave synergy to the disease. But also in Namibia we have a war involving exiled soldiers who, when they gained independence returned to their homeland carrying the disease with them. The speed with which infection rates grew in Namibia was startling to observers. Antenatal prevalence skyrocketed from 4% in 1992 to 21% in 2001. As early as 1996, AIDS became Namibia's largest single cause of death.

What we see in these two countries is relatively significant wealth, with great mobility, great income inequality, powerless and poor females, and a lot of sexually transmitted diseases. This led to rapid infection and high rates of infection. Also in southern Africa were Mozambique, Malawi, and Tanzania, poor countries and victims of war where infection spread with the movement of troops and refugees. However, concurrency was also a factor. Bonds of loyalty kept people in old relationships even as they moved on to new relationships. Especially if a couple had children together, it was expected that there would be an ongoing relationship even as one began a new relationship, and this included sex.

While the epidemic in southern Africa appears to have peaked, it remains the worst AIDS epidemic in the world. The reason it remains a disaster has much to do with the political response to it, especially in the Union of South Africa, which we will address later in the chapter.

West Africa

The region designated West Africa stretches from Cameroon along the southwest coast of the hump of Africa to Senegal on the northwest coast. It includes Nigeria, the most populous country in sub-Saharan Africa, as well as Benin, Togo, Ghana, Burkina–Faso, the Ivory Coast, Liberia, Sierra Leone, Guinea, Gambia, Guinea-Bissau, Niger, and Mali. This was the last region that the HIV-1 virus spread to and at least to date it has not experienced the high percentage of infections suffered in the south or east of Africa. This is a densely populated region with some unrest and social dislocation that one might expect to become highly infected, which of course could still happen. Why has the epidemic in this region been so relatively slow to develop?

There are factors unique to this area that offer some explanation. There are more Muslims in this area and their more disciplined approach to premarital and extramarital sex may be relevant. Male circumcision is also more universal, and as we have seen, this can reduce the risk of passing or acquiring the disease by 50%. It is also the case that women in most of West Africa have more economic opportunities and are not as likely to be trapped in the kind of dependency that leads to concurrency in East and South Africa. It is also the case that communications with eastern and southern Africa are difficult and there is less traffic from these regions than between southern and eastern Africa.

Another unique factor in West Africa is the existence of another form of HIV that appears to have been well established before HIV-1 entered the region. HIV-2 seems to have come from the sooty mangabee monkey, whose range does not extend beyond West Africa, or even include all of West Africa. It does not grant immunity from HIV-1 and it was not uncommon for West Africans to become infected with both viruses. In the long run it produces results just like HIV-1, a horrible wasting death from a variety of opportunistic diseases. What is unique about it is twofold: First, it is not nearly as virulent and therefore harder to catch, much harder than HIV-1. Second, after you catch it, the incubation period is usually much longer, perhaps 25 years. The social and economic implications of this difference are considerable. HIV-2 is about three times more difficult to pass on through sexual intercourse, and at least ten times more difficult to pass on from mother to child. In eastern and southern Africa, HIV-1 was causing not just physical pain, suffering and death, but also social and economic dislocation as people were dying during their most productive years. Sadly, tens of thousands of orphans were left to be raised by their grandparents or left on their own. A large hole was left in the workforce by people dying during their most productive years, and the family structure was severely strained by the death of so many young parents. HIV-2 might infect someone at the same age, and they might eventually die the same agonizing death. But because of the relative weakness of the virus and its long incubation period, death would most likely come in one's fifties, sixties, or even seventies. Orphans were less likely to be left behind, and death, while of a horrible sort, would come closer to the time frame normally expected.

HIV-1 first arrived in the Ivory Coast, probably in 1985, although possibly as early as 1980. By 2003, 7% of the adult population was infected, making it the worst epidemic in West Africa. The coastal city of Abidjan was especially hard hit. It is easier to explain why Ivory Coast had the worst HIV-1 epidemic in West Africa than it is to explain why the rest of West Africa did not suffer such a bad epidemic. Ivory Coast and especially Abidjan had many factors that encouraged the epidemic. The country was not developed until late in the colonial era in spite of the abundance of natural resources, especially vast forests. With independence from France came very rapid development with all of the consequences associated with growth and modernization. The country had been relatively sparsely populated, but now development attracted large numbers of immigrants. Abidjan became an important seaport and increased in population from 120,000 in 1955 to about 1 million in 1984. The country as a whole received about 2 million immigrants from Burkina and over 1 million from Mali as well as a large number from Niger. Many immigrants came to the cities and so overwhelmed the infrastructure and bureaucracy that cities such as Abidjan became lawless frontier towns. The city came to have a large transient male majority, which, as we have seen elsewhere in Africa, led to commercialized sex. Because of the relatively greater political and social power of women in West Africa, it did not lead to the degree of exploitation that women experienced in southern and eastern Africa, which is probably part of the reason that infection numbers never approached the horrible statistics of southern Africa, even in the Ivory Coast.

Abidjan was a coastal port and the center of a well-developed land transportation system. This was ideal for spreading the disease and a major factor in not only creating an epidemic in the city, but of spreading it to the countryside.

Besides the gender imbalance leading to prostitution, ease of communication between city and country, and large-scale immigration, there were two other factors that facilitated the spread of the epidemic. First there was the atmosphere of aspiring modernity that encouraged the rejection of group values and encouraged more individualistic choices. These choices included carelessness about condom use and sexual adventurism. Modernity also meant differences of wealth with the attendant possibilities of multiple sexual partners. By 1994, 51% of Abidjan's men confessed to casual sex and 56% said they never used a condom. This all led to sexual networks that created the phenomenon of concurrency that had been critical in epidemics elsewhere in Africa. Then during the 1980s a second factor appeared. Africa was and is heavily dependent upon markets for its raw materials in the developed world. As the world economy slowed, so did growth in the Ivory Coast. This led to mass unemployment, a decline in health services, and further commercialization of sex. The decline in health services meant that STDs went untreated and made HIV infection much easier.

By the late 1980s, Abidjan was in danger of an epidemic on the scale that existed in southern Africa. During this time HIV prevalence rose from 38% to 86% among sex workers, and 34% of the infected were infected with both HIV-1 and HIV-2. Because sex workers were the key infecting agents, men came to have five times the infection rate of women. As we have seen elsewhere, by 1993 the ratio was only about two to one as men infected their wives and girl friends. By 1994 it is estimated that 41% of West African AIDS cases were in the Ivory Coast. The mobility of the population, encouraged by the excellent transportation system, insured that the countryside was also heavily infected.

Abidjan was the key to the spread of HIV-1 to the east of West Africa. A critical factor was the mobility of West African sex workers. One important group spreading the virus was rural women who hoped to make enough money in the sex trade to establish themselves back home in business. Because their goal was to return to a conventional life, including marriage, they often left the country to ply their temporary trade, hoping to keep their sex work a secret. The predictable result was to spread the disease. Ghana, right next door to Ivory Coast, soon had its own epidemic. As of 2003, about 350,000 in Ghana were living with the disease. As early as 1986 nearly 50% of the sex workers returning to Ghana from Abidjan tested positive. As elsewhere in Africa these women were blamed for spreading the disease, but the evidence is that the spread came from other sources as well. It was not just sex workers who were mobile; several million immigrants had come into Ivory Coast, and of course, many of them returned home.

The Ivory Coast is the exception to the general pattern in West Africa. West Africa did not experience anything like the extreme epidemics of eastern and southern Africa. Even Ivory Coast was well below the percentages of infection in countries like Uganda and Namibia.

The best record came from Senegal, which kept its infection rate to about 1% of the population. HIV-2 had established itself in Senegal, but at a very low rate. The introduction of HIV-1 seems to have come from men who had traveled outside of Senegal, and there was also a homosexual and drug component. This disease did not spread into the general population in a significant way, with the exception of a tribal group, the Jola, who lived on the Guinea-Bissau border. Among the Jola, prevalence was two to three times the national average. The Jola fit a familiar pattern. Traditional values had broken down as a result of commercialization of the economy. The Jola had adopted risky sexual practices and had experienced high rates of STDs. The new economy made traditional marriage difficult and many left to go to places such as the Ivory Coast to seek employment. When the economy suffered in Ivory Coast in the 1980s, many returned home, bringing the disease with them.

The rest of Senegal did not experience a severe epidemic, and the Muslim religion was probably a key reason. Muslim attitudes toward marriage and extramarital affairs were strict. Women were closely guarded. Significant levels of condom use were also important and the response of Islamic leaders played a key role. Sermons were preached warning of the dangers and a compassionate approach to treating the sick was also a feature of the mosques. Some have argued that Moslem attitudes toward women that lowered their status was partly responsible for the epidemic, but the facts in Senegal and in northern Nigeria refute this contention, and point in the opposite direction. The quick and practical response of government leaders in Senegal should also be noted, and will be touched on again later.

The most populous country in Africa is Nigeria with over 120 million people. It is oil rich and fits the definition of a rich country with poor people. It has a history of dictatorship and massive corruption, but that is not unique in sub-Saharan Africa. By 2003, Nigeria had 3.6 million living with AIDS, the largest total number outside of South Africa. However, as a percentage of population that number was far lower than South Africa and lower than the Ivory Coast. The real question about Nigeria is why the numbers are so low. In spite of its wealth, Nigeria has a health system rated by the WHO as one of the worst in the world, and in spite of its national wealth, poverty is widespread in the country. These are the sorts of conditions that fueled the epidemic elsewhere. Finally, there are significant subgroups such as the Yoruba in southwest Nigeria, who engaged in a great deal of extramarital sex and still did not have high rates of HIV infection.

One argument explaining the absence of a greater epidemic is that Nigeria lacked a central city that connected to the entire country, such as Abidjan in Ivory Coast. The country is big and diverse and the parts are isolated from the whole. We have seen how Abidjan, a port with a strong road system, served as the epicenter of the disease in Ivory Coast. Lagos did not play a similar role in Nigeria.

Another argument is that Nigerian sex workers were largely from Nigeria and therefore did not carry the disease from somewhere else as was the case in Ivory Coast. Sex workers elsewhere in Africa were often, but not always, the first stage in an epidemic. In Nigeria, at least in the early stages of the epidemic, their infection rate was not as high as elsewhere.

Finally, as in Senegal, the Muslim religion seems to have helped keep the disease contained in the north of the country, a heavily Muslim area. Here women were commonly secluded, and sexual mores were enforced by the community. The result was much lower rates of infection than in the central and southern region of the country.

AIDS is not a disease that naturally runs its course and declines like a flu epidemic. Barring a cure, which seems unlikely anytime soon, the ebb of this epidemic will depend upon changes in human behavior. West Africa now seems to have escaped the severity of the devastation that afflicted southern Africa, but continuing success will depend upon cultural factors and the actions of governments. There is much good news from Africa; the decline in AIDS infections in Uganda is a good example of this, but at the same time a recent study indicates that the number of Ugandan adults engaging in risky behavior is once again on the increase. Among women there has been an increase in those who say they have had sex with someone they do not live with, from 12% to 16%, and among men an increase from 29% to 36%. The short-term and perhaps even the long-term hope for a victory over AIDS will come from permanent changes in human behavior.

The Role of Outside Forces

As the poorest region in the world and the politically weakest, sub-Saharan Africa is a region much acted upon by outside forces. Historically, these forces have been destructive, especially slavery and colonialism. Today many would-be benign forces have taken an interest in Africa, but not always with benign results. The United States and Europe have encouraged modernization in Africa but have not always acted to facilitate economic growth and modernization. The problem is that these governments are answerable to powerful interest groups at home that are part of the competitive world economy. A key issue is agriculture, where European countries and the United States all subsidize their farmers while insisting that Africans participate in a free world market. Africa as a developing country is still dependent upon its agriculture. In most of the developed world, industrial development was built upon a foundation of flourishing agriculture. Efficient agriculture meant capital accumulation, and it meant freeing up and being able to feed a population of workers. In spite of their advocacy of free trade, both the United States and Western Europe continue to maintain huge subsidies for their farmers, which makes it difficult for African farmers to compete.

Developed countries have also taken a big interest in Africa's considerable mineral wealth, including oil. Developed countries benefit from buying raw materials from Africa and processing them in their own factories. The problem is that, generally speaking, raw materials do not command as high a price as value-added products. Africa needs investment in manufacturing, so it can begin to exploit its own natural resources. Unfortunately, this runs counter to the interests of developed countries. Most recently China, with its enormous and expanding industrial base, has come into sub-Saharan Africa with an eye on its natural resources. The question is, what will Africa do as its resources are depleted if it has not created a modern infrastructure for producing and transporting value-added products? While we have seen that inside Africa it is not just the poor that are contracting AIDS, it is also true that good health care systems require wealth and that treatment of AIDS requires wealth. Even though modernization may have caused some of the cultural dislocations that have encouraged the AIDS epidemic, a modern economy will be a necessary part of a modern health system that can treat and help prevent the disease. A modern economy should also empower women and give them the independence to control their own bodies. As we have seen, in comparing the political power of women in West Africa and southern Africa, women's autonomy is a key variable in determining the severity of the epidemic.

Organizations such as the International Monetary Fund (IMF) and the World Bank, largely controlled by the United States and Europe, have taken an interest in the AIDS epidemic and have established funds to address the problem; but at the same time they have insisted upon a free-market approach as a condition for getting development funds that are critical to modernization. This has meant removing protections for African businesses and agriculture, and also getting rid of "socialistic" health systems. That health systems in Africa treat so few of the most needy means weakened immune systems and STDs that make people more vulnerable to AIDS. It also means less compassionate care for those already sick.

The Bush administration, after some hesitancy, finally committed a sizable amount of money to fighting the African epidemic. In 2003, Bush announced PEPFAR, The President's Emergency Plan For AIDS Relief. He appropriated $15 billion, most of it intended for sub-Saharan Africa. This figure was later doubled to $30 billion; 80% of the funds were designated for treatment, including payments for anti-viral drugs; 20% was committed to prevention, and this has caused controversy. Critics complain that Bush's religious views have prevented the most effective approach to AIDS education in favor of abstinence-only programs that are not effective. There have also been complaints that funding for AIDS has been used as a wedge to coerce acceptance of open markets for the United States.

The Bush administration defended itself by claiming credit for an increase from 50,000 people getting anti-viral drugs in 2003 to 1.45 million people getting treatment by September 2007.

Nongovernmental organizations such as the Bill and Melinda Gates Foundation have made impressive contributions to the fight against AIDS in Africa, contributing billions of dollars that have allowed more Africans to receive anti-retroviral drugs. They have also supported research looking for a cure. Formed in 1996 as an arm of the United Nations, UNAIDS has also appropriated money and supported programs to turn back the epidemic.

On the negative side, it is clear that much of the governmental dysfunction and poverty in Africa can be traced back to colonialism. This is most evident in southern Africa where a form of colonialism in Zimbabwe and South Africa is very recent and where the infection rates are very high. Just to cite one example, the mining operations in South Africa, which drew men from what were in effect reservations to separate them from their families and work in the mines, was a contributing factor to the South African epidemic.

The Role of Anti-viral Drugs

The year 1996 marked an important turning point in the African AIDS epidemic. This was the year that UNAIDS became active in coordinating the fight against AIDS, and it was also the year that anti-viral drugs became available in Africa. While anti-viral drugs were not a cure, they held out hope to alleviate some serious social problems. They could relieve suffering and extend life so that parents could raise their children and continue to work to support their families. It is important to remember that AIDS had produced approximately 12 million orphans in Africa. It threatened to destroy a family structure already weakened by economic change and the collapse of traditional values. The new drugs could help sustain a workforce hard hit by the epidemic. The people dying came from the age groups that contained the most productive workers. In a continent already struggling economically, this could be fatal.

The problem was that the drugs were produced by powerful Western corporations that held patents giving them monopolies. The cost was beyond the reach of most Africans, a significant number of whom survived on two dollars per day or less. In fact, early on it had been decided that because of cost, drugs could not be a practical solution to the African AIDS problem. This changed when it was shown that neurapine could reduce transmission from mother to child by 48% and at a cost of only four dollars per case of the drugs. Mother-to-child transmission was the second-greatest cause of HIV infection and was exacerbated by the strong African tradition of nursing. Transmission could take place either through carrying and delivering the baby, or through nursing. Unfortunately, neurapine did not stop transmission through nursing.

In 2000 the price of anti-retroviral drugs dropped 90% due to competition from generic drugs manufactured in India. As a result these drugs became a bigger part of the response to the African epidemic.

Also in 1996 the big breakthrough in drugs was the development of highly active anti-retroviral therapy, known by its acronym of HAART. This was based upon the discovery of drugs known as protease inhibitors that stopped the infected DNA cells from turning into an infectious virus. When combined with Azidothymidine (AZT) the disease could be arrested, if not cured. Unfortunately, as we will discuss later in the chapter, the government did not get behind this program in South Africa, the nation with the largest number of infections in Africa and in the world. When organizations like the Gates Foundation kicked in and Bush's PEPFAR program became available, anti-viral drugs became part of the war on AIDS in Africa. But in South Africa, the government got in the way of this solution.

The Role of Governments

Most governments eventually responded to the crisis, some sooner and more effectively than others. As we have discussed, absent a medical cure, the problem of AIDS has become largely a social problem. It is hard to solve modern social problems without the help of government. The initial response of many governments was denial. African governments had gained their independence from colonial rule after World War II, some very recently (South Africa, Zimbabwe). As one might expect, there was embarrassment about how AIDS spread. It played into Western stereotypes about black hypersexuality and uncontrolled behavior. Governments resented the seeming judgments rendered by former colonial masters. This response is not unique to Africa. In China embarrassing facts are considered state secrets and revealing them is a serious criminal offense. There too, the defensiveness caused problems, as witnessed by the SAARS outbreak and the failure by the Chinese government to acknowledge it and deal with it. This is just one example of the way colonialism continues to damage former colonies.

Even after recognizing the epidemic it was difficult to respond adequately. Most governments lacked resources. During the 1980s and early 1990s most of the funding came from outside Africa and it was inadequate to do the job. There were also those who saw AIDS as a diversion from more serious threats to public health. The World Health Organization (WHO), under the leadership of Halfdan Mahler, took this position. Diseases such as malaria were killing more people in the world than AIDS, so this was not an unreasonable concern. Of course what was not fully understood was the latent epidemic that was still hidden by the long incubation period.

Another issue was the threat to medical personnel. Accidental cuts were common and exposed nurses and doctors to contaminated blood. Surgery was a particularly big problem. Some surgeons refused to operate on AIDS patients or those who had not been tested; some nurses refused to care for AIDS patients.

Because of widespread fear and discrimination, there also arose the issue of privacy. Some in the community accused the infected of witchcraft; others condemned them for immorality. People with AIDS were commonly shunned by the community. Given the widespread discrimination, should it be revealed that someone had AIDS? Was there a right to privacy? Some doctors were uncomfortable giving the bad news, which was the same as a death sentence. Many doctors became demoralized in response to AIDS. Their identity as healers was challenged by an epidemic for which there was no cure.

Opposed to the privacy argument was the need to stop the spread of the disease. If someone was HIV positive should they be trusted to act responsibly and not spread the disease? What about the rights of potential partners? Shouldn't they be warned? On the other hand, if information was to be made public, wouldn't that discourage people from being tested if they then would be subjected to not only bad news, but the approbation of the community?

This dilemma was at least temporarily resolved in 1986 when the WHO recognized the seriousness of the epidemic and Mahler established a special program on AIDS headed by the American, Dr. Jonathan Mann. Mann, an extremely idealistic public health doctor, insisted upon the rights of the individual, the afflicted patient, which meant no forced testing and the maintenance of privacy. He was also a passionate voice for the afflicted, increasing funding from less than a million dollars to over 100 million. One of his priorities was to stem the tide of infection by screening blood supplies in countries too poor to do it themselves. He also made training new staff a priority, including counseling personnel. Finally, he recognized that in the absence of a medical solution, education had to be a priority.

As might be expected, his most controversial decision was his emphasis upon the rights of the infected. Undoubtedly this protected a great number of people against deep and widespread prejudice. But did it encourage the spread of infection? Some Africans regarded this as a kind of Western intellectual imperialism, growing out of a Lockeian emphasis upon the rights of the individual, a point of view not shared by much of the world. But what about the rights of the uninfected? Shouldn't they be safe from reckless carriers who, irresponsibly, had chosen not to be tested, or, worse yet, having been tested, used the cloak of secrecy to infect others? This is still a debate in Africa and not likely to be resolved soon.

Meanwhile some countries were taking action. Zimbabwe in 1985 was the first African country to screen all blood before transfusions. In Uganda, President Museveni insisted upon publicizing the epidemic, recognizing that silence was killing people. Under Museveni's leadership, Uganda became the first nation in Africa with an advanced epidemic to go public and use education and government's voice to stem the disease, and it worked. Nowhere in Africa has the disease been rolled back as effectively as in Uganda.

In Senegal in West Africa, President Abdou Diouf provided leadership that prevented HIV-1 from getting a foothold in his nation. He had some advantages in doing so. First, the disease was relatively late in arriving in West Africa. Second, nearly all of Senegal's males are circumcised, greatly reducing the risk of transmission. And finally, as noted earlier, the Muslim faith which oversaw the activities of women and frowned on premarital sex was important. The president used an already existing program to identify and treat STDs and to identify AIDS. He acted quickly to secure the blood supply, launch public education programs, and mobilize community leaders. As noted earlier, the result was a prevalence rate that never went much over 1%.

In contrast, South Africa did not face up to the disease and the consequences have been disastrous. About 5.7 million were living with the disease as of 2007, and it spread at an alarming rate. AIDS first came to South Africa as a white homosexual disease during the apartheid period of the 1980s. The minority government acted quickly and contained the disease. By contrast, when the disease struck the black heterosexual community after apartheid, the government's response was defensive, even though, or perhaps because a post- apartheid majority government was making the decisions.

Thabo Mbeki succeeded Nelson Mandela as South African president in 1999. Mbeki was faced immediately with protests from AIDS groups over the government's decision not to provide anti-retroviral drugs for infected pregnant women. The provincial government of the Western Cape, an area hard hit by the epidemic, challenged the central government by defying the ban on AZT for pregnant women. The program subsequently establish by Doctors without Borders was successful in cutting the transmission rate in half. When Mbeki became president in June, he surprised everyone by launching an attack upon the drug AZT as a toxin. The government had previously decided not to support anti-retroviral drugs because of the expense. In a system already overloaded it made the decision on the basis of priorities. Now Mbeki was questioning the efficacy of the drugs and even accusing the drug companies of producing poison. In fact, worldwide pressure on drug manufacturers plus market pressure from Indian generics had brought the price down to a reasonable level.

Dissident scientists, rejecting the mainstream scientific viewpoint about HIV/AIDS, had been active during the 1980s. After the success of anti-retroviral drugs in the 1990s, most of these critics had retreated. Now Mbeki turned to the remaining hard-core dissidents and invited them to a conference with African AIDS specialists. What Mbeki took from this meeting was that the real cause of AIDS was weakened immune systems caused by poverty. Malnutrition and other infections overloaded the immune system and caused AIDS. This formulation better fit his own pan-African nationalist sentiments, and shifted blame to the colonial world and all that it had done to weaken Africa. His own liberal press now attacked Mbeki as a scientific illiterate. Stunned by the attack, Mbeki announced that he was withdrawing from the scientific debate on AIDS.

Mbeki was soon brought back into the debate when AIDS activists filed a suit in August 2001, demanding that government institute a program using anti-retroviral drugs to save lives. Mbeki responded to the challenge and rejoined the battle. A speech given three years later to the national assembly suggests what was really behind his rejection of the scientifically demonstrated cause of AIDS:

> I for my part will not keep quiet while others whose minds have been corrupted by the disease of racism, accuse us. The Black people of South Africa, Africa, and the world, as being by virtue of our Africanness and skin color . . . lazy, liars, foul-smelling, diseased, corrupt, violent, amoral, sexually depraved, animalistic, savage and racist.

This outbreak suggested the deep bitterness about apartheid that was the basis of Mbeki's denial. The scientific explanation of what had happened with AIDS was deeply embarrassing to Mbeki and he regarded it as affirming white stereotypes about Africans. In fact, as we have seen, the cause of the epidemic in Africa was not behavior that was any more extreme than in the West; it was simply different. The pattern of concurrence that was significantly responsible for the size of the African epidemic did not mean that Africans were any more active sexually than Westerners; it just meant that the way they were active made them much more vulnerable to infection.

In December 2001, the high court of South Africa ruled against Mbeki and the government and ordered that a program to stop mother-to-child transfer be instituted. Mbeki had lost, but the real losers were the many who were infected because of Mbeki's obstructionism. Further pressure was put on the government when health officials threatened to resign. A commitment was made to increase the AIDS budget fivefold over a three-year period, while at the same time efforts were made to reduce drug prices even further.

The struggle over drugs to inhibit mother–child transfers was a turning point. It facilitated the organization of AIDS activists and put the courts on the side of AIDS activists. It also brought foreign attention to the problem and brought increased foreign aid.

Elsewhere in southern Africa the response was quicker and progress was being made. In Botswana, where the first program to prevent mother-to-child transmission was launched in 1999, there was success. By the end of 2002 about 34% of pregnant women with HIV were being given AZT and transmissions had fallen an estimated 22%.

The greatest success story was in Uganda, the most severely struck country in East Africa. In one Kampala hospital infection among pregnant women fell from 28.1% in 1989 to 16.2% in 1993. In Kampala the general rate fell from 29% in 1992 to 8% in 2002. UNAIDS estimates that the overall Ugandan adult prevalence rate fell from 13% in the early 1990s to 4.1% at the end of 2003.

There were many skeptics who did not trust the statistics, probably with good reason. One argument was that authorities were manipulating the figures to show success in hopes of encouraging more funding. Some questioned the accuracy of the tests. Others suggested that AIDS had simply killed off the most vulnerable and that preventive measures were not a factor. While some of this may be true, it became increasing clear that things were getting better. One indication was the significantly lower infection rate among 15- to 19-year-olds. These people, because of the long incubation period, rarely died before moving into a higher age category, making it unlikely that death was distorting the figures. The Masaka study, which looked at the long- term period of 1992 to 2003, was more definitive. It showed a 37% drop over a nine-year period among those over 13. Clearly there was real improvement, but why?

A number of studies showed a real decrease in risky behavior. The term "zero grazing," meaning being exclusive with one partner, was a phrase that reflected a new reality. There was a large drop in the percentage that said they had multiple partners. For instance, the number of men who claimed to have had three or more partners during the past year dropped by 80%. People were scared and it influenced their actions. Ugandans revitalized old narratives. One was a religious narrative emphasizing purity. Another was a return to traditional beliefs. Both helped discipline their new behaviors.

Three relatively unique factors characterized the Uganda battle with AIDS. Because the epidemic was so widespread, a very high percentage of people had firsthand experience of the disease. By 1995, 89% of Ugandans claimed to know someone with the disease. AIDS was for Ugandans, more than for most people, a personal and very scary experience. Watching people that they knew die a wretched death made a lasting impression.

It was also the case that Uganda's leadership set an example of talking openly about the epidemic. While other African leaders were embarrassed about the disease and tried to deny it, Museveni insisted upon publicizing the dangers and educating the public. This very public example convinced communities that it was not a taboo subject and that it needed to be addressed. As a result, Ugandans became active in organizing at the local level while women in other countries were doing such things as continuing to nurse their babies so no one would suspect them of having AIDS. This grassroots activism that was encouraged by the government was in sharp contrast to South African activism that came late and was opposed by the government.

Finally, Ugandans adopted the use of condoms. This is one area where Museveni did not provide unequivocal leadership. For religious reasons he initially opposed condoms, but under pressure from health care professionals, he changed sides and supported use that particularly targeted sex workers. Use of condoms with casual partners and prostitutes increased substantially and condom use in Uganda came to rank third in frequency among African nations.

Why should Uganda be so much more successful than other countries in addressing this crisis? One answer is leadership. Museveni's quick response and rational approach deserve a lot of credit. But it has also been suggested that part of the answer lies in Ugandan society. Even though it was colonized by the British, it was a less intrusive colonization than elsewhere. Traditional culture and traditional economic patterns remained in place. A real sense of community had survived. Perhaps this is what allowed the grassroots organizing to be so effective.

Other than South Africa, eastern and southern Africa began to see a leveling off of the disease during the 1990s, although not so dramatically elsewhere as in Uganda. Behavioral change was a factor, but so was increased condom use, especially in casual relations. There was an increase in distribution of condoms from 1998 to 2003 of from 150 million to 310 million. This gives cause for hope, but it is not yet clear that the changes are permanent or that they run very deep. In fact, there is evidence of backsliding even in Uganda. It seems clear that AIDS has not been defeated in Africa and that it will be around as a fact of life for a long time. In the United States the availability of drugs seems to have encouraged a return to dangerous behavior; it is a reminder that behavioral changes are conditional and conditions can easily be reversed.

As noted earlier, Merrill Singer makes much of the role of poverty in the spread of AIDS in the United States as the epidemic moves into the inner-city ghetto. No such easy generalization can be made about sub-Saharan Africa. While sometimes the disease attacks the poor, in other regions it is more prevalent among the more affluent, whose wealth and power encourage dangerous sexual behavior. Certainly the disease has no respect for national wealth, claiming its largest number of victims among the citizens of South Africa, the continent's richest country. Perhaps the most useful insight about the uniqueness of the African epidemic is Helen Epstein's idea of convergence. This insight seems to go a long way toward explaining why the disease has been so successful among heterosexuals in Africa. But to understand the disease as it exhibited itself throughout Africa involves many other variables that help to explain variations in the intensity of the epidemic in different parts of Africa.

For instance, circumcision plays a big role in determining the intensity of the epidemic. Among the Zulu, who had abandoned circumcision, the disease is particularly bad. Among the Senegalese, who are mostly circumcised, the epidemic is very small. However, this example highlights the difficulty of sorting out all of the variables, since Senegal also benefited from excellent leadership and from its Muslim faith.

Political leadership is very important. In South Africa where the leadership has been a disaster, the epidemic is also a disaster, although once again it is important to remember the other factors contributing to the South African epidemic, and also to remember that judgments about the failure of leadership there should be softened by an understanding of the impact of colonialism in shaping points of view. In Uganda progressive leadership helped stem the tide of an epidemic that threatened to be worse than the South African epidemic.

If we compare regions, we can surmise that one reason the West African epidemic has not gotten out of control compared with the epidemic in southern Africa is because of the relatively greater autonomy for women in that region. West African women generally have more economic freedom than women in southern or eastern Africa, although this is complicated by the Muslem societies in Senegal and northern Nigeria, who apparently have contained the epidemic partly by their strict controls over women.

Health care throughout the stricken regions of southern and eastern Africa is also an influence. Poor health care makes people more vulnerable to AIDS. Often international organizations such as the World Bank and the World Trade Organization have pressured countries seeking aid to economize and privatize health care. The result has been a decline in primary health care. One of the factors increasing the risk of heterosexual sex is STDs. Bad primary care means that there will be many more cases of STDs leading to higher risk of HIV infection.

Finally, there is a demographic issue. Because sub-Saharan Africa has such a high birth rate and such a low life expectancy, a very large percentage of the population falls into the age category where there is more sexual activity. Even if none of the other factors existed, Africa would likely have more AIDS than an area of comparable population but with a different age structure.

There is good news about the African epidemic. In West Africa the epidemic has been contained with relatively low rates of infection. Nigeria, a nation of 120 million people that looked like it would have an epidemic on the scale of South Africa, has stabilized at 3.1%. Still, as noted in chapter one, Nigeria is a place to keep an eye on. On one hand President Obsango appears to be addressing the problem aggressively, on the other hand Nigeria has a very poor health infrastructure with which to work, and a history of governmental corruption. In East Africa the epidemic is receding, with Uganda leading the way with adult prevalence down to 5.4%. Even in South Africa the epidemic seems to have peaked and the number of new infections is down.

The growing availability of cheap drugs means that more infected people will live long enough to raise their children, although a majority of infected Africans still do not have access to these drugs. Decreasing the number of orphans is good news for the stability of these societies.

Unless there is a cure developed, which seems unlikely in the foreseeable future, AIDS will remain a serious health, social, political, and economic problem in Africa. Human behavior remains the one big variable; it is the best hope in the near future for defeating the epidemic in Africa. It appears to have changed in significant ways, particularly in some hard-hit areas like Uganda. Unfortunately it can also change in the other direction, as reports of increasingly risky behaviors among gay Americans show.

The African epidemic became famous as a heterosexual epidemic, but recent research suggests that there is a significant homosexual aspect to it also. About 700 male prostitutes have been identified in the Kenyan city of Mombasa. Injection drug use, a major cause of the disease elsewhere, is reported growing within the turmoil in South Africa. Problems in the world economy also promise to increase turmoil throughout sub-Saharan Africa, a region already suffering from civil wars, extreme poverty, and administrative corruption. It is likely that in spite of recent good news, AIDS will continue to threaten the lives of Africans for some time.

Summary

This chapter traces the progression of the AIDS epidemic from beginnings in West Africa to epidemic status in central Africa (Kinshasa area) to the most devastating AIDS epidemic in the world in eastern and southern Africa. It looks at cultural differences in different regions that might explain why the epidemic is out of control in some areas and is a manageable problem in other areas. It discusses successful programs to curb the disease (Uganda) and looks at areas where lack of leadership has made the epidemic worse (South Africa). It also discusses both the positive and negative role of outsiders in dealing with the epidemic; from the residual effects of colonialism to the role of the the U. N., the World Health Agency, Western governments, and private philanthropists like Bill and Melinda Gates.

Name: ______________________ **Date:** ______________

Chapter 5 AIDS in Africa

Exercises

Exercise 1 Test Your Knowledge:

1. AIDS is just a disease of the poor.
   a. True
   b. False
2. Circumcision played a role in contracting HIV/AIDS. True or False?
3. Women often had no control over their sexuality because
   a. there were no men who wanted to have sex with them
   b. they were not allowed to have sex
   c. poverty led them to use sex as a form of income to survive
4. Authorities were never afraid to admit there was an epidemic in their country. True or False?
5. Unlike the US, African societies have more:
   a. People involved in multiple sexual relations during the same time period.
   b. Drugs available to treat AIDS
   c. Financial support in trying to fight AIDS
6. Immigration played no role in transporting AIDS from one area of Africa to another. True or False?
7. The disease often spread from:
   a. Children to adults
   b. The general public to sex workers and their clients
   c. Sex workers and their clients to the general public
8. In South Africa, like in the United States, the first serious outbreak was among:
   a. Infants
   b. Homosexuals
   c. Children

9. Anti-viral drugs:
    a. Were very inexpensive and could be obtained by anyone
    b. Ineffective at helping treat AIDS at all
    c. Helped relieve suffering and extend life
10. Those who had HIV/AIDS were faced with discrimination. True or False?

Study Questions

1. How does Merrill Singer's principle that AIDS follows poverty apply to sub-Saharan Africa?

2. What is the role of Kinshasa in the African AIDS epidemic?

3. Explain concurrency. How does this practice help to make heterosexual sex so dangerous?

4. What was the role of commercial sex in Rwanda and Burundi in promoting the African epidemic? Why did commercial sex play such a role?

5. What difference did circumcision make in infection rates in sub-Saharan Africa?

6. How do you account for the high rates of infection in the Union of South Africa?

7. What is meant when it is said that Botswana is a rich nation of poor people? How did this contribute to the epidemic?

8. What factors limit the extent of the epidemic in Senegal?

9. What is the relative status of non-Muslim women in West Africa compared to the status of women in southern and eastern Africa?

10. Why is the epidemic so serious in the Ivory Coast? Explain the various contributing factors.

11. Discuss Dr. Jonathon Mann and the issue of privacy. What are the pros and cons of maintaining the privacy of infected individuals?

12. What are the key factors causing the decline of the epidemic in Uganda?

Chapter six | HIV/AIDS and Commercial Sex

In many countries around the world, commercial sex workers are seen as reservoirs of infection or high-frequency transmitters, at the focal point of spreading HIV. What has been dismissed is the fact that sex workers who are HIV positive have contracted the virus through their clients who have not worn condoms and have engaged in unprotected sex.

Research of sex workers in developing countries has shown that in small towns, the suburbs, and large cities, sex workers with AIDS are shunned by many hospital doctors, brothel operators, and their own families (Stine 2007). Some are housewives working to make ends meet in their families. It was reported that in some towns in Africa, Vietnam, and India, between 50 and 90% of the sex workers are HIV positive. In northern Thailand, 72% of sex workers are HIV infected (Stine 2007).

UNAIDS has declared that "policy and program development is best served by language that is not stigmatizing and recognizes that many of those involved in sex work regard it as their source of livelihood. It should be noted, however, that no single term adequately covers the range of transactions taking place worldwide that involve sex work" (UNAIDS 2002, "Sex Work and HIV/AIDS").

UNAIDS has defined sex workers as "female, male and transgender adults and young people who receive money or goods in exchange for sexual services, either regularly or occasionally, and who may or may not consciously define those activities as income-generating (UNAIDS 2002, "Sex Work and HIV/AIDS"). Sex workers usually prefer the term "sex work" to "prostitution" because sex work is less stigmatizing and captures their experience as work.

In this chapter, I will first present feminists' diverse standpoints on sex and commercial sex. I will then introduce state policies on sex work around the world. Next, I will discuss HIV/AIDS and commercial sex in the context of Senegal and Asia. In the last section, I will scrutinize the power dynamics between sex workers and clients.

Feminists' Standpoints on Sex and Commercial Sex

Anti-sex feminists such as Andrea Dworkin and Catharine MacKinnon argue that messages of male power and female subjugation are inherent in sexual culture. They claim that the very meaning of sex is male domination. As Catharine MacKinnon argues, sex is constituted by male domination. Women, according to them, are no more than sex workers and objects for the pleasure of men. Women are caught in a passive condition within this social and cultural order. While other feminists contend that sex workers, like other workers and other women, engage in acts of negotiation, resistance, and subversion, anti-sex feminists believe that sex cannot be a tool for dismantling male supremacy because it is created by it and for it, thus implicated in it (see also Chapkis 1997).

Anti-prostitution activists argue that sex workers, because of the nature of their work, lack control in their lives. In selling the illusion of sexual desire, sex workers lose their abilities to experience sex in a noninstrumental, emotional, and intimate way. They argue that when sexuality becomes a commodity for exchange, it becomes an object, the means to an end. When sexuality is calculated and quantified for money exchange, its commodification destroys women's ability to experience real sexual intimacy outside of the marketplace, and leaves them with an impoverished sexual and emotional life.

Liberal feminists believe that sex workers have total control in their lives because it is men who feel powerless in the presence of women's sexuality and who have to pay for women's sexuality. Money, as they argue, crystallizes men's confession of their weakness when it is used to buy women's attention. Apart from anti-sex feminists who argue that sex is the root of men's oppression and abuse of women, liberal feminists believe that sex is benign whether it is an expression of love or pleasure, and that women's association with sex constitutes the source of their greatest power.

Romantic feminists tie sex to affection, intimacy, and love, and argue that love, relationships, and mutual pleasure are the only appropriate context for positive sex. They oppose sex work and pornography and consider them corrupting practices that undermine positive sex that is based on love. Cash in the context of sex work is a contamination of positive sex.

Romantic feminist Kathleen Barry argues that sex cannot and should not be purchased or commodified because positive sex must be shared between lovers through trust and sharing. She contends that the practice of sex work is not really sex, but an abuse of sex. She argues that the possibility of real, positive sexual experience is jeopardized and endangered by misrepresentations of sex via commercial sex work and pornography. Commercial sex is compared to a contaminating virus that is held responsible for both literal and symbolic violence against women.

Romantic feminists actively advocate a politics of cultural cleansing, and uphold the belief that pornography and sex work should be abolished, and their contaminating effect on sexual fantasy and practice must be actively challenged.

Feminists in the last camp represent a variation on the libertarian view. They argue that prostitutes threaten patriarchal control over women's sexuality and invoke sexual subversion through prostitution. They contend that the state regulates and punishes women's bodies by criminalizing nonprocreative sex and restricting access to birth control and abortion. Prostitution is a terrain of struggle where women, far from passive sexual objects, exhibit sexual agency and challenge the existing sexual order.

Political Policies and Prostitution

Overall there are four basic policies towards prostitution.

Prohibitionist Policy

The United States, with the exception of the state of Nevada, represents the prohibitionist policy, making the buying and selling of sexual services illegal. Some feminists argue that in this system, law enforcement targets prostitutes rather than those who profit from their income and morally condemn women who choose prostitution. According to these feminists, illegality drives prostitutes underground and makes prostitutes totally reliant upon pimps and police officers.

Prostitution is illegal in the United States except for the state of Nevada. In 12 counties of Nevada, there are over 30 licensed brothels and mandatory physical examinations are required of these registered prostitutes. Despite the prohibitionist policy, prostitution is common throughout the rest of the United States. Prostitutes may work alone, may be controlled by pimps, or may be associated with escort agencies. A common cause of prostitution is drug addiction. Escort prostitutes masquerade as entertainers or companion hostesses in escort agencies, bars, chiropractic offices, massage parlors, and so on. A relatively new source of prostitution in the United States is foreign-born women who are trafficked around the globe each year. It is estimated that around 20% of the over 1 million females who are trafficked are smuggled into the United States to work in brothels.

While the Democratic Party supports legalizing prostitution to end trafficking, the Bush administration adamantly opposed this approach. Bush stated that prostitution is inherently harmful to women and that no grants or funding will be given to groups and countries that support abortion or prostitution. The administration encouraged women to claim themselves as victims, under which condition they could receive cash compensations.

Researchers such as Jennifer Musto point out that because NGOs depend upon federal funding, organizations that accept sex work as a legitimate profession or argue against the conflation of voluntary prostitution with trafficking potentially run the risk of losing their funding (Musto 2009). Through investigating the history, organizational structure, and program offerings of a local NGO in Los Angeles, she argues that the anti-trafficking movement will not be successful unless the government changes its position on trafficking. She contends that the U.S. government's position and policy on trafficking directly influences the organization and leading ideology of NGOs and contributes to the asymmetrical power relations between NGO staff and clients.

Musto states that to ensure funding, NGOs must align their internal policies with the views of the U.S. government by claiming that all forms of prostitution are exploitative, equivalent of "sexual slavery," and are a "gateway" to trafficking. Such a biased and narrow definition of trafficking influences their identification practices, as they provide shelters to the involuntary trafficked persons and arrest the voluntary migrants. She argues that the organization fails to include trafficked persons' participation in the anti-trafficking movement. Since NGOs cannot use the U.S. government funds to promote or advocate the legalization or regulation of prostitution as a legitimate form of work, it prevents the staff from having any dialogues or developing any programs with clients who have worked voluntarily in the sex industries. Within this funding culture of fear, the staff feels obligated to exclude clients who may voluntarily choose sex work for survival.

Abolitionist Policy

Some European countries such as Sweden, the United Kingdom, and France have an abolitionist policy. This policy rejects the state's regulation of prostitutes, but makes it illegal for third parties such as brothel keepers or pimps to be involved with prostitution. This view holds it immoral and unethical for the state to regulate prostitutes, recognizing them as victims of social and economic hardships. By making third parties illegal, it pursues a policy of discouraging prostitution while not prosecuting prostitutes themselves, who are considered victims.

The abolitionist policy denies the possibility that women have willingly chosen sex work and categorizes sex workers as passive victims of trafficking and coercion. This system rejects them as subjects who are capable of assuming agency and responsibility and views them as women to be rescued and saved. This system negates individual choice and considers sex work morally evil. Abolitionism deploys this moral and ethical argument that sex work undermines family values against the involvement of the state or any other third party in the activity of sex work. Any involvement of a third party is regarded as encouraging moral decay.

For instance, in China, Chinese women in juristic and legal circles define it a violation of women's human rights to portray women as sexual objects and reduce women to the status of objects, chattels, or commodities. They construe any commercial sex–related activities as objectifying women's bodies and defaming and humiliating women. The laws promulgated in 1991 and 1992 represent the abolitionist policy that criminalizes the involvement of a third party in luring or trafficking women into prostitution: the 1991 Two Decisions on Strictly Forbidding the Selling and Buying of Sex and the Severe Punishment of Criminals Who Abduct and Traffic in or Kidnap Women and Children; the

1992 Law on Protecting the Rights and Interests of Women (Women's Law). The Criminal Law of 1997 continues this abolitionist thrust of UN Conventions. The 1999 Entertainment Regulations banned the resurgence of commercial sex–related activities such as striptease, "topless" and "bottomless" waitressing, table dancing, lap dancing, and so on.

Abolitionism, demonizing, criminalizing, and isolating prostitutes is believed to constitute the prime factor in perpetuating violence against sex workers as it pushes them to be completely dependent upon others such as pimps, procurers, and police officers. In reality, as a plethora of research contends, prostitutes, contrary to the victim script constructed in abolitionism, are agents who consider sex work a form of labor no different from other labor.

The abolitionist policy in China generates a violent and exploitative environment for women involved in the sex industry. Here we will draw on Zheng's three years of research on karaoke bar hostesses in urban China (Zheng 2009b). Female sex workers in China are camouflaged as female hostesses working in commercial sites such as nightclubs, karaoke bars, hair salons, sauna bars, and other leisure sites. Patrons are mainly middle-aged businessmen, government officials, policemen, and foreign investors. Clients can partake of the services offered by hostesses and at the same time engage in "social interactions" that help cement "relationships" with their business partners or their patrons in the government. Hostesses play an indispensable role in the rituals of these male-centered worlds of business and politics.

The Bureau of Culture and the Public Security Bureau represent the government's dual strategy of soft and hard administrative measures against these leisure sites such as karaoke bars. The Bureau of Culture is responsible for ensuring that karaoke bars are managed according to socialist standards of civility and morality. The main vehicle for the Public Security Bureau intervention was the anti-pornography campaign, itself a part of a wider comprehensive attack on social deviance known as "crackdowns" (*yanda*—literally, to strike severely). These campaigns lasted for spurts of three months at a time, to be repeated three times a year, strategically centering on important holidays (e.g., National Day and Army Day) and events (e.g., APEC conference). Crackdowns targeted a number of social ills, ranging from unlicensed video game arcades (said to corrupt the minds of the youth) to undocumented rural migrants (said to disrupt urban management).

Pornography is a mainstay in the list of crackdown targets. It includes a wide range of illegal behavior, such as pornographic media (e.g., magazines, laser discs) and performances (e.g., striptease). The behaviors that receive the most organizational resources and manpower, however, are the "erotic services" conducted in karaoke bars and other commercial establishments (e.g., saunas and hair salons). The Public Security Bureau employed a complex system of raids to attack karaoke bars. Their techniques were self-described as "guerilla warfare" (*da youji*) in reference to the heroic efforts of the communist revolutionaries against the Japanese invaders and nationalists. Raids were divided into several types, including: "regular raids and shock raids, timed raids and random raids, systematic raids and block raids, daytime raids and night raids." Those Public Security Bureau units and individuals who perform well—measured in the number of arrested hostesses and amount of fines levied—receive high honors and cash bonuses from the municipal government.

Police raids make hostesses both legally and socially vulnerable. If their sexual services are disclosed by the clients to the police, they would be subject to extreme humiliation, arrest, handsome fines, and incarceration. Indeed, in their everyday lives, the local police constitute daily fear and terror. Because the police wield arbitrary power, the hostesses find it obligatory to obey their sexual demands without monetary compensation. State policy is distorted and even derailed by the self-seeking behavior of local officials. Karaoke bars are an important source of their extralegal income. Local officials extract economic benefits from karaoke bars through a combination of bribes and fines. They not only sexually and economically exploit hostesses, but also keep "spy hostesses" as their personal harem. The anti-pornography campaign also allows the bar owners to impose more severe regulations and disciplines on the hostesses who otherwise would operate in a more laissez-faire manner. Because the state's anti-pornography policy is manipulated and usurped by local officials and bar owners for their own ends, leading to a violent working environment for the hostesses, hostesses do not disclose their real identities, which makes it more convenient for men (especially thugs and gangsters in the underworld) to be violent toward them and even to murder them (Zheng 2009b).

Regulatory System

In contrast to abolitionism, the regulatory system legalizes and regulates prostitution through registration and other forms of state control such as public health and tax collection. A regulatory policy exists in countries such as Germany, the Netherlands, and Senegal. These countries legalize and regulate prostitution through registration, collection of taxes, and regular physical tests. Prostitutes by law must register with the police and have regular STD tests, and face penalties if they fail to do so. Some women choose not to register to avoid the accompanying stigma. Some researchers argue that it is not the best way to manage sex work.

In the regulatory system, prostitutes have to apply for licenses and receive regular physical examinations. In the event that they carry any STDs, their licenses are confiscated and they are precluded from work until they have completely recuperated. On the surface, this system ideally promotes public order and public health. However, research in West Africa, England, and elsewhere points to its limitations. For instance, research in four British cities reveals that sex workers feel a lack of protection and respect from the police. Even sex workers who are physically and emotionally abused by their pimps generally prefer pimps to the police.

In West Germany, prostitution is legal, with the supply coming mainly from Eastern Europe. Hundreds of thousands of women from Russia and Ukraine sell themselves as prostitutes in Germany. Prostitutes usually work in streets, escort agencies, apartments, houses, or clubs such as sauna clubs, massage services, bars, and so on. Their income is taxed and they are free to advertise their services in public media. Although the law does not require physical examinations for prostitutes, many brothels do require them. In Amsterdam, even though non-European prostitutes without parents in residence are illegal, foreign women make up almost 90% of the prostitutes who are displayed in windows in the red light district. While this law is obviously not enforced, its intent is to provide economic protection for the Dutch prostitutes. In Western Europe generally, women are trafficked from Africa, Asia, South America, Iran, and the Caribbean. In Italy, for instance, 60% of all prostitutes are trafficked from Nigeria; in Belgium, the Netherlands, and Italy, Iranian women account for 10 to 15% of the prostitutes.

Decriminalization

Systems of decriminalization can be found in New South Wales and Australia, the only place that decriminalizes prostitutes and prostitution business. It asserts that it is the right of independent adult women to determine their lives by themselves. Elsewhere, it is favored by organizations supporting prostitutes' rights as workers. This system argues that criminalizing the sex industry creates ideal conditions for rampant exploitation and abuse of sex workers. Trafficking in women, coercion, and exploitation can only be stopped if the existence of prostitution is recognized and the legal and social rights of prostitutes are guaranteed.

State Policy and HIV/AIDS Prevention

According to UNAIDS,

"The legal status of sex work in a given region has significant bearing on the effectiveness of AIDS programs targeting sex workers. Where sex work is illegal, legislative frameworks are often oriented towards penalizing individual sex workers. In such settings, sex workers are less likely to seek health services and more likely to conduct their activities underground" (UNAIDS 2002, "Sex Work and HIV/AIDS").

Sex work is legal in most developed countries, where sex workers are able to enjoy the same rights and benefits as other workers. In these countries where sex work is legal, their legal standing helps protect themselves because the authorities are more likely to enforce laws against abuse and exploitation and hence minimize violence instances against sex workers. This legal situation can be juxtaposed to an illegal social context where authorities can be easily corrupt in terrorizing, abusing, and persecuting sex workers or enlisting briberies from them. However, legal sex work is often confined to specific geographic areas and sex workers are regulated by a system of registration and health checks. Although this sort of formal or establishment based sex work offers sex workers legal standing and health examinations, this system still cannot reach informal sex workers who refuse to register and remain clandestine. In addition, the system, while constraining legal sex work geographically, has benefited public health from the public health perspective, but perpetuates and encourages social stigma against sex workers (UNAIDS 2002, "Sex Work and HIV/AIDS").

UNAIDS declares that discriminatory laws have made it almost impossible for sex workers to successfully bring charges against someone who rapes them. "In contrast, laws, policies and policing methods that perpetuate poor working conditions for sex workers and encourage unscrupulous behavior by third parties are common. This combination of circumstances makes both sex workers and their clients more vulnerable to HIV infection. In some countries—for example, most of the United States of America and parts of the Middle East—selling sex is forbidden and has been made both illegal and punishable. In the face of oppressive laws and policies, sex work is likely to become increasingly clandestine, making HIV/AIDS and STI prevention and care activities nearly impossible to implement.

Countries as diverse as Australia, Bangladesh, Brazil, Greece, Guatemala, Kenya, Peru and the Philippines, among others, allow or tolerate commercial sex under certain conditions. These conditions may include registration and medical testing for sex workers, confining sex work to specific geographical areas, and banning advertising, public solicitation and/or the involvement of third parties. Despite existing protective legislation, however, the police and other authorities or interest groups have been known to choose to take punitive or more restrictive actions. Punitive and restrictive regulations can violate sex workers' right to voluntary and confidential medical testing, alienate them from available health services and discourage them from seeking safer sex-related information and education" (UNAIDS 2002, "Sex Work and HIV/AIDS").

Case Study of Registration System: Urban Senegal

Below is a case study represented in Michelle Renaud's book *Women at the Crossroads: A Prostitute Community's Response to AIDS in Urban Senegal* (Renaud 1997).

Cultural Background

In the book, Renaud depicts the cultural backdrop against which women choose sex work (Renaud 1997). During the time when Senegal was under the reign of the Europeans, it was a male-dominated world where women did not have a say in political issues. Women did not gain the right to vote until the twentieth century. Despite the fact that the religion of Islam warranted women new privileges of complete control over their own earnings, there is still little representation of women's interests in government institutions and organizations that control economic resources of the society.

Renaud points out that individuals are located at the center of three circles: mainstream culture, community, and family. These three circles carry the overarching beliefs and expectations that are enforced by Islam and other nonreligious cultural factors. Individuals' lives are shaped and gauged by these beliefs enforced by families and communities.

The dominant beliefs represented by these three circles are patriarchal in nature. For instance, if a married man commits adultery, he is only punished if the act takes place in his home, and his partner is not punished. If a married woman commits adultery, both she and her partner are punished. The overarching beliefs also grant men the right to legally forbid wives to work outside the home.

Traditional Islamic law also allows men to marry up to four women as long as they treat their wives fairly and equally. The law also bestows men the right to divorce their wives at will. A woman, however, cannot get a divorce unless she goes to the court and proves that her husband is irresponsible.

The dominant values deem women's primary domain to be in the household. Their major duty is to perform domestic tasks and receive an allowance from their husbands. Led by this dominant value, fathers do not allow girls to go to school, and force them to marry against their wishes.

Marriage does not occur across caste or ethnic groups, and rarely involves love. It is economic and social benefits that families are concerned about, not love. During the courting period, the male suitor offers a bride price in the form of gifts and money and the bride lists a number of objects she wants. The bride price is considered essential security to guard against possible divorce or desertion in the future. More than half of the marriages in Senegal are polygamous and the age gap increases as husbands marry younger and younger wives. To Renaud, marriage in Senegal is symbolic prostitution (Renaud 1997).

In urban areas, divorce is tragic for women. A woman gets divorced usually for the following three reasons: her husband beats her, her husband marries other wives with whom she does not get along, or her husband is dead. After divorce, ex-husbands are not required by law to pay mandatory child support and grown-up sons are not obligated to financially support their widowed or divorced mothers. Hence a divorced woman is on her own in assuming the responsibility of bringing up the children and making ends meet. If she is lucky, she can depend upon the safety net provided by her family and community for the compensation of the loss. If she lacks such a support net or cannot access it, especially when she lives in an urban area far away from her family and relatives, she is forced to make a living and feed her children on her own. Since women traditionally do not receive education, they usually find themselves unable to gain employment and shoulder the responsibilities for their children because of little or no education or skills. In this case, a woman would turn to prostitution as a last resort and distance herself from her community and family, which were the focus of her life.

AIDS and Sexual Relationships

Due to the nature of their work, sex workers rely heavily on the STD clinic for medical care and shelter from a society that shuns them. They have an altered, new value system that comes from women with whom they live and work, rather than from their families or clinic staffs. The women form alliances and families within their coterie to communally solve disputes and build a communal spirit and solidarity that helps them survive in a society replete with criticism against them and the stigma attached to their profession.

They regularly attend health classes and learn about information on HIV and STD transmission. They are advised to exert control over their health and apply behavioral changes. They attach a lot of value to the advice given them and try to incorporate it into their decisions about sexual behaviors with clients. AIDS prevention education has forced these women to drastically shift their sexual relationships with clients by taking power and control over sexual behaviors.

For instance, when the women do not want to argue with a client about condom use or have pain from frequent intercourse, they will use their thighs to stimulate intercourse until the client ejaculates. They have learned not to trust clients' use of condoms because they have witnessed that clients deliberately insert holes in condoms so that they break during the intercourse. For the women, maneuvering ways around clients' schemes through use of their thighs achieves the goal of deceiving clients and precluding semen from entering their vagina, ultimately avoiding potential HIV infection.

Although the women are skillful in deceiving clients and circumventing possible HIV infection, they are willing to put themselves at risk for HIV infection with their boyfriends. As Renaud asserts, in this sense they are no different from women who are not prostitutes.

Renaud points out that in a male-dominated society, education about AIDS can result in changes in sexual behaviors and power imbalance. Renaud describes a list of options that the women choose in order to gain more leverage in their relationships with clients. She argues that they are cognizant of the fact that a wrong decision could result in infection and an early death, and they are extraordinary agents in constantly weighing the costs and benefits of their behaviors and making a significant difference in their lives and others'.

Reconciling Profession with Religion

Believing that God has power over life, death, and eternal fate, prostitutes conceive AIDS as the worst punishment from God. Hence they resort to a series of behaviors to reconcile their profession with their religious beliefs.

First, they try very hard to play the roles expected of them as good Senegalese women and mothers. They remain single so that they can care for their parents, siblings, or other relatives' children. They reconcile their beliefs that God might punish them for their work with the conviction that they are exerting their best efforts to take charge of their lives and that they serve as good, caring women and mothers. They assert themselves as good mothers. They rationalize prostitution by telling themselves that it is the only way for them to care for children when leaving a husband. "God will forgive me—not let the babies starve and succeeding on my own."

They believe that God should forgive them for engaging in shameful sexual practices because their practices enable them to act responsibly in other aspects of their lives. Indeed, participation in the stigmatized profession of prostitution allows them to be more financially independent and more powerful than other women, as they can survive and take care of children on their own, despite the absence of support by their families and communities.

Second, these women pray for forgiveness for those behaviors that their families, friends, and communities disdain. They believe that they will not receive God's blessing if they have provoked divorce, been involved with many men, or have not practice Islam regularly. They pray to make their dreams more likely to come true. They pray to God every morning and evening asking him to forgive them for the sin of prostitution so that they can enter paradise after death.

They believe that God will be more forgiving to them because they will be judged according to all their behaviors, not just those sinful ones. They hide their work from family and friends; they move hundreds of miles away from children to live among strangers and pray daily for a way out.

Third, while wrestling with forgiving themselves and criticizing prostitution from a Muslim perspective, the women choose to believe that God will forgive them if they prove themselves to be good Muslims. They feel they are prostitutes because it is the wish of God. They define good Muslims as those who pray and observe religious rituals. To them, real worshipers—good Muslims who pray—are less likely to contract HIV, whereas those who do not pray are more likely to receive HIV infection.

The women assert that they are good Muslims. Good Muslim also means engagement in "normal sex." The women refuse oral and anal sex because both are considered abnormal and highly stigmatized in Senegal. It is said that the clients might eat them during oral sex. They are also cautious not to appear naked because this is the best time for devils to prey on victims, weaken and kill them.

Being a good Muslim also means adherence to ritual practices. They make pilgrimages to Mecca, walking on the ground where the prophet once walked and praying in the mosque where millions of Muslims pay homage to the prophet. They stay away from the mosque during menstruation. They observe all the religious rules including never eating pork and never smoking or drinking. They observe Ramadan during the holidays, when they fast not only on food but also on the pleasure of the flesh. During the fasting period, they remove themselves physically and emotionally from other prostitutes. They also consider it offensive to God to change what God has given them.

They believe that prostitutes who do not go to the mosque or observe religious rituals have a questionable faith and integrity, and hence will not be pardoned by God for their sins and will not enter paradise after death. A prostitute may convene and discuss with others where she may end up after death. If she lacks faith in God, God will not listen to her after her death, but instead, will ask her family members and neighbors about her conduct during her lifetime.

Political Economy of AIDS: Registration System, Poverty, and Stigmatization

Prostitutes fear legal registration because registration discloses their profession to their family and friends. Therefore, as Renaud relates, 80% of prostitutes remain clandestine for fear of marginalization and humiliation as a result of public registration.

Clandestine prostitutes outside of the legal system have the advantage of not only keeping their profession secret from their families and friends, but also easily exiting prostitution without residual effects. Registered prostitutes, on the other hand, have to endure a long process before clinics and police take them off rosters. Even then, despite the fact that their requests are approved and their registration is relinquished, their files are eternally kept in clinics and police stations. This means that their future husbands could potentially access these files and learn about their previous profession. In the book, Renaud relates one instance where an ex-prostitute was going to get married. Before the wedding ceremony, her finance visited his friend who happened to be a policeman; here he had a chance to access her file and learned that she used to be a prostitute. He immediately called off the marriage after that.

In the registration system in Senegal, prostitutes are entitled to police protection. As long as they register with the local police and a health care clinic, they have the right to practice prostitution without any harassment or disruption.

Renaud recounts that as early as the 1980s, health clinics in urban Senegal started educating registered prostitutes about the AIDS virus, testing them for infection, providing free condoms, and encouraging condom use. Since 1987, their health has been monitored by foreign researchers and donors. However, as Renaud states, the clinics at all levels in all areas are deprived of adequate equipment and medicine. For instance, she relates that needles and other equipment that come into contact with blood are reused without sterilization. Clinics at the lower levels lack alcohol and the necessary equipment for boiling water.

Prostitutes visit the clinic for a short appointment twice a month. Every 45 days, they have a longer visit where they have to go through a physical examination that includes laboratory tests. Each time when they have a long visit to the clinic, they receive 28 free condoms.

If they are sick, they receive the medication for free as long as it can be directly provided by the clinic or the dispensary pharmacy. However, if certain medication is a gift granted by a medicine salesman, they will be obliged to pay some money for it. If the medication cannot be supplied either at the clinic or the dispensary pharmacy, they will have to travel to a pharmacy in town and purchase very expensive ones.

Unless they are fully cured of an STD, it is illegal for them to practice prostitution while taking the medication and waiting for recuperation. Their registration cards are revoked during this time and will not be returned until they are fully cured. They are also required to turn in their registration cards to the clinic during menstruation, since the presence of blood increases their chance of HIV infection during sexual intercourse.

In this registration system, for women who have contracted HIV, their registration cards will not be confiscated or revoked. Instead, they are allowed to continue working as a prostitute. This policy is established to prevent these women from leaving the city to practice prostitution covertly.

Renaud accounts that the system uses fear to scare the women about AIDS in an effort to assure that they will avoid sexual risks. As a result, women have developed paranoia about AIDS and they refuse to take care of their sick colleagues and friends no matter how much they need them.

Political Economy of AIDS: Power Dynamics between Clinic Staff and Registered Prostitutes

Renaud unravels the power dynamics between clinic staff and registered prostitutes. She reveals that the staff members in the clinic are controlling, judgmental, and critical of the prostitutes. They are also indifferent to the prostitutes' plight. Despising the prostitutes for their profession, they show little concern about their health.

Prostitutes feel powerless dealing with staff members because staff members dictate their health. Renaud discusses how staff members withhold tons of condoms, and how they would rather let them expire in the warehouse than give them to the prostitutes for free. Their rationale is that they are afraid that prostitutes will sell additional condoms for money. While the staff members attend the AIDS conference in Dakar, they close the clinic and leave no condoms for the prostitutes. Renaud comments that their behavior reveals their nonchalant attitudes toward, and little concern about, the women's welfare. Without access to condoms, it is extremely difficult for women to practice safe sex. Prostitutes' dissatisfaction about condom distribution leads to a tension between themselves and the clinic staff and draws them apart from each other. While the prostitutes resent staff for withholding condoms from their reach, the staff members consider the prostitutes rebellious children warranting parental control.

The prostitutes also dislike the laboratory technician because of his blackmail. The lab technician demands a bribe from the prostitutes each time they come in for a physical examination. He threatens them that unless the bribe is in his hand before their urine and vaginal smear samples are tested, he will lie about their health. He also sells them condoms that are supposed to be free. Often times he will order the prostitutes to sell several boxes of condoms for him and turn in the earnings. The prostitutes will risk not having any condoms at all if they fail to submit to him the earnings. Prostitutes have no alternative but to obey his orders because it is essential for them to receive a negative test report in order for them to continue working with the registration card. They certainly know the stakes in their dealings with the technician.

Case Study of Sex Work and HIV/AIDS in Asia

Similar to the case in Senegal, many prostitutes in Asia choose the profession because they need to support their children, siblings, and parents, or because they are divorced or disowned by their families. Some children are even sold into prostitution by poor parents. Throughout Asia, youth is an essential prerequisite for sex workers, and young girls between the ages of 10 and 16 are in high demand by clients.

Many of these countries are both the source and destination for trafficking of women. For instance, it is reported that women are trafficked from Burma, Laos, Cambodia, and China to Bangkok in Thailand; from Nepal to East and South Asia, and the Gulf; and from Thailand and China to South Africa. Because prostitution is illegal in many countries in Asia, it is forced into camouflaged brothels such as massage parlors, hostess bars, karaoke bars, nightclubs, teahouses, and so on. Prostitutes are subject to police harassment, incarceration, and HIV infection. It is reported that condom use is inconsistent among sex workers due to financial concerns and the power hierarchy between sex workers and clients. While HIV-prevention programs have been very successful in countries such as Thailand and Cambodia, most countries in Asia are experiencing an increase in HIV/AIDS infection due to the secret nature of sex work and political inertia.

Political Economy: Economic and Social Inequality

In China and Thailand, there is a tradition that parents sell their daughters for prostitution to help the family survive. In Thailand, prostitutes believe that since they are filial to their parents and support their rural parents, they can earn a good karma. In many countries, rural women's low social status and unequal access to economic resources make them easy targets for exploitation in the sex industry.

In Zheng's research on karaoke bar hostesses in urban China, the vast majority of the hostesses came from the countryside. The hostesses or escorts who work at karaoke bars are referred to by the Chinese government as "*sanpei xiaojie,*" literally, "young women who accompany men in three ways." These "ways" are generally understood to include varying combinations of alcohol consumption, dancing, singing, and sexual services. Mainly 17 to 23 years of age, these women form a steadily growing contingent of illegal sex workers. Their services typically include drinking, singing, dancing, playing games, flirting, and caressing. Beyond the standard service package, some hostesses offer sexual services for an additional fee.

Of the 200 hostesses with whom I worked, only four were from cities. These women carried heavy cultural and historical baggage with them when they migrated to the urban areas, which made them easy prey to the sex industry. Historically, rural–urban relationships have evolved from equality and co-dependence to drastic inequality and a rural–urban apartheid system.

Although late imperial China was characterized by a high degree of integration between the city and countryside, the Maoist state and the emergence of a new bureaucratic structure eviscerated rural social institutions and stripped away the power base of the former elites. From 1949 to 1978, the state policy of "segregation between city and countryside" made the Mao state stagnant and static—a place where rural residents were cloistered in "cellularized villages and inward-looking work units" and experienced immobility. It also exacerbated the urban–rural divide, with most resources concentrated in the urban areas.

In 1958, the Maoist state initiated the household registration system, a method for controlling population movement through the management of resource distribution. Under this system, every household was required to register its members with a local public security bureau. The national population was classified into mutually exclusive urban–rural categories possessing unequal political, economical, social, and legal access. Rural residents found themselves on the losing end of a heavily lopsided distribution of social wealth.

Concomitant with the communist broad-based restructuring of society, the "peasantry" as a derogative cultural category and revolutionary mainstay was further refined and concretized. The Maoist government portrayal of the countryside in terms of peasant administrative categories involving the house registration system and mobility restrictions reinforced the cultural stereotypes of rural identities and segregated and branded the peasants as the reservoir of backward feudalism and superstition and a major obstacle to national development and salvation.

In the post-Mao era, relaxation of state mobility controls has allowed rural residents to migrate to urban regions, where they are labeled as the "floating population." In search of job opportunities and adventure, these migrants have become the "vanguard" in China's largest population movement since the establishment of communist rule, and in China's economic reforms as the harbingers of the market economy. As China's engagement with the global economy and experiments with economic reform continue, cities highlight the deepening disparities between permanent urban "citizens" (those with urban residence permits) and migrant populations without the residence permits.

Although the post-Mao state tolerates a higher degree of population mobility than the previous government, the urban–rural gap is still the main fault line between rich and poor in Chinese society. Inequalities are perpetuated and even aggravated by post-Mao state policies that transfer the brunt of the state and collectives' tax burden onto poor rural households (Khan 1998). This situation has not gone unnoticed by peasants, themselves. Since 1985, peasants have launched collective protests against taxes, fines, cadre corruption, and the drastic urban–rural income gap. This unrest points to their discontent with local authorities and constitutes one of the major threats to the Chinese Communist Party's power and stability (Li 1996).

With 100 million rural migrants on the move in post-Mao China, China's urban landscape is faced with the management of individuals who by definition are "outsiders." Despite their contributions to local and overall economic growth, migrants encounter severe institutional and social discriminations (Kipnis 1998). Blamed for blemishing the appearance of cities and contributing to overcrowding, migrants have become the scapegoats for a multitude of social problems, ranging from crime to urban pollution. As the "losers" in the market reforms, migrant workers are denied civil, political, and residential rights.

Women account for over 30% of the total number of rural–urban migrant laborers (Tan 1996). They are the providers of labor power for the state and important social and political actors. Institutional (such as the household registration system) and social discrimination (such as the derogative category of migrants) forces the vast majority of female migrants onto the lowest rungs of the labor market, where they commonly work as garbage collectors, restaurant waitresses, domestic maids, factory workers, and bar hostesses.

The above illustrates the intersection between power dynamics, rural–urban inequality, and sex work in China. Migrating from rural areas, these women shoulder the responsibilities for the survival of their parents and family members. Indeed, in many parts of Asia, forces of poverty are one of the reasons that young women choose the profession of sex work.

Urbanization and Consumer Culture

Urbanization and the consumer culture have also facilitated the commercialization of sex. In Japan, for instance, the highly advanced economy gives rise to a proliferation of consumption sites where sex work is provided—brothels, clubs, bars, health and fitness clubs. Japan is a major destination country into which many women are trafficked from China, Russia, Eastern Europe, Cambodia, Thailand, and other countries to work as prostitutes. During my fieldwork in urban China, pimps often came to each sex work site to enlist sex workers to work in Japan. Indeed, it is a high aspiration of hostesses to work in Japan as a sex worker. Each woman has to turn in 20,000 yuan and pass the interview in Japanese before being permitted to go through the visa process.

The Japanese consumer culture, or, to be more precise, cutie culture, has a great impact on the Japanese teenage schoolgirls. In Japan, teenage schoolgirls aspire to achieve the cutie style. They shop for the trendy gadgets, latest-style cell phones, and other modern and cute accoutrements such as Hello Kitty decorations. Young girls consider it their ambition to achieve anything cute, or kawaii. This young generation is mired in pursuing fashion and studying the industry of cute gadgets. They frequent stores that are designed for young, modern shoppers. They dye their hair different shades of brown, red, yellow, blue, and purple. They darken their skin color until pitch back. They create their own styles that are rebellious against the conservative tradition.

The consumer culture in Japan allows compensation dating, or enjo cosai, to be prevalent. It is extremely common, and popular, for high schoolgirls to offer sexual services to middle-aged businessmen in return for gifts and extra pocket money. Sometimes schoolgirls will perform sexual service just for a cute, trendy backpack. Also, since there are mushrooming stores that specifically sell schoolgirls' panties, they also bring their panties to the stores for sale.

These teenage schoolgirls usually meet middle-aged businessmen through Japan's many telephone dating clubs. In the telephone dating clubs, men pay to sit in booths and wait for girls or women to call in. Phone conversations sometimes lead to dates, and dates lead to sex for compensation.

Tokyo also has several hundred image-clubs where Japanese men pay about $150 an hour to live out their fantasies about schoolgirls. In this club, male customers can choose from 11 rooms, including classrooms, school gym changing rooms, and imitation railroad cars wherein men can molest girls in school uniforms to the recorded roar of a commuter train.

It is said that in Japan, the center of sexual fantasies is shifted from office ladies in their twenties to college women, and then from college women to high school and juniorhigh school girls. There is a clear demand for increasingly younger aged girls.

From Direct to Indirect Prostitution

In many countries in Asia, prostitution is indirect instead of direct. In other words, sex workers are camouflaged in some other kind of work such as hostesses working in entertainment places such as saunas, karaoke bars, and hotels, and providing erotic services. The clandestine nature of their work makes it extremely difficult to target them in the HIV prevention work.

Another impediment to HIV prevention work is that these women do not identify themselves as sex workers. If we define prostitution as the exchange of sex for some form of material rewards, then sex work involves a substantial proportion of the general population. However, although many women exchange sexual intimacy and love for resources such as food, shelter, clothing, social capital, and so on, they do not perceive themselves as sex workers because it is not their primary occupation.

For instance, in my previous working unit in China, there was a mass-scale lay-off of employees. At this moment, only those who either had a network with the superiors or had high qualifications were able to stay. A 21-year-old female migrant clerk was on the brink of being laid off. She had no network to pursue and no money to bribe her superior with. In the end, she had no alternative but to choose to become the mistress of the superior of the company, and thus stayed employed. Everybody in the company knew about this and they would gossip about how, at such a young age, it was very unusual for her to possess such a large sum of money.

In this case, the migrant woman exchanged sexual intimacy and love for material rewards and security of her job, but she would not have to identify herself as a sex worker because she had a legitimate job in a company. The widespread indirect prostitution in Asia has created a major obstacle in disseminating HIV-related information to those engaged in risky behaviors.

International and Domestic Market

In some countries in Asia, the sex industry is organized with one market for domestic men and another market for foreign men. For instance, in Thailand, the sex industry is bifurcated into two markets, with one market for Thai and immigrant workers who pay in local currency and another market for foreign tourists who pay in foreign currency.

Sex tourism and prostitution is a huge business that helps generate a high GDP in Thailand's economy. Researchers have stated that far more people are employed in Thailand's local sex trade than the tourist trade. It was a long-held tradition that Thai men perceived visiting brothels as a pastime and leisure. Fathers would introduce their sons to brothels, as prostitution is regarded as an accepted form of entertainment. Wives are culturally expected to tolerate their husbands' infidelities. According to a recent study by the Ministry of Public Health, roughly three quarters of all Thai males regularly visit prostitutes and prostitutes initiate almost half of all teenage boys into sexual activity (Brown 2001).

Since countless young girls, at least a third of all Thai sex workers, are under the age of 18, prostitution in Thailand has a devastating effect on them (Brown 2001). It can be considered as child labor. However, teenager girls are the most in demand with clients, and the majority of adult prostitutes started as children themselves. Brown notes that children are much more likely to be victims of debt bondage, trafficking, physical violence, or torture (Brown 2001).

The international sex market caters to male tourists and business travelers from around the globe. These foreign men fly to Thailand to indulge themselves at bargain prices and engage in sex with teenage children without suffering from legal consequences such as arrests. The money they spend on sex, hotels, meals, gifts, transportation, and other tourist-involved miscellaneous costs is a major source of Thailand's foreign currency exchange (Brown 2001).

Power Dynamics between Sex Workers and Clients

Condom Use and Clients

In Zheng's research on hostesses and clients in China, Zheng observed that female sex workers who were informed about the dangers of HIV/STDs and the risk-reduction benefits of condom use were nonetheless unable to convince their clients to use condoms. This is because male power is amplified in the case of sex–money exchanges where the female sex worker directly depends on the man for her economic livelihood. Given the intractability of the unequal economic relations that weaken female sex workers in relation to their clients, it is essential to scrutinize male sex consumers' perceptions of condoms as the point of departure for STD/HIV research and intervention.

Among the client group Zheng interviewed, comprised predominantly of well-educated government officials and entrepreneurs, 100% understood that condoms offered protection against sexually transmitted diseases and HIV. Among all the groups Zheng has interviewed, including male and female university professors, students, hostesses, hotel workers, clients exhibited the highest level of knowledge of HIV and condoms. One would expect the clients to consistently use condoms to protect themselves. However, many clients wrote directly on the survey that they did not use condoms because condoms dulled the sensation.

Zheng's subsequent interviews suggested that clients perceive condoms as the unnatural control over their natural sexual expression; they perceive contraceptive use as the women's responsibility; and they perceive non-use of condoms as being brave in the peer group (Zheng 2009a). Zheng's research revealed that clients strove for complete freedom from any kind of control over their sexual expression through unleashing their sexual desire and pursuing maximal sexual pleasure. Meanwhile, men believe that it is women who should take care of contraceptive responsibilities. Also, men who do not use condoms are highly regarded by their peer group.

This finding resonates with research in Tanzania, Thailand, and South Africa. Research in Tanzania reveals that men complain about condoms because condoms dull their sexual sensation and defeat the purpose of sexual encounter. Men compare sex with condoms to having sex with oneself. To them, it is unnatural, wasteful, and irresponsible. They regard achieving multiple ejaculations within one sexual encounter as an ideal. Non-use of condoms can maximize their pleasure and demonstrate their prowess through reproduction (Calves 1999; Knodel 1994; Plummer 2006).

Research in Thailand (Knodel 1994) contends that the major obstacle to common use of condoms is that most Thai men dislike using condoms, whether in the context of commercial or noncommercial sex relations, and whether for prophylactic or contraceptive purposes. He argues that in general, Thai men believe condoms detract from the pleasure of sexual intercourse. The fact that men dislike condoms surfaced in almost all the male focus group discussions and in most of the interviews with in-depth male respondents. He notes that if condoms are used, it is because there is a compelling reason to do so, in spite of the fact that it detracts from sexual pleasure. Furthermore, no one indicated that he or other men liked using condoms, and no one explicitly denied that condoms reduced at least somewhat the pleasure of sex. He points out that the fact that Thai men believe condom use reduces the enjoyment of sex has been documented in numerous studies using both qualitative and quantitative methodologies. For instance, among samples selected in 1992 of three different groups targeted for a study dealing with issues related to HIV/AIDS in Thailand, 63% of male truck drivers, 74% of low-income urban adult men, and 72% of low-income urban male adolescents agreed that condoms reduce the pleasure of sex. Many men agreed that "condoms reduce sexual sensitivity and pleasure," and that "during sexual intercourse condoms are an interference."

Research with gold mine workers in South Africa (Campbell 1998: 52) also reveals that gold mine workers stress that a man must have flesh-to-flesh sex. The emphasis on non-condom sex, according to Campbell, is a response to the loneliness in their migration and a loss of masculinity. As Campbell states, before these workers migrated, they lived in patriarchal rural communities where their masculine identity was defined and manifested in their participation in homestead and family leadership. After migration, however, these men experience untold loneliness, reduced opportunities for intimate social relationships, and the loss of masculinity that traditional patriarchal family provided. In response, they develop and formulate an aggressive and macho masculinity to compensate for the loss of masculinity amongst them. Non-condom or flesh-to-flesh sex provides not only a sense of closeness and intimacy, but also a reformulation of masculinity. To the male migrants, such sexual behavior is beneficial in the stressful and socially impoverished living and working environments of the gold mines.

Condom Use and Female Sex Workers

For sex workers, condom negotiation during sex exchange encounters involves economic and survival considerations. Facing the cultural pressure that flesh-to-flesh sex is necessary for men's sexual pleasure, women's demand for safe sex will jeopardize the relationship they have built with customers.

In Zheng's research of female sex workers (karaoke bar hostesses) in China, the hostesses wish to stay ignorant about HIV. The same research finding is discovered in Hillbrow sex workers in Britain, who wish to be uninformed of their HIV status (Henrickson 1990). Researchers have observed that some Hillbrow sex workers have chosen not to test for HIV, and others chose not to return for the results because they were not interested in learning their HIV status. In Hillbrow, sex workers fear that if they were tested HIV positive, their lives would be more miserable. They would be depressed, and forced to leave work. Staying ignorant is their coping strategy to better handle the stressors in their lives: poverty, violence, and discrimination in a tense, dangerous, and difficult world.

In the case of hostesses in Zheng's research, since they do not have control over condom use in their sexual relationships with male clients, information and knowledge about sexual means of transmission of HIV would only contribute to their already high levels of stress. Indeed, due to a variety of factors including gender hierarchy and culturally prescribed sex roles, HIV sentinel surveillance with female sex workers found that a national average level of consistent use of condoms with male customers was only 17% (Qu 2001, 2002). This rate was extremely low compared to that found among female sex workers in other Asian countries, such as 48% in Vietnam (Thuy 2000) and 89% in Thailand (Mills 1997). The main reason for the low consistent use of condoms in China was clients' refusal of condom use. Researchers across the globe have maintained that due to the power hierarchy between male clients and female sex workers, clients are the key determinants of decisions about condom use during sex exchanges (Aral 2002; Elifson 1999; McMahon 2006; Vanwesenbeeck 1993).

Hostesses in Zheng's research are at a disadvantaged position vis-à-vis male clients not only because of power hierarchy, but also because of economic dependency and survival strategies in a highly competitive environment. This research finding resonates with research of female sex workers elsewhere around the world.

In order to perpetuate their relationships with the regulars, hostesses resort to specific tactics to deal with the competitive market with other women, such as beating up other women and passing negative remarks about the looks of others. They act hastily to satisfy clients' desires, please them, seduce them, and win them over. In other words, fear of poverty is greater than fear of AIDS. Men and sexual partnerships are central and prioritized as the survival strategies of the women.

Research on female sex workers in Johannesburg has demonstrated the same kind of competition tactics (Maria 2001). Sex workers in Johannesburg deal with the competition by beating up other women, and either passing or explicitly saying negative remarks about the looks or behaviors of other sex workers to clients. In both cases, hostesses and sex workers in Johannesburg strive to satisfy clients' desires. They are fully aware that they must please clients, and they must be aggressive in their "game" to win with clients—to get them to give up their money. They deploy alcohol to loosen them up and become more forward with clients. The environment in both places is a competitive one wherein women try desperately to seduce clients (Maria 2001).

In Zheng's research, the competitive environment wherein clients are critical for hostesses' survival has profound ramifications for condom use. In the competitive environment of sex exchanges for money, women find it difficult not to engage in condom-less sex and capitalize on clients' reluctance to use condoms in sexual exchange (Maria 2001). Attracting clients is an extremely competitive business for hostesses. They are aware that some women may be willing to have sex at lower prices or sex without a condom. They are also sensitive to competition from younger girls and other entertainment places. They perceive the sexual relationships with clients from a work perspective and with a goal of economic gain. Like any workers in any job, they strive for the most money possible for their efforts. If some women are willing to accept clients without condoms, it is increasingly difficult for other women who require condoms to attract clients. Since many clients resent condom use and pursue absolute pleasure, the lure of not using condoms is great. It is not surprising to learn that some hostesses, like female sex workers in Johannesburg, choose to have condom-less sex in order to cope with a difficult environment and survive in a competitive market.

According to the hostesses in Zheng's research, despite the fact that some clients would refuse condom use, they would still propose condom use with strangers. However, after first-time sex, clients were not strangers any more. Rather, they became embroiled in a lover relationship and relinquished condom use in subsequent sexual intercourses. Hostesses rationalized this change from request of condom use to rejection of condom use as imperative to enter a romantic and intimate relationship with clients to guarantee themselves a constant financial source and social network.

Research on female sex workers elsewhere has also demonstrated that sex workers exhibit low condom use with intimate partners to demarcate commercial from private sex, and with clients to elicit more money to support their boyfriends (Macaluso 2000; Van den Hoek 1988; Waddell 1996; Warr 1999). Women are more likely to engage in riskier sexual practices with regular sex clients because of the more intimate nature of their relationships (Roche 2005). For instance, female sex workers in Australia engage in condom-less sex with boyfriends and husbands to demarcate work sex from non-work sex (Pyett 1997; Waddell 1996). Condoms thus become a marker that separates commercial from intimate sex.

Indeed, it has been proven on a global scale that the nature of the relationship influences condom use. Condoms are much less acceptable by couples involved in cohabiting or romantic relationships, and non-condom use is justified by trusting relationships (Blecher 1995; Campbell 1995; Campbell 2001; Cohen 1996; Worth 1989). In fact, condom use decreases as a relationship grows more stable and more intimate over time. For instance, studies in South Africa, Cameroon, and Zambia have demonstrated that interviewees exhibit strong negative attitudes toward condom use in these kinds of relationships (Agha 1997; Calves 1999, 2004a; Maharaj 2004b). In Zambia, trusting partners is the most commonly cited reason for non-use of condoms (64 percent) (Agha 1997). In London, Manchester, Tanzania, and Khutsong, interviewees classified their new relationships as serious and incorporated issues of trust to justify their non-condom sex (Campbell 2001; Holland 1990, 1991, 1994a, 1994b; Klein 1999).

Around the globe, condom use has been reported the lowest with regular clients and love mates (Basuki 2002; Bloor 1995; Day 1988; Morris 1995; Oladosu 2001; Tran 2006; Walden 1999; Wilson 1990; Wong 2003). In Nigeria, for instance, studies of clients showed that the reasons for non-use of condoms were related to the level of intimacy shared within the relationship (Messersmith 2000). In the Dominican Republic (Kerriga 2003), research on female sex workers has shown that the courtship-like process between sex workers and clients by which trust or affection are established over time leads to decreased condom use. In Zambia, women's desire to satisfy their sexual partners to retain their loyalty and faithfulness was an important reason for non-use of condoms (Kapumba 1991).

Because regular clients occupy the fuzzy middle ground, sex workers in southern Africa (Maria 2001) do not use condoms with them. They state that although they may not take a stranger who desires sex without a condom, they will agree to condom-less sex with regular clients, as regular clients provide a steady stream of income. Many sex workers feel that the more familiar they are with a client, the less risky it is to have condom-less sex with him.

Cohabiting together in the same apartment signified the closeness and intimacy of their relationships, and hence influenced non-use of condoms (see Cusick 1998). Studies have found that sex exchange encounters at prostitute's homes were less likely to involve condom use because it indicated special relationships and arrangements between the clients and the women. A similar finding was also reported by Hansen, Lopez Iftikhar, and Alegria (Hansen 2002), in a qualitative study of Puerto Rican sex workers.

Female sex workers sometimes also go through health sacrifices for the sake of men (Civic 1996). The Bulawayo women in Africa, for instance, to satisfy men with dry sex, applied drying agents to their vaginas, from which they suffered lower abdominal pain and internal infections. Other side effects included sores on female genitals, bruised skin, vaginal swelling, cuts and abrasions. They were also reluctant to use condoms because condoms would block the "love potion" effects of the agents and stopped their magic. Despite these health sacrifices, women continued to use drying agents because of the positive effect on men's libido. They believed that the effects of drying agents attracted and kept a sexual partner (Civic 1996).

Similarly, hostesses in Zheng's research sacrifice their health and endure all sorts of physical problems. The underlying reason was their economic dependency upon men. Studies have pointed out that economic dependency involved in sexual relationships has a profound ramification for condom negotiation and condom use (Calves 1999). In addition to love, trust, and intimacy, economic and survival considerations are crucial to condom-less sex (Oladosu 2001).

Many sex workers in southern Africa (Maria 2001), for instance, insisted that they chose not to use condoms out of economic desperation. Baganda women ascertained that economic needs constituted an important factor for non-use of condoms (Mukasa 1992). Indeed, if sexual partnerships involve financial gain or increased financial security, then it is difficult for them to request condoms because they recognize the potential economic harm. It is axiomatic that the economic context within which risky behaviors occur is critical (Rwabukwali 1991; Schoepf 1988; Schumann 1991).

In Zheng's research, hostesses used abortion and STD infection as a bargaining tool to procure additional money from their client lovers. Elsewhere, sex workers also used non-use of condoms as a critical bargaining tool to obtain extra money from their exchange partners (Wojcicki 2001). Although their sexual relationships with clients vary in the amount of financial gains and the stability of relationships, the hostesses' goal of establishing a long-term, intimate, and romantic relationship with their clients is constant. The economic dependency involved in the sexual relationships between hostesses and their client lovers constitutes an invariable barrier to condom use.

Researcher Teela Sanders (Sanders 2004), in her ethnographic study of female sex workers in a large British city, argues that sex workers construct a continuum of risks that prioritizes certain kinds of dangers. Although health-related matters are a real concern to many women, because they generally have comprehensive strategies to manage health risks at work, this risk category is given a low priority compared with other risks. The risk of violence is considered a greater anxiety because of the prevalence of incidents in the sex work community. However, because of comprehensive screening and protection strategies to minimize violence, this type of harm is not given the same level of attention that emotional risks receive. Indeed, the emotional risks of selling sex and chances of being discovered by their families and boyfriends is prioritized in the hierarchy of harms, followed by the risk of violence from clients, and finally, health-related risks.

Sanders (Sanders 2004) argues that sex workers rationalize the outcomes relating to non-condom use by relying on the excellent health care services available, their knowledge of what to do should such an occasion arise, and peer support. The legalities around selling sex place women's mental as well as physical well-being at risk. Pressure to hide their work, live a "double life," and fabricate stories to their families and partners in order to avoid stigma and marginalization result in significant psychological stress. By legitimating sex work as a profession the structural inequalities that leave many women vulnerable could be addressed, enabling women to organize themselves in public and private without fear of committing an offense. Protective relationships with the police could also be established and resources could move away from criminalization, fines, arrests, court appearances, probation and imprisonment through anti-social behavior orders.

Similar to sex workers in Britain, hostesses also use a continuum of risk to prioritize and understand different risks in their lives. Indeed, hostesses encountered a range of risks in their everyday lives, including criminalization, physical violence, exploitation by managers and owners, arrests, fines, and imprisonment (Zheng 2007). They need to cope with a difficult environment and survive in a competitive market. Violence, discrimination, and psychological stress are the constant risks to them. For instance, police, madams, waiters, managers, thugs, and so on, inflicted physical violence on hostesses' bodies, such as slapping their faces, kicking their chest and stomach, pinching or raping their bodies, and so on.

Different from sex workers in Britain, many hostesses' families and boyfriends were not only aware of their profession, but also appreciative of their financial support (see Zheng 2009b). Therefore, unlike British sex workers, hostesses prioritized financial risks over emotional risks. Their economic dependence upon clients and intra-competition with other hostesses precipitated hostesses to establish long-term, intimate, and romantic relationships with their regular client lovers. Going condom-less was one of the strategies to ensure such a relationship, and the financial benefits that come with it.

Summary

This chapter illustrates the cultural, political, and economic factors that affect sex workers' vulnerability to HIV infection. The chapter begins by presenting feminists' diverse standpoints on sex and commercial sex. It then discusses different state policies on sex work around the world. Following that, the chapter examines the cultural, political, and economic factors of HIV/AIDS and commercial sex in the context of Senegal and Asia. In Senegal, since women traditionally do not receive education, divorced women are usually unable to gain employment and must shoulder the responsibilities for their children because of little or no education or skills. In this case, they may turn to prostitution as a last resort and distance themselves from the community and family, which were the focus of their lives. Similar to the case in Senegal, many prostitutes in Asia choose the profession because they need to support their children, siblings, and parents, or because they are divorced or disowned by their families. Some children are even sold into prostitution by poor parents. Throughout Asia, youth is an essential prerequisite for sex workers, and young girls between the ages of 10 and 16 are in high demand by clients.

Name: ______________________________ **Date:** ____________________

Chapter 6 HIV/AIDS and Commercial Sex

Exercises

<u>Exercise 1</u> Discuss with your partner your knowledge about commercial sex workers. What do you think about them? What do you think about their lives? Where did you acquire the knowledge about them?

<u>Exercise 2</u> Reading Comprehension:

1. What are the common perceptions about commercial sex workers in relationship to HIV/AIDS in the world?

2. Why do anti-sex feminists oppose sex?

3. Why do liberal feminists believe that sex workers have total control?

4. Why do anti-prostitution feminists argue that sex workers lack control in their lives?

5. Why do romantic feminists oppose sex work and pornography?

6. How do you compare prohibitionist policy with abolitionist policy in terms of advantages and disadvantages?

7. How do you compare the regulatory system with decriminalization in terms of advantages and disadvantages?

8. What is the cultural backdrop wherein women conduct sex work in urban Senegal?

9. How do sex workers deal with HIV risks in urban Senegal?

10. How do sex workers reconcile their sex work with their religion that opposes it in Senegal?

11. What is the political economy of AIDS in Senegal?

    Registration system and stigmatization:

Power dynamics between clinic staff and registered prostitutes:

12. How do you compare and contrast sex workers in Asia and Senegal?

    Cultural Factors:

    Political economy—political policy and social inequality:

    Political economy—power dynamics between clients and sex workers:

Exercise 3 Discussion Questions:

1. Why do you think there is so much stigma attached to sex workers in the world?
2. Which standpoint do you agree with: anti-sex feminists, anti-prostitution feminists, liberal feminists, or romantic feminists?
3. What do you think of sex work and pornography? Should they be banned? Why or why not?

4. Do you think sex workers in Senegal and Asia enjoy a certain amount of power? Why or why not? If yes, what kind of power is it?

5. In your opinion, what would be the best intervention to convince the clients to engage in safe sex with sex workers?

Exercise 4 Test Your Knowledge:

1. In many countries around the world, clients of sex workers are blamed as reservoirs of infection of HIV and STDs.

   a. True

   b. False

2. Research of sex workers in developing countries has shown mounting stigma against sex workers with AIDS.

   a. True

   b. False

3. Liberal feminists believe that sex workers lack control in their lives.

   a. True

   b. False

4. Romantic feminists believe that sex workers have total control in their lives.

   a. True

   b. False

5. What differentiates Senegal from many parts of Asia is that child prostitution is prevalent in Senegal.

   a. True

   b. False

6. Senegalese women believe that they are forgiven by God because their practices enable them to be caring women and mothers.

   a. True

   b. False

7. Japanese teenage schoolgirls engage in enjo cosai because they are too poor to pay for school tuition.

   a. True

   b. False

8. This chapter discusses the power dynamics between sex workers and clients that inhere in condom use in China.
    a. True
    b. False
9. This chapter illustrates the cultural, political, and economic factors that affect sex workers' vulnerability to HIV infection.
    a. True
    b. False
10. This chapter discusses economic and social inequality that drives sex work in China.
    a. True
    b. False

Chapter seven | HIV/AIDS, Ethnicity, Women, and Young Adults

This chapter will scrutinize the population of women, ethnic women, and young adults in their relationships with HIV/AIDS. For each population, I will provide both the alarming statistics and the complex factors of culture and political economy to explain each group's specific vulnerabilities to HIV infections.

HIV/AIDS and Women: Statistics

According to the UNAIDS, in 2002, half of the AIDS cases worldwide were women. By the end of 2005, women above the age of 15 comprised over 50% of the 41 million people living with HIV/AIDS worldwide.

According to the World Health Organization, each year from 2002 to 2005, half of the annual AIDS deaths of 3 million around the world were women. That was about three female deaths per minute, and five women became infected with HIV every minute (Stine 2007).

In sub-Saharan Africa, women make up of 58% of the HIV-positive adults and the ratio of women to men infected with HIV/AIDS is currently 7:5 (Scalway 2001: 9). In parts of Latin America and the Caribbean, women take up 45% of the HIV-infected population, and this percentage is on the rise. In Sao Paulo, Brazil, the female-to-male ratio shifted from 1:42 in 1985 to 1:2 in 1995 (Stine 2007). In rural districts of Uganda such as Rakai and Masaka, the ratio of women to men infected with HIV/AIDS is 6:1 (Stine 2007).

The median age of women infected with HIV is 35 years, and women from ages 25 to 44 account for 85% of female AIDS cases. In the group of youths, young women and girls ages 15 to 24 have made up 64% of the young people in developing countries living with HIV/AIDS. It was reported globally that young women and girls are 2.5 times more likely to be HIV infected than their male counterparts. In sub-Saharan Africa, three quarters of young people living with HIV are young women ages 15 to 24, and in parts of Africa, the HIV infection among teenage girls is five times the rate among teenage boys (Scalway 2001).

In Trinidad and Tobago, the number of girls between ages 15 and 19 living with HIV is five times higher than the number of adolescent boys (UNAIDS 2004). In rural districts of Uganda such as Rakai and Masaka, 70 percent of the women from the ages of 15 to 25 were infected with HIV. In Rwanda and Tanzania, the ratio of girls and boys below the age of 25 living with HIV is 2:1. In Ethiopia, the teenage girls-to-boys ratio living with HIV is 3:1, and in Zimbabwe, the ratio is 5:1 (Stine 2007).

These alarming figures indicate the pressing situations concerning women and HIV/AIDS. The reason that increasingly more women are vulnerable to HIV transmission worldwide lies in the biological, cultural, political, and economic factors. In order to curb the HIV spread, it is critical to address women's needs for HIV prevention.

HIV/AIDS and Women: Biological Factors

As illustrated in the first chapter, women are biologically more vulnerable to infection. This is because semen conserves higher concentrations of HIV virus than vaginal and cervical secretions, and the vagina area has a much larger mucosal area for exposure to HIV virus than the penis. Hence, male-to-female transmission is 2 to 10 times more effective than female-to-male transmission.

HIV/AIDS and Women: Social Factors

Blame on Immoral Women

Leclerc-Madlala points out that women are paradoxically both targets of protection and agents of pollution. Because women's sexual purity is considered essential to the family and moral social order, women's sexuality can potentially become a threat and menace to the rubric of political and social order (Leclerc-Madlala 2001a).

Women, especially immoral women, are blamed for causing and spreading HIV/AIDS because of a range of social and cultural factors (Bujra 2000; Leclerc-Madlala 2001a; Schoepf 1993, 1998). Blaming immoral women as vectors and transmitters of HIV/AIDS confirms Paul Farmer's theory of "geography of blame," and Carol Vance and Leclerc-Madlala's argument about the danger of women's sexuality and women as the agents of pollution (Farmer 1993; Leclerc-Madlala 2001b; Vance 1982). In many countries around the world, immoral women have been blamed for the spread of sexually transmitted diseases. Among certain peoples in Thailand and Uganda, STDs are known as "women's diseases" (Stine 2007). In the language of much of East Africa Swahili, the word for STD means literally "disease of women" (Stine 2007). In other parts of the world such as South Africa (Leclerc-Madlala 2001a, 2001b), Brazil (Goldstein 1995), and South Korea (Cheng 2005a), there is invariably a fear of women beyond control, especially at times of rapid social transformations. Hence each country has an array of distinctive strategies such as purity campaigns and virginity testing to manage women's sexuality and put it in check.

Below I will discuss the intersection of immoral women and foreign men as the object of blame at the time of HIV/AIDS in China. As studies of gender and nation have shown, women bear the burden of representing the nation's future and honor (Yuval-Davis 1997). The female body is an important historical symbol of social and national boundaries in various societies, including colonizing powers (Stoler 1991), autonomous nations (Mosse 1985), and the colonized (Chatterjee 1993; Cheng 2005a; Jager 1996).

Immoral Women and Foreign Men in China

In China, women with immoral values are perceived as the mediums of transmission. The intersection between foreign men and Chinese women is especially a highly contentious issue in China. The Chinese state has striven to police Chinese women's bodies to protect national integrity. For instance, the 1984 criminal law defined women who "seduce foreigners and have intercourse with foreigners" as "female hooligans." In one popular movie, female "hooligans" who seduced and slept with foreign men were tracked down by government agents (Zheng 2009a).

This first film on AIDS was titled "AIDS patient" and was released in 1988. In this mystery, Tony, a foreign teacher at a university on the east coast, died of AIDS. The police organized an investigation unit to collect Tony's relics and track down the three Chinese females who had had sexual relationships with him. This investigating unit also included the female secretary from the foreign affairs department, Xiaoyu Wang. The unit screened the blood samples of all the teachers, staff, and students under the pretext of physical examinations. The result showed that two women were infected. The first infected female student was found immediately. The unexpected blow made her desperate to commit suicide, but she was stopped by the police. She told the unit that Tony used to know a woman at a restaurant, but it was impossible for the unit to locate this woman. The second woman infected had used a fake name on the name list, so the investigation was stranded. At this time, more relics of Tony's were shipped from abroad, including a picture and a shopping receipt from a Friendship store. From the picture, the unit located the woman, who had married a rich Japanese businessman and had gone to Japan. The second piece, the shopping receipt, showed that Tony had bought a record of *Madam Butterfly*. It so happened that Xiaoyu Wang, the female secretary in the foreign affairs department, also had the same record. Was it a coincidence? After a thorough investigation, the truth was revealed: Xiaoyu was the infected female they had been looking for. Xiaoyu went to a room at the seaside where she had had intercourse with Tony and committed suicide by setting herself on fire.

The film targets women who might be tempted to have sexual relationships with foreigners and portrays how they are doomed as a result of their "immoral" behaviors. This cautionary tale is intended to warn women against getting too close to foreigners because the foreigners will corrupt them and infect them. While the mass media stress that foreigners are the vectors of disease, they also show the catastrophic consequences of women's immoral behavior.

Women with corrupted morals were depicted as the major source of HIV/AIDS transmission. Categorized as "female sex criminals" (*xingzuicuo funu*) or "clandestine prostitutes," they were reported as "the most dangerous group" that spread the disease to the general population. Media illustrated how the infected prostitutes endangered the society by deliberately transmitting their disease to the general public, although the results of the national sentinel surveillance surveys continued to show that HIV-infection prevalence was very low in these selected populations (Qu 1997).

Underlying this discourse of HIV/AIDS is nationalism and male dominance. The national superiority is confirmed in condemning the infiltration of foreign corruption and identifying foreigners as the sources and transmitters of the HIV virus. The national pride is heralded in the Confucian morality and chastity that is deemed as the most effective and superior Chinese weapon to fight HIV/AIDS. The national purity is presented as embodied by virtuous Chinese women.

The official media stress the necessity of women's moral conduct to protect the nation's purity. In the current social and cultural climate, women are targeted and held responsible for maintaining social stability and safeguarding national morality. This attitude toward women is not unique to China.

Researchers have argued that women's bodies have historically been used to demarcate national boundaries (Chatterjee 1993; Mosse 1985; Stoler 1991). For instance, the rape of Chinese women by foreigners has historically been considered as the rape of the Chinese motherland (see Cook 1996). It is commonly believed that women's sexuality and bodies must be kept under strict control because women, as the bearers of national virtue and tradition, metaphorically mark the boundaries of a nation (Clarke 1999; Finnane 1996).

In South Africa, the African solution to the HIV/AIDS epidemic is to support virginity testing, that is, periodically inspecting girls to see if they are chaste (Leclerc-Madlala 2001b). Virginity testing is seen as "the only way to reinstill what they view as the lost cultural values of chastity before marriage, modesty, self-respect, and pride. For them, imbuing girls with these lost values represents the surest way to repair the frayed moral fabric of society that has led to the ever increasing problems of teenage pregnancies, STIs, and HIV/AIDS" (Leclerc-Madlala 2001b: 535). Leclerc-Madlala argues that virginity testing is South Africa's gendered responses to HIV/AIDS that places women at the epicenter of blame for the epidemic (Leclerc-Madlala 2001b: 537). Similar gendered responses occur in China where women and girls are the target of control and the center of blame in the current HIV/AIDS epidemic.

In China, prostitutes and immoral women are blamed as the vessels and transmitters of HIV/AIDS, and teenage and adult women are placed at the center of education and training. The assertion of power and control upon women's sexuality is meant to maintain a national purity. As Jeffrey has observed, "Prostitution is a particularly rich ground for the investigation of the links between gender identity and national identity because the centrality of prostitution involves identifying correct and incorrect sexual behavior on the part of women, and distinguishing between good and bad women. Women's correct sexual behavior—usually within the bonds of marriage and family—grounds the categories of gender (what men and women should be and do)" (Jeffrey 2002: 127).

In this time of dramatic social and cultural change, controlling women's sexuality is key to the national project. Chatterjee has stated that the nation is situated on the body of women as "chaste, dutiful, daughterly, or maternal" (Parker 1992: 6). Women's sexuality and bodies must be kept under strict control because women, as the bearers of national virtue and tradition, metaphorically mark the boundaries of a nation (see Clarke 1999; Cook 1996; Finnane 1996).

In China, women's sexuality is strictly regulated within the conjugal relationships, and women's special nurturing and reproductive role is considered crucial in the transmission of virtues to the next generation, and to the moral well-being of the nation.

HIV/AIDS and Women: Factors of Culture and Political Economy

HIV is mainly transmitted through heterosexual contact. In the United States, from 2002 to 2008, women comprised about 40% of those newly infected with HIV infections through heterosexual contact. Among women from ages 13 to 24 who were newly infected with HIV, about 76% were infected through heterosexual contact.

Gender is a crucial factor in determining individuals' vulnerability to HIV infection. It is usually men who determine when and how often to have sex, and whether or not a condom is used. It is also men who usually have multiple sexual partners, which enhances the opportunity that they will transmit HIV to their partners. Global research has proven that gender norms, gender inequality, and poverty intensify and fuel HIV transmission for women.

Gender Norms and Impact on Sexuality

Gender is culturally structured and inscribed in men and women's social and sexual experiences. Gender comprises socially constructed beliefs, expectations, customs, and practices that define femininity and masculinity. That is, the meanings of manhood and womanhood are created by culture. Culturally defined gender norms constitute the social and cultural factors that make women more vulnerable to HIV infections.

Masculine values are instilled by society as a whole, internalized by individuals, and reinforced by peer pressure (Scalway 2001: 10). Across the world, masculinity is associated with bravery, physical and psychological strength, independence, and sexual activity (Scalway 2001). Some cultures, such as in parts of Africa, emphasize circumcision rites where young men are expected to tolerate high levels of pain. In some African countries, a woman is not a woman until she has gone through genital mutilation. In many parts of Africa, manhood is also bolstered if their wives have many children. That is, a woman's fertility determines her man's manhood. As a result, men avoid contraceptives such as condoms to assure a woman's fertility so that the man's manhood is not compromised. Similarly, in many parts of Latin America, fathering many children is seen as proof of virility (Scalway 2001).

Sex and masculinity are closely intertwined. In many developing countries, especially Asia, the Middle East, and Africa, it is culturally believed that men are both biologically and naturally determined to be lustful and assertive, and women to surrender and be conquered. Cultural norms favor multiple partnerships for men, and women cannot control risks of infection.

In a report on seven developing countries that included Costa Rica, Cameroon, Zimbabwe, Chile, Cambodia, India, and Papua New Guinea (Dowsett 1999: 32), there is a convergence that the cultural environment encourages young men to perceive women as sex objects whose personalities and wishes are subordinate to the demands of men. While women's key qualities are defined as virginity, fidelity, and fertility, men's key qualities are identified as bravery and aggressiveness; having sex with sex workers and multiple sexual partners, and engaging in coerced sexual activity and rape of women (Scalway 2001: 10).

In these developing counties, cultural values deem young men's sexual needs to be beyond their control and demanding immediate satisfaction. Because they are culturally regarded as needing sexual experiences, young men are encouraged to take risks and be sexually aggressive. Once they are pubescent, they are facilitated by older males, families, or peers to seek sex workers or older women to engage in sex. These practices are culturally predicated upon the belief that young men are sexual beings upon puberty.

For instance, in Cambodia, young men regard deflowering young women as the "ultimate sport" (Dowsett 1999: 35). They are also allowed and approved of by traditional values to visit sex workers to satisfy their sexual needs (Dowsett 1999). Similarly, in Latin America and Thailand, it is tradition that an older relative takes a young man to a sex worker to initiate his sexual experience, symbolizing his entry into manhood. In Thailand, young men often celebrate their payday by drinking and visiting brothels.

While young men are under cultural pressure to have sex with multiple sexual partners to express their virility and manhood, women are expected to refrain from sexual activity and keep themselves purely virgin. Gender norms dictate that women and girls should be ignorant and passive about sex, because women are considered to have natural inclination to marriage and childbearing. Sexually active women face derogatory and degrading labels such as slut, whore, sick, or shameful (Dowsett 1999: 35).

Young women are forced to understand and experience their sexuality in this cultural milieu of "double binds" (Dowsett 1999). Virginity can guarantee them a potential marriage partner, and a testament to their character, virtue, and worthiness in the eyes of the partner, family, and community (Dowsett 1999: 36).

Since cultural norms expect women to be docile and obey their partners, many young girls experience forced sex and rape at an early age. Violence against women such as rape and coerced sex increases women's vulnerability to HIV infection because forced vaginal penetration causes abrasions, tears, and cuts that allow the virus to cross the vaginal wall more easily.

In many developing countries, a significant number of young women experience rape or forced sex at an early age; 20% of young girls in Kisum, Kenya, and Ndola, Zambia, said their first sexual encounter involved physical force (UNAIDS 2004). Around 25% of 15 to 24-year-old girls in KwaZulu-Natal, South Africa, said they had been tricked or persuaded into the first sexual experience (UNAIDS 2004).

As we have seen, in many parts of the world, cultural norms demand that young women maintain sexual abstinence and encourage young men to experience sexual adventures. The cultural imperative leaves young women vulnerable with inadequate knowledge about sex, STDs, and HIV/AIDS.

Cultural Norms and Sexual Practices

In many developing countries, certain sexual practices such as dry sex, widow inheritance, and ritual cleansers enhance both women and men's vulnerability to HIV transmission.

Dry Sex

Throughout southern Africa where the AIDS pandemic is beyond control, dry sex is a very common, traditional sexual practice, which can damage genitals and increase chances of transmission of STDs and HIV.

Many African women, including Bulawayo women, apply drying agents to their vaginas to satisfy men with dry sex (Civic 1996). The drying agents include detergents, salt, cotton, shredded newspaper, or soil mixed with baboon urine, which can be obtained from traditional healers. It was reported that a woman from Zimbabwe uses herbs from the Mugugudhu tree. After grinding the stem and leaf, she mixes a pinch of the powder with water, wraps it in a bit of nylon stocking, and inserts it into her vagina for ten to fifteen minutes. The herbs swell the soft tissues of the vagina and dry it out (Stine 2007).

These women concur that dry sex hurts, but they believe that the effects of drying agents help attract and keep a sexual partner (Civic 1996). The Bulawayo women reported that from dry sex, they suffered lower abdominal pain and internal infections (Civic 1996). Other side effects included sores on female genitals, bruised skin, vaginal swelling, cuts and abrasions. Yet women said: "The man keeps coming back. It will be hurting you, but he will be enjoying it." "The man wants sex all night which will cause you to have a swollen vagina."

Civic (1996) states that group participants in all groups responded that condoms frequently break when used in conjunction with drying agents. The women reported that they were reluctant to use condoms because condoms would block the "love potion" effects of the agents and stop their magic. As an interviewee said, "If you use condoms, the magic doesn't work right—you need skin to skin contact." Several participants noted that drying agents are used more often with steady partners, where condoms tended not to be used, so that the agents could "work their magic."

Researchers in Zimbabwe had trouble finding a control group of women who did not engage in some form of dry sex (Stine 2007). They pointed out that dry sex causes vaginal lacerations, suppresses the vagina's natural bacteria, causes condoms to tear more easily, and increases the likelihood of HIV infection.

Widow Inheritance

Some countries, especially eastern and southern Africa, practice home guardianship or widow inheritance (Stine 2007). This cultural practice deems it imperative that a widow marries one of her dead husband's brothers or cousins. The underlying logic of the tradition lies in the fact that it not only ensures the children's membership in the clan of the husband but also guarantees that the widow and her children are provided for. The dead husband's brother or cousin is perceived as the guardian of the widow. It is believed that he cleanses the widow of the devils of death by taking her and engaging in sexual intercourse with her. If a widow refuses the guardian, she is considered bringing down chira, that is, bringing ill fortune onto the entire clan.

This cultural tradition provides a convenient avenue for the transmission of HIV. If the widow's husband died of AIDS, widow inheritance makes it possible that she will pass it on to her guardian. A public health worker from the Red Cross said, "We have homes where all the males have died of AIDS because of this widow inheritance" (Stine 2007).

Ritual Cleansers

It is a tradition in some rural African villages that a woman whose husband has died and an unmarried woman who has lost a parent or a child must sleep with a ritual cleanser. Village elders in Gangre, Kenya, proclaim that this custom is necessitated by the guarantee of good crops in the community, as the lack of this custom would leave the community vulnerable with a curse of bad crops. This tradition, which dates back centuries, is rooted in a belief that a woman will be haunted by spirits after her husband dies. If she abstains from sex and remains unmarried, she is considered to be unholy and disturbed. Thus, unless the widow sleeps with the ritual cleanser, she is not allowed to attend her husband's funeral or be inherited by her husband's brother or cousin (Stine 2007).

This practice is found in rural Africa in Uganda, Tanzania, Congo, Angola, and across West Africa, specifically in Ghana, Senegal, Ivory Coast, and Nigeria. Hundreds of thousands of men work as ritual cleansers. Although they are perceived as being at the low range of the society, they are considered essential to purifying women. Payment to cleansers are in the form of cows, crops, and cash. Researchers state that these areas that practice this tradition have the highest rates of HIV/AIDS (Stine 2007).

Poverty and Cultural Norms of Sex

Due to poverty and rapid social transformations, transactional and intergenerational sex is prevalent in many developing countries. In these relationships based on power and economic inequality, young women are caught in a vulnerable position and susceptible to abuse, exploitation, violence, and HIV (UNAIDS 2004).

It was reported from Zimbabwe, Papua New Guinea, and Cameroon that, with the ascendancy of a cash economy and economic modernization, young women were encouraged in their cultures to demand favors, commodities, and cash in exchange for sex (Dowsett 1999: 33). In Papua New Guinea, for instance, the drastic shift to a cash economy has transformed traditional patterns of exchanging sex for goods, such as bride price in marriage, to an increased number of female and male sex workers (Dowsett 1999: 40).

In Papua New Guinea, the cultural pattern of young women exchanging sex for goods has left unemployed young men desperate. The pressured and distressed young men respond to it with a widespread and institutionalized rape (Dowsett 1999: 38). In many country reports, coerced sexual activity is ubiquitous, especially in the institutionalized pack rape of young women in Papua New Guinea.

In sub-Saharan Africa, cross-generational relationships make it difficult for girls to resist pressure of unsafe sexual practices. In this region, sexual partners of girls between 15 and 19-years-old tend to be six or more years older (UNAIDS 2004). The underlying reason is not only that poverty and hardship drive girls into transactional sex with older men, but also that some girls perceive older men as good marriage partners and providers of a better life, offering education or work opportunities. Gifts of perfume, clothes, and jewelry help enhance their status among peers and in their own self-esteem. This cultural phenomenon makes abstinence-only before marriage unsuccessful for these girls because they marry early and their older husbands may have already carried the virus (UNAIDS 2004).

Both transactional sex and intergenerational sex have become the norm in many countries. For instance, in Zimbabwe, nearly 25% of women in their twenties are in relationships with men at least 10 years older (UNAIDS 2004). It is also apparent that these relationships are a major factor in the feminization of AIDS in Africa. As the report states (UNAIDS 2004), because African men are expected to have multiple sexual partners, on average, they become infected in their mid- to late twenties. However, girls usually stay in a long-term sexual relationship with one partner. Despite their relative fidelity, many girls get infected after having sex. A study in Zambia revealed that among the HIV-infected women, 18% of them have been sexually active for a year or so. In South Africa, 20% of the girls between 16 and 18 were infected.

Young women are not only vulnerable in the power-infused transactional and intergenerational relationships, but also are defenseless in forced rapes by poor men. Young men in impoverished communities are divested of educational and employment opportunities and control over their working conditions or job security. Some work in the mines of southern Africa, some conduct seasonal work on farms, and some work as truck drivers' assistants (Scalway 2001: 13). Poor men, deprived of employment and livelihood, feel frustrated that they do not fit into the cultural ideals of manhood that define men as strong, powerful, and resourceful to support a family (Scalway 2001: 13). Emasculated by their economic conditions and failure to uphold the cultural masculine ideals, poor men assert their masculinity through sexual intercourse and other escapist behaviors such as alcohol and drugs. Many of these young men enforce sexual intercourse on women via coercion, disregarding whether the women consent to it or not (Scalway 2001).

Gender and Condom Use

In general, inconsistency in condom use stems from men's dislike of condoms and the negative cultural meanings associated with condoms.

In the broader contexts of American constructs of black masculinity, women are reluctant to use condoms considering the need or desire to maintain an ongoing relationship. They fear that men would leave them because of the strong male dislikes for condoms. Men also associate practices of initiating condoms with a woman being sexually loose, dirty, and diseased.

Similarly, research in Cameroon revealed that cultural norms expect Cameroonian women to be docile and obey their partners not to use condoms (Calves 1999). Among the youth in urban Cameroon, young women exhibit great shyness purchasing condoms and a lack of confidence in their ability to correctly use or put on a condom. Hence it is not surprising that exposure to condom advertising did not have an effect on their confidence to convince partners to use condoms (Calves 1999).

Researchers pointed out that in South Africa, condom use is seen to undermine South African men's notions of masculinity that valorize flesh-to-flesh sex with multiple/numerous sexual partners (Holland 1994; McGrath 1993), fertility (Abdool Karim 1992), and pleasure (Preston-Whyte 1991). As researchers indicated, masculinity in southern Africa is tied with flesh-to-flesh sex (Maria 2001; Webb 1997). Campbell argues that workers view it as necessary for a man's good health to maintain balanced levels of blood/sperm within the body (Campbell 1998). Informants spoke of the way in which the build-up of sperm led to a range of mental and physical problems. Flesh-to-flesh sex was regarded as the only pleasurable way of meeting male sexual desires, with condoms being seen as cold and unpleasant.

Masculinity is associated with physical strength and bravery, and serves as a key coping mechanism whereby miners deal with the harsh and dangerous working conditions of underground mining (Campbell 1998: 52). South African men who refuse this dominant masculine notion by using condoms or avoiding sex are taunted, teased, and ridiculed as stupid (MacPhail 2001). Rural Tanzanian men reject condoms and believe that conception defines masculinity (Plummer 2006). Researchers have also observed the pervasive *machismo* culture among Latino men that defines machismo behaviors as having multiple sexual partners, imposing physical abuse and restrictions on women's mobility, and so on (Inciardi 2000; Singer 1990). Being *macho* also means being passionate and irrational during sexual intercourse, and not disrupting the sexual flow with condom use (Carrillo 2002; Ibañez 2005; Marin 1996).

Among the clients in China, Zheng's research revealed that a similar concept of machismo is manifested through engaging in illicit sex with multiple sexual partners, not wearing condoms and not fearing STDs, while imposing control over hostesses. Previous studies in South Africa and Thailand have shown that peer norms are powerful in impacting the behaviors of groups (Campbell 2001: 1614; Maticka-Tyndale 1997). Peer norms can either facilitate discussions of safe sex and generate safe sexual behaviors, or function to promote unsafe sexual behaviors and encourage risk (Campbell 2001). For instance, research on Thai men showed that peer pressure prompted them to participate in risky activities during group partying and consumption of alcohol (Maticka-Tyndale 1997). In Zheng's research in China, peer norms among clients valorize macho display of a fearless spirit and the pursuit of absolute sexual pleasure, and prevent them from protecting their health.

Indeed, because condoms are culturally associated with promiscuity, infection, infidelity, and a lack of trust in a partner, women initiating condoms are interpreted as being sexually loose, dirty, and diseased. It was also reported that many young men perceive condoms as signaling a lack of trust in a partner, although sometimes they abjure condoms because of other reasons as well, such as conducting sex secretly and in a hurry, without parental consent (Scalway 2001: 22).

In general, men consider condoms as reducing male sexual pleasure and sensation. In many countries, preserving male comfort is an important task for women. Contraception is considered primarily a woman's responsibility. Women or wives are expected to employ many alternative means of contraception that are viewed as not interfering with male sexual pleasure.

Since men control the sexual decision-making, they generally do not use condoms, in order to assert their male potency by achieving multiple ejaculations without condoms, facilitating what they believe as the healthy exchange of bodily fluids, and assuring many children. In some African cultures, men believe that exchanging bodily fluids with their sexual partners can improve their health.

Older Women

Starting from the year 2008, women aged 50 and older accounted for 10% of all female AIDS cases. The major route of HIV transmission for these women is through heterosexual activities. One of the main reasons for older women's vulnerability is that older women do not request their male partners to wear condoms because they have passed the fertile age and do not need contraceptives. It was reported that most seniors are first diagnosed with HIV in the hospital after they've already progressed to AIDS (Stine 2007).

Lesbian Women

There is ample evidence that demonstrates the existence of HIV among lesbians. This is because lesbians engage in behaviors that put them and their partners at risk for HIV infection. It was reported that 80% of lesbian women have had sex with men during their lifetime (Stine 2007). Certain common sexual behaviors among lesbians can possibly subject women to HIV transmission through vaginal fluid, menstrual blood, sex toys, and cuts in the vagina, mouth, and on the hands (Stine 2007). In a nutshell, it is an erroneous assumption that lesbians are immune to HIV.

Ethnicity and Women: Factors of Culture and Political Economy

The number of women of color living with HIV has dramatically increased. In the United States, at the end of 2008, African-American and Hispanic women accounted for more than three-fourths (78%) of AIDS cases despite their representation of less than one-fourth of all U.S. women. In 2000 alone, African-American and Hispanic women comprised an even greater proportion—80% of HIV cases reported in women.

FIGURE 7.1 Race/Ethnicity of U.S. Women Diagnosed with HIV/AIDS in 2005

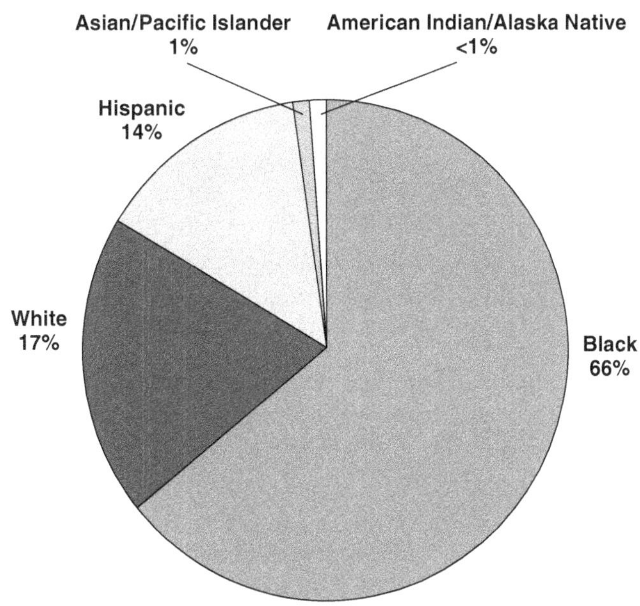

Source: Centers for Disease Control and Prevention. HIV/AIDS Among Women. *Revised June 2007.*

While HIV/AIDS was the fifth leading cause of death for U.S. women from ages 25 to 44, HIV/AIDS was the third leading cause of death for African-American women in the same age group in 1999.

Researchers state that several factors expose women to HIV transmission through heterosexual contact. These factors include racism, the sex-ratio imbalance, low levels of condom use, multiple partners, and bisexuality among African-American men (Peeler 2006a, 2006b).

Racism and the sex-ratio imbalance have been identified as two culprits causing the high prevalence of HIV in African-American women. The African-American community distrusts the American health care system due to the history of the exploitation of their people during the Tuskegee Syphilis study. Researchers point out that even in the contemporary United States, there is substantial evidence that demonstrates disparities in health care related to racism and bias throughout the health care system. It was reported that due to racism, African-American women tend to receive less follow-up care, are considered noncompliant, and are prescribed therapies less often than white women (Peeler 2006a; Stine 2007).

Not only racism, but also the lopsided sex ratio constitutes the cultural backdrop against which the phenomenon of low levels of condom use and low levels of health information take place. Researchers point out that due to high rates of homicide, suicide, and imprisonment among African-American men, black women outnumber black men by roughly 19 women to 17 men (Peeler 2006a: 98).

The reasons for low levels of condom use among African-American women have been identified as the following: perceived obstruction of spontaneity, perceived obstruction of sexual enjoyment, and perceived lack of trust in condom use (Peeler 2006a: 99). African-American women reported that request of condom use conveyed and insinuated a suspicion and mistrust that their partners engaged in infidelity. They believed that their male partners would be hurt, insulted, and angry about their suspicions of them. As a result, they would inflict violence and abuse upon the women. Studies of African-American girls ages 13 to 19 reported that 26% felt little control over condom use during intercourse (Peeler 2006a: 99).

African-American culture also equates masculine virility with making decisions of [non-] condom use and having multiple sexual partners, which exposes both men and women to HIV transmission. In the African-American community, if a woman suggests condom use, it implies a situation of gender equity where a woman is asserting her power and her needs. This is unacceptable to the African-American men. Despite the fact that men engage in more risky sexual practices, men believe that they have the right to make the decisions about condom use, not the women.

African-American women often turn a blind eye to their unfaithful male partners due to the shortage of African-American men. There is a consensus in the culture that sharing a man is the price to pay for being in the community. This cultural ideal leaves both younger women and older women at high risk. There is a disproportionately high percentage of sexual unions between younger women and adult men in the community. Older women who are widowed, divorced, or separated are put back in the dating game and realize the difficulty for them to have a male partner. In both cases, younger women and older women find themselves at high risk due to their ignorance of their sexual partners' sexual history and HIV status, and their compliance and concession with non-condom use (Peeler 2006a: 100).

African-American women have internalized the male-dominant and female-subordinate gender roles and uphold their men as the "head of the house." Researchers have stated that they are socialized to make their partners feel in power and to suppress their own knowledge, wisdom, and expertise (Peeler 2006b: 115). This culture of gender inequity is co-opted by women themselves, leading them to vulnerability of HIV transmission. African-American women feel pressured to reduce their assertiveness and directness, minimize their accomplishments, and even endanger their own health to maintain the relationship and not upset the balance of power. The power differentials in gender relationships have exerted a great impact on women's ability to make informed decisions.

Researchers also believe that the high prevalence of HIV in African-American women is also because many African-American men are bisexual, or on the down-low. According to researchers such as Richards (Richards 2001), many African-American men negotiate racism, sexism, and homophobia by living a life on the down-low. That is, they call themselves straight but have secret sexual intercourse with men. Their clandestine bisexual behaviors and lack of condom use leave their African-American women partners ignorant and vulnerable to HIV transmission.

The high prevalence of HIV in African-American women not only stems from the above factors, including racism, the sex-ratio imbalance, low levels of condom use, multiple partners, and bisexuality among African-American men, but also arises from the sociopsychological elements. Below I will enlist two studies to illustrate how the sociopsychological factors influence non-condom use in ethnic women's relationships with men.

Ethnicity and Women: Religious Factors

Lorraine Peeler (2006b) identifies religious belief as one of the factors that have a significant impact on African-American women's compliant attitude toward their male sexual partners. Peeler argues that the interplay between religion and culture both cultivates and reinforces gender beliefs in the African-American community.

Peeler maintains that gender roles and norms in the African-American community are inseparable from the religious context. The religious tradition of the African-American community instills the ideology of "the man is the head of the household" in everyone's minds and is internalized by the women. This ideology prescribes the man as the one in power and in control, regardless of his merits or fidelity. In this religious tradition, women who are assertive, independent, or strong are not supported or encouraged.

Peeler observes that women in the black church are encouraged to submit to their men and get validated by their men. Women are expected to obey their husbands or men without question. Submission opens up the chances of abuse and violence upon the women (Peeler 2006b: 117–118).

Ethnicity and Women: Sociopsychological Factors

Studies of ethnic women in Baltimore and Cleveland have shown that women comply with unsafe sex with their male partners for sociopsychological reasons. While ethnic women in Baltimore submit to their male partners in unsafe sex to maintain their long-term relationships, ethnic women in Cleveland appropriate unsafe sex to feel good about themselves because their status and self-esteem are predicated upon relationships with men.

Research in Baltimore, Maryland, has shown that a number of low-income African-American women were reluctant to request condom use from their male partners (Wiutehead 1997). Their reluctance was based on their need or desire to maintain their ongoing relationships, and the fear that men would leave them because of their strong dislike of condoms. Women were also very cautious about initiating condom use in their sexual practices because they feared that men would associate such practices with a woman being "sexually loose." If a woman initiated discussions of condoms, she ran the risk of being suspected of promiscuity. Men interpreted this action as an insinuation that the women had been sleeping around and carrying diseases (Wiutehead 1997). Therefore, women were afraid to bring up condom use for fear that it could threaten the survival of the relationship. Research in Greece has also revealed the same findings: that a woman who introduces condoms into marital relations could be seen as shedding doubt on her own or her spouse's sexual fidelity.

In a study with ethnic women in Cleveland, Ohio (Sobo 1995a), Sobo argues that unsafe, condom-less sex provides women, especially those women who depend upon relationships with men for status and self-esteem, with a way to feel good about their lives. Among the group of ethnic women, women harness barrier-less and condom-less sex to assure themselves that their relationships are committed, close, and intact, as only women with faithful partners can have the freedom to have condom-less sex.

Sobo maintains that these women's dream of faithful monogamy and long-term relationship originates from TV soap operas, popular songs, and women's magazines. This romantic rhetoric promoted in mass media depicts an idealized and monogamous long-term relationship. Because their status is partly based on the loyalty and other qualities of their sexual partners, realization of this romantic ideal will bring the women both status and esteem.

Women deny the possibility of adultery in their relationships because they emphasize that they have the ability to judge men. They believe they are well-versed in identifying responsible and irresponsible men. Through unsafe sex their partners are deemed worthy in a committed, stable, monogamous conjugal relationship that validates not only the women's status and esteem, but also the model that the culture recommends.

Unsafe sex helps the women maintain the belief that they are in a faithful, caring, and satisfying relationship that fits the popular U.S. conjugal ideal. The purpose of sex, to the women, is to feel loved, needed, and wanted. Women proclaim that their partners and their relationships are ideal, and unsafe sex makes them feel close to their partners both emotionally and physically.

Condom-less sex is directly described as "a sign of trust," "honesty," and "commitment." Using condoms announces that partners are not sexually exclusive and signals infidelity and a lack of mutual trust. The strength of the association between condoms and extra- conjugal sex means that condom use denotes failure in a relationship. Women actively use unsafe sex to demonstrate to themselves that their men do not stray sexually. They do so as part of a psychosocial strategy for building and preserving an image of themselves as having achieved the conjugal ideal. Women can build status and self-esteem by presenting themselves to others as having attracted loyal, honorable partners and as having attained perfect, intact unions.

Poverty and Lack of Education

Economic necessity, limited access to preventive health care, and lack of access to education are all factors that lead to poor people's susceptibility to HIV infections. This is because poverty contributes to poor nutrition and chronic stress, which compromises the immune system and increases susceptibility to new infection.

Globally, feminization of poverty and gender inequity has heightened women's vulnerability to HIV transmission. In many countries around the world, women and girls have limited access to education and health care services. Statistics reveal that the countries where women's status is low are generally those where HIV is now spreading fastest via heterosexual contact.

Poor women not only have inadequate access to health care and information about prevention of HIV and STDs; they also feel so overwhelmed by the stress in their daily lives that risks of HIV infection is not on the priority list. Research has also shown that poor women are more likely to engage in risky sexual activities to cope with their stress (Raffaelli 1998: 11). Poor women also lack the resources to leave a relationship with a high-risk partner and others may depend on sex as a survival activity (Margillo 1998; Raffaelli 1998).

Member states of the United Nations, at the 2006 High Level Meeting on AIDS, pledged to "eliminate gender inequalities, gender-based abuse and violence and increase the capacity of women and adolescent girls to protect themselves from the risk of HIV infection, principally through the provision of health care and services including sexual and reproductive health, and the provision of full access to comprehensive information and education."

Women need to be empowered via health knowledge, health care, and education. They need to know that they can and should protect themselves against HIV infection. They need knowledge about HIV and AIDS, self-confidence, and the skills necessary to insist that partners use safer sex methods and good medical care.

HIV/AIDS and Young People

Worldwide, the rate of HIV infection among young people is soaring. In the developing world, 67% of newly infected individuals are young people between the ages of 15 and 24. Among these young people living with HIV, young women and girls ages 15 to 24 make up 64% of the population.

In sub-Saharan Africa, among the young people, the main mode of transmission is heterosexual intercourse. The sub-Saharan Africa contains almost two-thirds of all young people living with HIV, approximately 6.2 million people, 75 percent of whom are female (UNAIDS 2003).

In the United States, every year since 2002, young adults under age 25 comprise 50% of the population newly infected with HIV (Rosenberg 1994; Stine 2007). The youth population amounts to 21,000 new infections or two infections every hour. About two-thirds of them are contracted sexually, and three-quarters of them are ethnic minorities. Statistics show that young people are the group most vulnerable to HIV infection.

FIGURE 7.2 Young People (15–24 Years Old) Living with HIV, by Region, End 2003

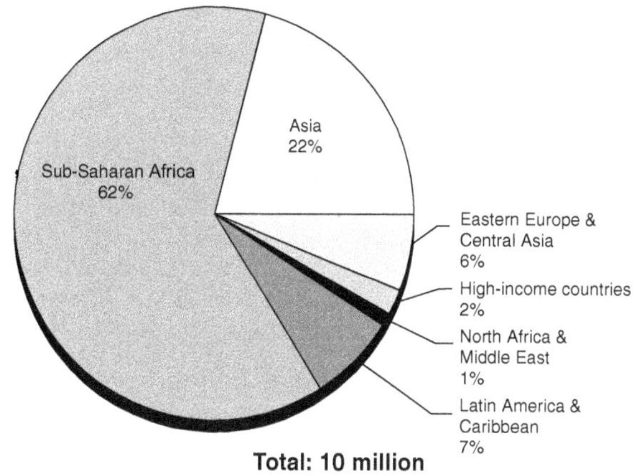

Source: UNAIDS/UNICEF/WHO, 2004.

Factors of Culture and Political Economy

Cultural Factors

Many factors have been identified to explain why young people are exposed to HIV infection. Researchers maintain that young people are undergoing a rite of passage to adulthood. This liminal stage is one replete with exploration, rebellion, and independence. Young people are more inclined to take risks and experiment with new experiences, including involvement in sexual behaviors. In the United States, statistics show that half of American college students have unprotected sex (Stine 2007).

Research of American college students (Cohen 1998) has also shown that institutionalized rules in colleges have increased students' desire to rebel against authority via heavy drinking and unsafe sexual practices. These rules and regulations, however, do not address unsafe sexual practices that threaten students' health. Students tend to follow their peer groups and engage in heavy drinking and taking sexual risks (Cohen 1998).

These American undergraduate students' rebellious sexual acts and alcohol use resonate with their peer groups elsewhere around the globe. A report of seven developing countries (Dowsett 1999) reveals that many young people resisted exhortations to abstinence or delayed sexual activity (Dowsett 1999: 32). This was mainly due to widespread premarital sex as a result of delayed marriage and prolonged educational training (Dowsett 1999). Middle-class young people contested the "infantilization" of their bodies and persisted with their sexual pursuits (Dowsett 1999: 32).

Young people are caught in a cultural milieu that valorizes virginity in girls and active sexual behaviors in boys. They also encounter a contradiction between the abstinence education and a sexualized culture that is suffused with sexual images and appropriates sex in the sale of commodities.

Factors of Political Economy: Lack of Health Education and Services

Young people are not only confused by a cultural dilemma, but also are disempowered by the cultural denial of their right to health education, including understanding the risks of sexual behavior and ways to self-protection.

Worldwide, poor, out-of-school young people are more vulnerable to HIV than others. These young people include those who live in dire situations, drop out of school, live on the streets, share needles with other injecting drug users, engage in commercial sex, or are sexually and physically abused (Stine 2007).

In sub-Saharan Africa, only 8% of out-of-school youth and slightly more in-school youth have access to prevention education (UNAIDS 2004). The concomitant figures in Eastern Europe and Central Asia are 3% of out-of-school youth and 40% of in-school youth; and in the Caribbean and Latin America, 4% and 38%, respectively.. Globally, 44 out of 107 countries did not include AIDS in their school curricula (UNAIDS 2004: 95–96).

Even in some countries where AIDS is included in the curriculum, the information is usually perfunctory and inadequate, or only emphasizes purity and abstinence prior to marriage. For instance, in India, although sex education is part of schools' education programs on AIDS, the messages are diluted and some topics are avoided by the teachers. Young people are often reprimanded if they seek information or services. Girls often seek illegal services since sexual health services offer little privacy or confidentiality (UNAIDS 2004: 94).

It was reported in seven developing countries that young people demanded and needed sex education, yet sex education was sadly inadequate (Dowsett 1999: 33). In the report, sex education in the seven countries is described as "patchy and partial, delayed or deferred, and generally inadequate" (Dowsett 1999: 37). Many young people have little knowledge about HIV and STDs. As a result, young people are in a desperate quest for knowledge and information in the cultural silence about sexuality. Caught in the double bind, young men experience an immense amount of sexual confusion and distress. Often, fathers defer the responsibilities for sex education to older sons, sex workers, pornography, or their own adventures (Carrillo 2002; Dowsett 1999: 37).

The report reveals that young people have no or little access to information or health services in these developing countries (Scalway 2001: 23). It is worrisome that young people possess such a poor level of knowledge about STDs and HIV/AIDS. They are situated in a cultural and socioeconomic context that circumvents their sexual understanding and sexual behaviors. Hardly any young men have ever received comprehensive sex education. Instead, they depend upon their peers or older men to draw up an inaccurate and, at times, erroneous picture of the sexuality of their own and the women's experiences. Because of the culture pressure that expects them to be knowledgeable, many young men try to appear informed about sex and are afraid to admit their ignorance and lack of knowledge. The outcome is that a significant number of the youths remain misinformed about sex (Scalway 2001: 19). As Scalway maintains, in Paraguay and Mexico, where the most common method of contraception is the rhythm method, only a quarter of young men and women can identify a woman's fertile period. In a study of adolescents in Pakistan, a quarter of them are ignorant of the routes of HIV transmission. Only 5% of male university students in Ilorin, Nigeria, know that they can carry STDs and HIV and show no outward evidence of their condition (Scalway 2001: 19).

In some Asian countries such as South Korea and China, sex education centers on purity and abstinence before marriage and associates sex with conjugal practices, reproductive responsibilities, moral obligations, and nationalistic commitment (Cheng 2005a: 11).

In China, for instance, in 2004, despite the call from the Beijing and Hubei Hygiene Departments to prevent venereal diseases, no universities allowed them to install condom vending machines or distribute free condoms on campus (Jing 2004; Zhang 2006). During Zheng's research in two local universities, one of which was a medical university, local professors were very careful not to "corrupt" their students with discourses on sexuality. When I showed them my survey on HIV knowledge, they crossed out all the questions that contained the word "sex" before distributing the surveys to the students. As a result, half the survey was deleted. When I asked for the reason, the professors looked at me as if I came from another planet, saying: "We can't expose the students to these sexual ideas. They are too young to know this stuff. Knowledge about sex can only arouse their curiosity and encourage them to try it out. It's too dangerous for the students to know about this stuff."

Some professors at the local universities rejected proposals from local NGOs to educate the students about condoms. They contended that the school was different from society and that condom distribution or education on campus was inappropriate because very few students engage in sexual activities, hence the program would only initiate and encourage their sexual practices.

Professor Wang Wei from National Executive College spent ten years completing a book titled *Sex Ethics*, arguing that despite the importance of condoms, they are, after all, special merchandise that should be available for purchase, but not seen everywhere in the society (Rong 1999). Professors such as Wang Wei believed that using condoms to prevent AIDS had turned what should be a moral issue into a technical issue. They argued that sexual morality, rather than condom use, should be emphasized on TV.

At times, these university professors' stance was co-opted and reinforced by foreign Christian groups who preached in Chinese universities on abstinence only. For instance, three American "sex-education experts" arrived in Beijing on October 10, 2004, and spent a week delivering speeches on abstinence only at middle schools, colleges, universities, and other community locations. They warned China not to relive the errors that the United States had committed for 30 years, that is, emphasizing condom use and not emphasizing abstinence as the sole safe choice. They stressed that "sex is only beautiful when it happens within a marriage" and that condom use is only applicable to prostitution (Li 2004).

Some training lessons specifically targeted female teenagers. In Chongqing of Sichuan Province, doctors in City Family Planning Hospital brought in 47 female students ages 9 to 17, accompanied by their parents, to visit the abortion operation rooms (Qu 2005). They intended to educate the young girls by confronting them with the harsh reality of abortion. They told the female students that "if you engage in premature intimate contact with men, one day you may have to suffer the damage of this operation." Doctors explained in much detail how the sharp instruments are inserted into the uterus and stir and then suck out the fetus. After the visit, these girls claimed that "I do not want ever to enter this room again in my life. After school starts, I will tell my classmates about it so that the girls will know how to love and respect themselves (*zizunziai*)." Some parents considered it a violent education that extinguished the girls' rosy hope for the future. According to them, these terrible scenes were very cruel for adults, let alone for little girls. They argued that teenage girls should not have reproductive education as their psychological state of mind is not mature, and it has the potential to generate negative feelings toward future sex life, making them not want to get married at all.

The fact that education and training centers on young female students and not male students shows that women are used as barricades against the HIV transmission. Women are made to shoulder the responsibility of keeping the society clean and embodying and demonstrating the superiority of the nation. They are the weapons the state uses to fight HIV/AIDS.

In general, young people around the world are suspended in the cultural rhetoric of abstinence only and a sexualized socioeconomic context. Compounding this frustrating and confusing situation is the fact that they are often deprived of the rights to health education, health information, and health services. Lacking the appropriate knowledge of self-protection, many of them engage in unsafe sex and expose themselves to a high likelihood of HIV infections.

Summary

This chapter scrutinizes the population of women, ethnic women, and young adults in their relationships with HIV/AIDS. For each population, this chapter provides both the alarming statistics and the complex factors of culture and political economy to explain each group's specific vulnerabilities to HIV infections. Gender is a crucial factor in determining individuals' vulnerability to HIV infection. It is usually men who determine when and how often to have sex, and whether or not a condom is used. It is also men who usually have multiple sexual partners, which enhances the opportunity for them to transmit HIV to their partners. Global research has proven that gender norms, gender inequality, and poverty intensify and fuel HIV transmission for women. In many parts of the world, cultural norms demand that young women maintain sexual abstinence and encourage young men to experience sexual adventures. The cultural imperatives leave young women vulnerable with inadequate knowledge about sex, STDs, and HIV/AIDS. In many developing countries, certain sexual practices such as dry sex, widow inheritance, and ritual cleansers enhance both women and men's vulnerability to HIV transmission. Due to poverty and rapid social transformations, transactional and intergenerational sex is prevalent in many developing countries. In these relationships based on power and economic inequality, young women are caught in a vulnerable position and susceptible to abuse, exploitation, violence, and HIV. Young people are caught in a cultural milieu that valorizes virginity in girls and active sexual behaviors in boys. They also encounter a contradiction between abstinence education and a sexualized culture that is suffused with sexual images and appropriates sex in the sale of commodities.

Name: ______________________________ **Date:** __________________

Chapter 7 HIV/AIDS, Ethnicity, Young Adults, and Women

Exercises

Exercise 1 Discuss with your partner whether you and your lover engage in safe sex. How long have you and your lover been in a relationship? What are the reasons for you and your lover to choose safe or unsafe sex? Under what conditions do you engage in safe sex with a sexual partner? Under what circumstances do you engage in unsafe sex with a sexual partner?

Exercise 2 Reading Comprehension:

1. What is the biological factor that makes women more vulnerable to infection?

2. What are the social factors that stigmatize women in the current HIV pandemic?

3. Why is women's sexuality regulated and controlled?

4. What are the gender norms across the world? Which are associated with masculinity and which are associated with femininity? How do these associations affect sexuality?

   Gender norms:

   Masculinity:

Masculinity's impact on sexuality:

Femininity:

Femininity's impact on sexuality:

5. Describe the practice of dry sex in relationships with HIV infection.

6. Why do women engage in painful dry sex throughout southern Africa?

7. How is the cultural practice of widow inheritance related to HIV infection?

8. How is the cultural practice of ritual cleansers related to HIV infection?

9. Why is cross-generational sex so prevalent in sub-Saharan Africa?

10. Why are transactional and intergenerational sex related to HIV infections?

11. What are the cultural factors that impact ethnic women's vulnerability to HIV infection?

12. What are the sociopsychological factors that impact ethnic women's vulnerability to HIV infection?

13. What is the political economy of AIDS in the population of ethnic women?

14. What are the cultural factors that impact young people's vulnerability to HIV infection?

15. What is the political economy of AIDS in the population of young people?

Exercise 3 Discussion Questions:

1. Research has discovered that unsafe sex provides women with status and self-esteem. Through barrierless sexual contact, women assure themselves that their relationships are committed, close, and intact, for only women with faithful partners have the freedom to have condomless sex. What is your position on this?

2. College students have a rate of HIV infection 10 times higher than the general heterosexual population. Are college students less informed than the general heterosexual population?

3. Some societies believe that HIV transmission can be curbed by controlling and regulating women's sexuality. First, virtuous women can nurture and educate moral children—the next generation of the nation. Second, by controlling women's sexuality, men's sexuality can be controlled. What do you think of this intervention strategy? Can it work? Should it be carried out? Why or why not?

4. Do you think societies should change the associations with masculinity and femininity in relationships with sexuality? Why or why not? Can they be changed?

5. In your opinion, how can we change the situation where young people are vulnerable to HIV infection?

<u>Exercise 4</u> Test Your Knowledge:

1. It was reported in many developing countries that young people received ample sex education.
   a. True
   b. False
2. In many developing countries, young people learn about sex through older men, sex workers, pornography, or their own sexual adventures.
   a. True
   b. False
3. Young people around the world have the appropriate knowledge of self-protection, but they refuse to engage in safe sex.
   a. True
   b. False
4. Studies have shown that ethnic women in Cleveland, Ohio, find comfort and satisfaction in safe sex.
   a. True
   b. False

5. Studies of ethnic women have shown that racism constitutes the only reason for unsafe sex in the African-American community.
   a. True
   b. False
6. Studies have shown that African-American women believe that safe sex would hurt their male partners.
   a. True
   b. False
7. Studies have shown that African-American women are held in high esteem as the "head of the house."
   a. True
   b. False

Chapter eight | Intravenous Drug Users and Prevention

In this chapter we will address two major issues: intravenous drug use as a means of transmitting HIV, and strategies for prevention of HIV infection. Understanding these two problems is crucial to the containment of this disease, and as you will see, there is little consensus as to the right approach to either problem.

Prevention is complicated because there is no cure for the disease, so the only way to stop it is to prevent infection in the first place. This is a social problem, not a medical problem; the answer lies in finding ways to change human behavior, including behaviors driven by powerful elemental instincts. Because it is a social problem, the solutions will have to be culture specific. We can state fairly specifically what behavioral changes are necessary to stop the epidemic; the desired outcomes are general across cultures. The means to achieve these outcomes, however, must take into account the unique social and cultural patterns of behavior in different societies.

Intravenous drug use has spread across the globe. In the United States it is now responsible for about 25% of new infections. Around the world it is the second-largest cause of infection. In some areas, China for example, it is the leading cause of infection and it is primarily responsible for the beginnings of epidemics in Russia, the Ukraine, and elsewhere in Eastern Europe.

The Basics of Intravenous Drug Use and AIDS

Intravenous drug use (IDU) is a relatively recent phenomenon. Not until 1960 were there cheap disposable needles. The injection of illicit drugs followed shortly after this innovation. It is the best means of getting drugs directly into the bloodstream and obtaining the maximum high. Intravenous drug users (IDUs) are often identifiable by "tracks," scars left by the repeated use of needles to inject drugs. There are many potential dangers from this practice, including drug overdoses, since injection puts the drugs directly into the bloodstream as opposed to, say, smoking it. The problem is that because the drugs are illegal, users must depend upon unregulated criminals to deliver them. Drug dealers "cut" the drugs, that is, reduce their potency by mixing them with non-narcotic substances (which may themselves be dangerous). Users cannot be sure of the strength of the drugs they use, and therefore it is easy to use too much and overdose.

The problem we will be concerned with is not overdose, but infected needles. IDUs had to worry about infected needles long before the AIDS epidemic. Hepatitis was and is a common and serious problem for drug injectors. However, our concern is with the transmission of HIV and, as was mentioned earlier, this is now the second-leading cause of HIV infection. Infections occur when drug users share needles with HIV-infected people. It is not enough to wash needles with water; they need to be thoroughly disinfected, since remnants of infected blood in the needle can pass the disease. Recent experiments have demonstrated that these remnants can maintain their virulence for up to six weeks. A short-cut way of disinfecting the needles is through the use of bleach, which is now given to drug users in some programs to prevent infection. This is not foolproof, especially since people craving a fix cannot be counted upon to be careful and thorough. The best solution, short of not injecting drugs, is that everybody has their own needles and do not share. A supply of needles is necessary since needles become dulled with repeated use and need to be replaced. If everybody had their own needles, transmission of AIDS through drug injection could be stopped.

What are the barriers to providing IDUs with clean needles? There are two issues: first, financial and second, moral/legal. The cost of providing needles in poor countries is a serious problem. In sub-Saharan Africa, for instance, where many live on two dollars per day or less, the resources, without outside help, are just not sufficient. In these poverty-stricken areas there is great competition for very few health dollars. Malaria, for instance, still kills over a million people annually. In the early stages of the AIDS epidemic in Africa, some even suggested that the AIDS epidemic should be ignored in favor of other serious diseases such as malaria. Understandably, clean needles for drug users was not a priority.

The second consideration, which often overlaps with the cost issue, is the moral issue, which is often also a legal issue. Drug users are generally regarded in Western society as moral miscreants. Their activities are regarded as immoral and almost always as illegal. The question asked is whether government should, in any way, give support to illegal activities. To provide clean needles used to shoot dope seems to sanction an illegal activity. Not only is there opposition to government providing clean needles; there are laws in many American states forbidding even the sale of needles to ordinary citizens who are not licensed health care professionals or diabetics.

Historically, we can see here the collision of two American myths. One tradition of laissez-faire would free the individual of all restraints, allowing any activity that did not directly harm others, an extreme libertarianism that allows the individual almost complete personal freedom. The other great American myth or tradition comes out of America's Puritanical heritage. It sees American society as a community, bound by moral duty to God. In this tradition we are our brother's keeper; it is our duty to regulate public behavior or face the wrath of God. Important to the Puritan perspective is that immoral behavior is not necessarily regulated for the good of the sinner, but rather to prevent an offense against God's sensibilities. Neither of these traditions is helpful in providing a foundation for useful action on the needle issue. The libertarian position would probably not restrict drug use, but would not feel compelled to help those who had made the choice to use drugs with any form of government handout. The Puritan tradition would make laws against drugs, but would not support what it would consider sanctions for immoral behavior. Another American myth is probably also relevant to understanding the antagonism toward supporting programs like clean needles. This is related to the libertarian position but with some added twist:. American ideology was shaped when America was an agrarian society. The ideal was the strong individual standing on his own two feet. Government's role in rural society was less necessary. It is taking Americans a long time to realize that there is a necessary role for government in managing large populations crammed into big cities, particularly in the area of public health.

Another context for understanding the drug problem in America involves the issue of criminalization. Until legislation passed in the 1930s, narcotics were not illegal in America. One could purchase drugs such as opium at the drug store. When they were made illegal it created a market that could only be met through criminal activity. Those who, from libertarian impulses or from pragmatic considerations, favor decriminalization, point to the history of Prohibition. When alcohol was made illegal in America, the illicit, but very lucrative market, gave rise to organized crime. Al Capone made a fortune in one illegal activity, selling alcohol, which allowed him to invest in a variety of other activities such as gambling and prostitution. It also led to loss of respect for the law and to massive corruption of government.

Those favoring decriminalization can also make their argument solely on the basis of drugs. Clearly, demand for drugs has created a huge criminal empire outside the United States in places like Mexico, Columbia, and Afghanistan, which threatens to destabilize those countries, and in the case of Afghanistan has even been used to support terrorism. In the United States it has led to a huge criminal infrastructure and crowding of prisons with many offenders who would not otherwise be in jail. Our purpose here is not to argue for or against criminalization. Drugs constitute a serious danger to the American population and many fear that legalization would lead to a massive epidemic. However, those favoring decriminalization argue, and recent research supports them, that in the case of alcohol there is no evidence that prohibition decreased consumption. While there is a need for more studies of this subject, what is clear is that driving alcohol underground meant there was no regulation of this dangerous substance and often deadly results. Here the parallel with drugs is obvious.

Whether decriminalization of drugs is a good idea or not, it is not likely to happen given current political attitudes. A first practical step toward a policy that recognizes some of the complexities of the drug problem might involve de-escalating the war on drugs, or at least the way in which it is being conducted. President Nixon declared the war, and every president since has accepted the war metaphor. The problem with declaring war is that it traps us in a situation where any change in strategy can be considered a defeat. The war from the beginning has focused on the supply side of the problem. It is politically easy to proceed in this way, since drug dealers, especially foreign ones, make such good villains. This is reinforced by popular media with their plethora of crime dramas that thrive on a manichean struggle between good cops and evil drug dealers, the stuff of exciting if not very sophisticated drama. The problem is that this ignores the other half of the problem, which is the overwhelming demand for drugs coming from consumers. Dealing with drug consumers is not as attractive, since it requires some admission that there is a problem, and the problem is in our society. The war metaphor does not work as well here either, since the solution to the demand side of the problem must involve attempting to get people off drugs and keeping them from starting in the first place. This involves the hard work of trying to understand why people do drugs and how the conditions leading to them using drugs can be altered. One approach to the demand side has been locking up drug offenders, which has put hundreds of thousands in jail who would not be criminals on the basis of any other activities. This has cost a fortune and has ruined the lives of many otherwise harmless people. It has also made the problem of dealing with drugs and AIDS more difficult by defining drug users as criminals and undeserving of society's help. Some ultra-right religious groups have picked up on this and declared AIDS as God's retribution for society's sins: homosexuality and drug use.

The practical reality is that narcotics are illegal and drug use is spreading AIDS. The only practical way to stop this is to stop needle sharing. Education is important, but it only goes so far. Ethnographic studies of drug users show that they are generally aware of the dangers of contaminated needles, and that they are worried about it. Unfortunately, the addiction to drugs makes it difficult to make good decisions. An addict in the throes of withdrawl does what ever is necessary to get a fix.

An important point of view among social scientists is "rational choice." Rational choice is based upon the assumption that if people have adequate information they will most of the time make a decision that is best for them. This perspective is heavily influenced by the discipline of economics with its original emphasis upon "enlightened self interest." Even in economics this point of view has been heavily challenged, especially in recent years. Making the rational choice is dependent upon good information, so anthropologists who support this perspective advocate education and see a big role for government in publicizing necessary information. They can point to Uganda where government used the media and supported education to get the message out on AIDS. As we have seen, Uganda is a big success story. On the other side, they can point to South Africa where the government failed to dispense appropriate information and where the epidemic has gotten much worse.

Few would argue that education and information are unimportant, however; the success in Uganda is much more complex than is suggested by the above illustration, and it is not clear that it will continue to be a success story since, as we have seen, there are surveys indicating that there is a significant increase in risky behavior. As we have said before, it is also true that every culture is unique and requires tailored solutions. In Uganda there was an intact social community at the grassroots level that allowed the community to pull together. It seems also to be the case that the very severity of the epidemic in Uganda probably played a role in scaring people into better behavior. Most people had seen a relative or acquaintance die of this horrible disease. In much of sub-Saharan Africa the lingering effects of colonialism and the disarray created by modernization and urbanization make people less able to act rationally, even when they have good information.

In inner-city America rational behavior is not always viable. This is especially true for inner-city minority women; their economic and emotional dependencies make them especially vulnerable. Although there is disagreement on this point, some observers see in needle sharing more than just a convenience or a lapse in judgment brought on by the demands of addiction. Some see it, as is the case with other shared objects or procedures, as a kind of binding ritual. This may be especially true between couples. In any case, needle sharing, even between people who are aware of the risk, is a fact of drug life.

An added complication in understanding the risks of HIV from IDUs is the sexual factor. Besides sharing needles, IDUs have sex. What is happening in many epidemics, Russia and Eastern Europe for instance, is that AIDS starts out as an epidemic among IDUs who share needles. At this stage the epidemic is limited. The next step involves these infected people spreading the disease through sex with their husbands, wives, and other partners, moving the infection into the general population.

For those who see AIDS as a moral issue, this should be an important consideration. Even if one defines drug users and those engaged in promiscuous or nontraditional sex as miscreants, it is hard to blame vulnerable spouses or children for the disease they may get as a consequence of our failure to address the social realities of HIV transmission.

There is a parallel between the problem with needle sharing and the problem with sexual transmission. In both cases there is a relatively efficacious way of preventing the spread of infection. In the case of drugs, the problem is in avoiding needle sharing. In the case of sex, it is using condoms. This is generally understood by all involved parties; the problem comes when applying this to specific partners with whom one may have emotional involvement or when the needs of the moment cancel out good sense. As we have seen, most IDUs are at least generally aware of the risks in both areas. Given this, how do they assess specific risks when making decisions about whether to share needles or engage in unprotected sex?

Two important factors play a role. First is the idea of the other, meaning what is different, strange, unknown, threatening, apart from, not part of our community. Overlapping with this is a second factor, the unclean or morally tainted. Clean and moral are linked in our consciousness, as are immoral and unclean. Filth comes from outside and invades us. It is the other and associated with the other. Venereal disease is a kind of filth that invades the body; to have it is not just to be unclean but also to be immoral. Study after study shows the disjuncture common in our consciousness when the known and the unclean appear together. It violates our instinct as to the way things are supposed to be. When someone in our community has AIDS, it creates just this sort of cognitive dissonance. In other words, it is hard to associate something like an STD with someone with whom we are intimate. Recalling the previous chapter on Africa, it is instructive to remember that very few people saw themselves as vulnerable to AIDS, even though as outsiders observing the situation and knowing the statistics we would make a very different judgment. The comments of those interviewed in Africa mirrored comments in the United States: I know the person well, she seems very clean, and so on. This is the language of community, not the other. Historically, threats come from outside, in this case threats come from inside.

When we look at the data on condom use and needle sharing, we see that they reflect this principle. Intravenous drug users feel safe sharing needles with people they know and not safe with people they don't know. This may seem like common sense, but their sense of safety with people they regard as part of their community is not based upon specific knowledge of what behaviors that person has engaged in; it is rather with a sense of comfort with that person because of familiarity. Feeling triumphs over reason. In fact, while the vast majority of those participating in questionnaires in a New York City study were able to link AIDS with drug use and sex, most were not able to understand the specifics of risk. Commonly, risk was associated with other groups than the one they belonged to, such as gays. This was true in spite of having heard campaigns warning many different kinds of communities as being at risk. Again a kind of cognitive dissonance seemed to be at play, making it hard to rationally analyze the risk in their own specific circumstance. Even though nearly half (43%) shared needles at least some of the time, they did not regard themselves as at risk.

What is evident is that knowledge of risk, although admittedly imperfect in the study just cited, does not automatically translate into safe conduct. In the case of needles, both the need driven by addiction and assessment of the potential partner play a role, and their decision is often not rational. Even those who responded by saying they never shared needles admitted under further questioning that they had made exceptions when driven by extreme needs. These needs often focus upon feeling sick, described as feeling a general pain and anxiety that is associated with heroin withdrawal. Under these circumstances, people who say they do not share needles will share.

Among the large number of intravenous drug users who say they sometimes share needles, the assessment as to whether to share or not is based largely on familiarity with their potential partner. The New York study describes a woman in a stormy relationship with a frequently abusive husband. During periods of reconciliation they would share drugs and he would inject her. This woman clearly regarded this as a romantic act that brought them together and helped to preserve their marriage. When this happened her husband had chosen to be with her instead of his "running buddies." It seems likely that her emotional needs were masking a serious risk from a man who spent a lot of time with his "running buddies" doing drugs. In her world, the need for the affirmation of a loving gesture from a man dangerous to her health was too important to allow her to clearly evaluate her risks. Among inner- city drug users, her feelings are not unique.

Another story from the New York survey describes a group of friends, "running partners," who for nearly two decades had gathered at a friend's house to share dope and listen to jazz together. The informant describes the experience with obvious affection for the event and the people. This is clearly a description of a community that has been created around drugs, but goes much further than the convenience of getting dope together. The informant knew of the risks of needle sharing, but justified his behavior on two grounds. He claimed to have known all of the members of the group for a long time and there had never been a problem, such as hepatitis infection. Second, he justified the sharing by pointing out how difficult it was to get needles and how risky it was to carry them, since possession of needles was illegal. Neither of these arguments passes the test of rationality. His argument that it hadn't been a problem up to this point is based upon risky behavior that happened to have worked out so far. As to the difficulty of getting needles and the risk of carrying them, it is hard to see how this outweighs the danger of AIDS, although it also highlights the importance of legalizing the purchase of needles and making them easily available. The most important point in this is the pull of community. His friends were not the other, the cops, the landlords, the people who made life hard for him. What he got from these ritualistic gatherings was more than just a high from dope. He also obtained membership in a community, a sense of belonging. His group provided a sharp contrast with the other, those outside his community who controlled and made life difficult in his community.

When we consider the importance of community and ritual in normal lives, it should not be difficult to understand the irrational choices sometimes made by intravenous drug users. Inner-city minorities who have been cut off from or have cut themselves off from the traditional sources of community, such as work or church or clubs, must find these things where they can.

Smoking dope and listening to jazz with friends or having a wayward husband return and lovingly inject you fulfills deep human needs for emotional bonding with others. The term "running partners" is also expressive of the need to bond in a common experience. After all, the whole psychology of the local tavern thrives on this human need to bond and share. The popularity of the television show *Cheers* was at least partially based on a vicarious friendship with the cast of characters in that show and the sense of community it advertised: "a place where everybody knows your name." Taverns that just dispense alcohol are soon out of business. They must make the customers feel that they belong and are part of a community.

The Other Risk Factor from Intravenous Drug Use

The catastrophe of AIDS is happening in two stages in many places around the world. In China, and Southeast Asia, in Russia and Eastern Europe the AIDS epidemic is growing rapidly. The first stage is infection through needles shared by intravenous drug users. The second stage is when these intravenous drug users infect the larger society through sexual transmission. Once again it is important to remember that AIDS is a stealth killer. HIV may be dormant for ten years or more before becoming AIDS. During this dormancy the virus is at its most virulent stage. As happened in Africa, it is possible to create widespread infection without any alarm. By the time people are noticeably sick there is an epidemic.

Russia is a good example of how drugs and sex can deliver a one- two punch to a society. It is believed that the first AIDS case in Russia was transmitted through homosexual activity, probably around 1987. By the mid-eighties intravenous drug use was spreading the disease rapidly. The Russian government under Vladimir Putin was very slow to recognize the danger of this disease and has provided minimal funding for treatment and prevention. Gerald Stine, in his book "AIDS Update 2007," quotes UNAIDS director Pater Piot as saying that Russia has the fastest-growing epidemic in the world. In 2006 there were about 1 million cases, but if the current rate of infection were to continue, by 2015, ten million will have died from the disease. There is little reason to believe the disease will abate soon, given the lack of attention shown by the Russian government. If this is the case, then more than personal tragedy will follow. Russia, occupying the world's largest land mass with an already shrinking population of 145 million, will see devastation to its most productive age group. Given the likely political and economic impact it is hard to see how Russia could remain a viable state.

What is happening in Russia is different from what happened in Africa. Russia is a modern state that has politically and economically collapsed with great demoralization of the population. Perhaps it is not surprising that the AIDS epidemic began because of the widespread use of drugs. The critical period of incubation of the epidemic came during the disarray and economic decline of the late eighties and early nineties. While Russia suffered from the economic downturn beginning in 2007, it now has a stable if less than democratic government. The current increase in oil prices may be bad news for non oil producing developing countries, but for oil rich Russia it offers hope that funding will be available to stem the tide of this developing epidemic. President Medvedev has promised action. He faces opposition from a conservative health care establishment, and also from a revitalized and powerful Orthodox church that sees a moral issue in urging condom use and in providing clean needles for drug users. It is not yet clear whether action will follow rhetoric.

While there are hopeful signs, the disease remains a serious threat in poor areas such as sub-Saharan Africa and poverty stricken Haiti. Russia, with oil revenues exploding, still has failed to address an epidemic that has moved from prostitutes and drug users into the general population. Ukraine, without Russia's oil wealth, is at a similar stage. In China, where the lax response of the government in the past allowed expansion of the disease, it is not clear that they are controlling the spread from the very large number of prostitutes into the general public. These cases also make the point of those who advocate Freire's theory that we must have social justice growing from an awakened grassroots consciousness if we are going to change the conditions leading to AIDS.

What are the dynamics of sexual relations between intravenous drug users and their sex partners in the inner city in America, where the disease is now growing fastest? The problems of sexual transmission are very similar to the problems of IDU transmission. In both cases there is significant general knowledge about risk among the most at- risk members of the community. They may be wrong about specifics, but there is general knowledge that shared needles spread the disease and that prophylactics can provide good if not perfect protection. For sexual partners the problem is assessing their partners and having the power to avoid sex or at least to make sure it is protected sex.

As with needle sharing, the irrational attractions are the problem. Because sex is more intimate and more powerful symbolically, the difficulties are even greater than with needle sharing. The problem comes in assessing the risk with a partner, that is, in assessing the partner. In some cases this is easy, for instance, in the case of prostitutes where the exchange is strictly monetary and it is easy to demand the use of condoms. The key is the lack of emotional involvement in this kind of exchange. However, it should be remembered that condoms provide safer sex, not safe sex. Surveys in New York City verify that it is easier for prostitutes to demand the use of protection. Typical comments by prostitutes were: "If they don't want to use a rubber I won't date them," "I worked the streets for a long time and I always used one[condoms], even before I learned about AIDS. Most of them [clients] cooperate in the end"; "I'd say 'you don't want to catch something, I don't want to catch something."

Clearly this is the language of matter-of-fact commercial exchange, not the language of romance. However, even with sex workers condoms were not universal. Drugs were sometimes an issue, especially when sex workers were also addicts, which was not uncommon.

When a sex worker was in a hurry to get a fix and when the client was resistant to a condom, exceptions were made. As one former sex worker observed:

> There was pressure from the guys. [They] said they couldn't feel anything, they say it is no good with a rubber, but if they'd pay enough I'd do it without, sure. Women junkies who are in a hurry, it takes longer to get a guy off [with a condom], they won't use them. They just want to get it over with, get the money so they can get a hit.

In this case we can see how commerce can play a negative role in safety. Since this woman refers to junkies as the other, she presumably is not one. She affirms that drugs lead to unsafe sex, even for professionals, but goes on to admit that she too will take the risk of unprotected sex if the client is willing to pay for her risk.

When we move from professional sex workers to those involved in romantic relationships, the problem grows more complicated. First there is a category of women who may be involved with more than one man and may be somewhat, if not wholly, dependent upon them for financial support. We saw this problem in Africa and it exists in the inner city in American also. Because these relationships are romantic more than commercial, the rules change. To understand this it is useful to review the revolution in the role of condoms. Before the development of the birth control pill and the intrauterine device (IUD), the condom was the major means of birth control. This made it easier for a woman to insist upon the use of a condom, because it was understood that the alternative was possible pregnancy. Since the development of the pill and the IUD the role of the condom has changed dramatically, and so has the symbolism. Condoms are for the prevention of disease. Disease, uncleanliness, is associated with the other, not the intimate. It suggests mistrust and classifies the would-be loved one as the other. The entire emotional content of the relationship is destroyed. In the case of women who are economically dependent, the results can be a threat to their material lifestyle.

More common than this category of semi-professional sex workers, are women involved in solely romantic relationships, although even here an economic aspect may be part of the relationship: wives who depend upon husbands, for instance. In a harsh world where traditional values have broken down, a woman may be faced with an ambiguous situation. Because of the economic blight of the inner city, where male employment is difficult, what is called serial monogamy is common. Women may live with men but not necessarily in formal marriage, and the tenure of any one man may be short. Still, the relationship requires trust. The demand that he use a condom is a violation of trust. Condoms are not only undesirable because they detract from the pleasures of sex, but also because they signify mistrust. As one respondent confided, if I ask him to use a condom he either thinks that I don't trust him, or that I have been "fooling around." The frequency of drug use in the inner city is a complicating factor. As we have seen, most drug users, while recognizing the dangers of needle sharing on the one hand, seldom see themselves as personally at risk. Undoubtedly this involves a huge element of self-deception, but nevertheless, this is their perspective. When this person, who believes they are not at risk from drugs and perhaps not at risk from sexual encounters, is confronted by a spouse or loved one insisting on the use of condoms what is he to think?

Yet, 25% of the new AIDS cases in America are coming from drug use, or through sex by people who are infected from drug use. Chances are this percentage will increase as the American epidemic comes to be centered among minorities in the inner city. It is significant that the fastest-growing infected group in America is black women, the group most at risk from the behaviors we are discussing.

It is not by chance that this epidemic is coming to rest in the blighted inner city. As was discussed in an earlier chapter on the political economy of AIDS, this is a space where economic blight has much to do with political and business decisions, often contaminated with conscious or subconscious racial attitudes. Discrimination involving employment, education, credit, and housing create vulnerability. Minority women are at the bottom of this social order and are highly dependent, both economically and emotionally. They are both the victims of and the unwitting accomplices to a socially constructed system that marginalizes them and limits their ability to make rational choices. Even when they are able to break through this construct and make an affirmative choice, there is still the good chance that their choice will be negated by violence, outright rape, or more subtle coercion.

Not only are these women physically vulnerable; they are psychologically fragile. Like all humans they need to be loved, need to fit in and be accepted in the community in which they find themselves. Perhaps these needs are heightened by the precarious economic and social situation in which they exist. When confronted by a partner who wants to have unprotected sex, to say no is to destroy the trust that an emotional relationship is built upon. Undoubtedly the conflict between their knowledge of risk and their emotional needs leads to rationalization. Rationalization falls back on the idea of the familiar and the other. Because I know him, because he is part of my community, he must be clean.

This rationalization is not limited to vulnerable women. Men also use the concept of clean versus tainted, of familiar versus the other as comments of male intravenous drug users indicate: "I just thought she was clean"; "I know that the woman I know is clean"; "depends on who I pick up. If she looks like she takes care of herself; I wouldn't bother"; "when I do have sex with a female I tend to know the female."

There is a defensive tone in these statements, the concept of cleanliness and familiarity allow them to rationalize convenient, but still risky, behavior.

Beverly Sillthrope, in an article entitled "The Social Construction of Sexual Relationships as a Determinant of HIV Risk Perceptions and Condom Use Among Injection Drug Users," sums up the problem as follows:

> Cross-cultural studies have long confirmed that social bonding through sexual behavior is a universal human phenomena; sexual exchanges in conjugal and para-conjugal relationships constitute one of the bases of human social relations. In this context, the attribution of both sexually transmitted disease and (in the case of HIV) life threat to a sexual partner may be

> profoundly dissonant. It is incompatible with other components of important relationships such a respect, trust, support and protection, and thus has the potential to undermine the foundation of such relationships.

Conjugal relationships contain even greater degrees of significance, symbolizing the most important building blocks of human society. The hearth, sacred symbol of the family, represents warmth and safety from outside forces. It is almost inconceivable that it could harbor the filth and corruption associated with the other. In a world where modernization and urbanization have destroyed many familiar and traditional values, people feel more and more alienated and lonely. Ironically, the need to establish trust and a sense of community with others may be threatening people's lives.

Prevention

With most diseases, science is one of the keys to prevention. Since there is no scientific cure for AIDS, prevention must focus on altering human behavior. Because there are several ways in which people can be infected with HIV, prevention must be addressed in several ways. AIDS is passed through homosexual and heterosexual sex. It is passed through drug injection with contaminated needles and through transfusions, which have been especially hard on hemophiliacs; and from mother to child through birthing and through nursing. Other than abstinence, we know the best way to prevent transmission is through the use of condoms and the practice of monogamy, although a program of universal circumcision would certainly reduce transmission, as would rapid treatment of STDs. With drugs, the key is clean needles. As for mother-to-child transmission, anti-retroviral drugs can reduce transmission dramatically and transmission through nursing can be stopped by providing baby formula for mothers in poor countries. Of course blood supplies need to be monitored adequately. Even though none of these approaches is perfect, except clean needles for drug addicts, they could reduce the epidemic to a matter of rare contagion.

As we have seen, the biggest problem is not knowing what behaviors will end the epidemic, but rather getting people to adopt the appropriate behaviors and getting government to assist in these efforts. As we have also argued, programs to change behavior must do more than publicize the dangers of certain behaviors. These programs must be tailored to account for the specific cultural traits operating in various cultural communities. In the remaining pages of this chapter we will discuss various approaches to prevention, both in the United States and elsewhere. We will discuss what has worked and what has not worked and the reasons for success and for failure.

The first epidemic in the United States was in the gay community, centered initially in large cities such as San Francisco, New York, and Los Angeles. This epidemic was ignored by the Reagan administration until a well-organized gay lobby was able to bring political pressure. The leadership of Everett Koop, the Surgeon General, was important in publicizing the problem and in helping pressure the Reagan administration. Two lessons can be drawn from this experience: first, the importance of government leadership in educating the public and second, the importance of grassroots organization to lobby government, but equally important, to educate and inform those most vulnerable.

This experience is reinforced by what happened in Uganda. The Uganda epidemic, like the gay American epidemic, began as a stealth attack. Infection was widespread before people were aware of the presence of the disease. But in Uganda the epidemic was finally stemmed by strong grassroots community organization that educated people thoroughly and put social pressure on people to change risky behaviors. The Ugandan government was faster in responding than the Reagan administration and was forthright in talking about the cause of AIDS and the necessary social changes to stop the epidemic. In both Uganda and the American gay community the severity of the epidemic was critical in scaring the community into action, and in both cases there was a cohesive community that was capable of addressing frankly the social situation, although in the gay community it took a lot of sickness and devastation to get the community to recognize the need for behavioral change.

These were the two factors: a cohesive grassroots community that ultimately rejected bigotry toward the infected and worked together to change behavior, and, although belatedly in the United States, good government leadership. This was exactly what was missing in southern Africa, especially in the Union of South Africa.

President Mbeki became an AIDS denier and grassroots organization was slow to form (except in the white gay community). This scenario has been repeated again and again. When government provides funding for publicity and education and when grassroots organizations work at the local level, the epidemic is brought under control. Thailand provides a positive example of this and Russia a negative example. In Thailand what looked like an African-scale epidemic has been contained and rolled back. Intravenous drug users from the Golden Triangle area and a thriving sex industry catering to foreigners in Bangkok had given impetus to the epidemic. As a result of the anti-AIDS campaign visits to prostitutes fell by 60% and condom use skyrocketed. We have already discussed how the failure of the Russian government to act has allowed the disease to move from intravenous drug users and sex workers into the general population.

Abstinence Only versus Condoms

The only absolutely safe way to avoid AIDS from sex is to abstain. Next best is to have only one partner. Finally, the use of condoms, while not foolproof, is reasonably safe. Beyond this there is considerable risk. To review, anal sex is riskier than vaginal sex because the anal lining is more fragile. Oral sex is hard to pin down with percentages. HIV is passed through oral sex, but because oral sex is often not done in isolation it is hard to calculate the degree of risk. STDs greatly increase risk because they cause genital abrasions that allow mixing of blood and weaken the immune system. For some reason, circumcision seems to cut risk in half. A key risk factor is concurrent sex as frequently practiced in sub-Saharan Africa and to a lesser extent in inner-city America. Concurrent sex is especially dangerous because it not only increases exposure, but increases exposure at a time when the virus is likely to be most virulent.

Critical to stopping the epidemic is expansion of the health care system where it is deficient. In America over 45 million people do not have health insurance. Because health insurance is usually tied to employment, inner cities with high unemployment rates are especially hard hit. This is a major factor in sub-Saharan Africa also. Adequate medical care for individuals means several things: clearing up STDs that weaken the immune system and cause genital sores; identification of nutritional deficiencies that weaken the immune system; testing for HIV so that the disease is not passed on; administration of anti-viral drugs that lessen the chance of passing HIV to children and mitigate some of the worst consequences of AIDS such as poverty from unemployment; and leaving orphans behind, an especially serious problem in sub-Saharan Africa.

There is a policy debate in the United States pitting abstinence- only education against broader sex education that focuses on the use of condoms. Those arguing for abstinence-only education insist that only abstinence is 100% safe and they are correct in this. Because the impetus behind their arguments is usually religious, they are not often open to compromise on this issue. It is possible to teach both abstinence and the use of condoms. The trouble with abstinence-only programs is that teaching abstinence often doesn't result in abstinence. Sex is a powerful drive, especially for teenagers. Brain studies have shown what experience had already taught us: that brain development is not complete until the mid-twenties. One of the last things to develop is the frontal cortex that controls risk assessment and judgment. The statistics for abstinence-only education strongly suggest that there needs to be a backup when powerful physical and emotional urges overpower not yet fully developed judgment. Teaching abstinence and the importance of condoms when you do have sex are not mutually exclusive. Because we are often dealing with children whose judgment is not yet as fully developed as their physical urges, this is critical.

When it comes to sex education, ignorance is not bliss. One of the consequences of the AIDS epidemic is a huge increase in oral sex among teenagers. One survey conducted in 2005 by the National Center for Health Statistics showed that over half of American teenagers aged 15 to 19 had engaged in oral sex. While we do not have good data as to how effective transmission of HIV is through oral sex, we do know it is a way to get AIDS. Since it involves a transfer of bodily fluids, it is reasonable to assume it is very dangerous. Good sex education is critical, because a high proportion of people will engage in premarital sex. It is necessary to apply what works to stop the epidemic, not what we wish to believe will work.

We will discuss only briefly the problem of transmission through intravenous drug use, since we addressed this earlier in the chapter. As we saw, the key issue with intravenous drug users is hung up on a moral issue that has become a legal issue. As with abstinence in sex, the safest solution is to abstain from using needles to inject drugs. Unfortunately, abstinence of needle use is as problematic as sexual abstinence. In the case of drugs there is a backup solution that is more effective in preventing AIDS than the use of condoms; in fact it is 100% effective. Clean needles do not pass on AIDS. Recent experiments have shown that the HIV virus in blood residue in used needles remains contagious for up to six weeks. Clean needles solve the problem. Perhaps the first step is to get rid of remaining laws that forbid buying or possessing needles. But to really stop HIV among intravenous drug users it will be necessary to have clean needle programs that make sure that nobody is sharing needles.

Up to this point we have only been discussing what people need to do to ensure that they will not get AIDS, or at least reduce the odds that they will get AIDS. As we have emphasized, education alone is not sufficient. An education-alone strategy assumes that people who have knowledge will act rationally. We know that this is not universally true, that emotional needs and cultural habits often outweigh reason. The question is then: How do we change habits? How do we change culture? It seems that in San Francisco and Uganda the very horror of the disease has been effective in changing people's actions, but this is clearly not an acceptable solution, nor is it apparently a permanent solution, as there seems to be an increase in reckless behavior among both Ugandans and American gays.

One approach to prevention has been the application of advertising techniques to changing behavior. In 1986 in New York City the advertising firm of Saatchi and Saatchi volunteered its services to the city to conduct campaigns designed to warn the heterosexual community of the danger of AIDS. At this time the public perceived AIDS as a disease of marginal groups, primarily gay men and intravenous drug users. The purpose of the ads was to make clear that heterosexual sex was also a risk factor. Its approach was educational; it did not attempt to address the irrational causes of risky behavior common among the economically marginalized elements in society. Its key slogan was: "If you don't think you can get AIDS you are dead wrong." The message was clear and stark. Where the campaign ran into trouble was in its frankness about the disease and its advocacy of condoms. The intent was to get people's attention by being frank and shocking; inevitably there were venues that found it too frank and too shocking. Some television and radio stations refused to run the ads, as well as the *New York Daily News*. In spite of these problems, the campaign seemed to succeed in getting the message out to the heterosexual community. In light of the difficulties we have seen in changing behavior in poverty communities, one can say that these ads were most effective in informing middle-class heterosexuals more likely to act on information. The ads did not use the more powerful techniques of identity appeal that get people to drink beer or buy jeans. They were primarily, if shockingly, informational.

The Love-life program in South Africa does try to do more than educate. It has a strategy to change behavior and relies on more sophisticated ad techniques that have been successful in selling commercial products to kids. Over a thousand Love-life billboards dot the South African landscape and they use what has worked to sell soda and jeans, sex. The ads feature beautiful young people in provocative poses, but being smart about sex, that is, using condoms. Here the appeal is identity appeal. Emulate these images of kids who are beautiful and cool and you too will be beautiful and cool. The Love-life campaign rejects the idea of scaring kids into smart behavior, arguing that positive images are more powerful than negative images. The idea is to create alternative cool models with which the kids can identify.

Perhaps the approach that takes most seriously the disjuncture between information and action is a program based upon peer counseling. This approach uses Paul Freire's concept of critical consciousness as a guide to educating youth about how to control their own lives and make healthy decisions regarding sexual activity. This program has been used in South Africa among poor township youth whose incidence of HIV infection is very high. An analysis of this program in a black community outside of Johannesburg is reported in a paper by Catherine Campbell and Catherine MacPhail, in the journal *Social Science and Medicine.*

The social environment they describe is typical of what we have witnessed elsewhere in southern and eastern Africa: poverty is the norm; young girls grow up in a socially constructed environment in which they are at the bottom of the pecking order. They are coerced into sex, sometimes through rape. As Campbell and MacPhail report: "young people's sexual encounters were negotiated within a context where dominant social norms of masculinity portrayed young men as conquering heroes and macho risk takers in the sexual arena, and where the social construction of femininity predisposed women to use the response of passivity or fruitless resistance in the face of male advances."

Obviously the problem is to change this environment to give young women a stronger negotiating position. Through peer counseling the program's administrators hope to change the consciousness of both men and women. Freire calls the initial stage of consciousness intransitive thought. He argues that at this stage individuals do not understand how their social condition shapes their personal well-being. They feel helpless to act to change their condition.

The function of peer counseling is to lead them as a group to an explanation of their condition that connects their personal life to the larger environmental context which has shaped them and continues to control them. If successful, they will reach the final stage of "critical transivity," having learned to understand themselves and how they have been shaped by larger historical and social forces. Because the group has worked together to reach this stage, they are now able to work collectively to change the social conditions. The key is that the group now has an empowering analytical tool, in a sense, a whole new vocabulary for understanding how they have been shaped and for understanding the forces that have shaped them. They have reached a fuller consciousness that allows them to understand that things don't just happen, but rather that there is a logic to how things come about, a logic that they now understand. This new narrative clarifies a concept of justice and thereby enhances their own sense of self-worth.

Critical to the success of this process is that everyone, male and female, is able to move to the final stage of critical transivity; that is, to transcend to this new level of awareness that gives clarity to the entire group's situation and places it in a larger historical and social perspective. There are obvious obstacles to this, particularly for young men. Since males seem to be advantaged in the status quo, why should they embrace change? It is necessary that they understand that while they may have authority over the young women, they are also trapped in a social structure (and a political economy) that provides no outlet for them other than bullying the young women. The most obvious sign of their entrapment is that the likely actions taken by them, given this social structure, will not allow them to escape the prison of poverty, but will cause them to continue the behaviors that will likely lead to AIDS and an untimely death. They must be convinced to renounce concrete and immediate status and power in order to advance the interests of all of the community, including their own long-term interests.

One should not underestimate the power of the romantic narrative with which the boys identify. The devil-may-care, macho hero image is universal around the world. It is a fundamental staple of male identity, and is particularly compelling to young men who have no real concrete hopes for advancement in the world, a description that fits these young men perfectly. It gives them a way of conceptualizing themselves that gives them more dignity than the larger world is likely to grant them.

What does critical transivity mean? It means that the individual and the group have now arrived at a state of consciousness where they understand the cause and effect of their own condition. Part of this is just understanding that there is causation, that things don't just happen. There is a logic to their condition which they should now be able to collectively deconstruct and understand. Instead of being reactive, they now actively and collectively work to create a new narrative and a new social structure based upon justice for all. Now understanding what justice is, they can begin collectively working toward it.

This takes us back to the chapter on political economy. Young township blacks in South Africa live in a political economic structure not of their own making. What are the implications of understanding this larger world in which they live? The point is to allow them to act collectively on what they now understand. South Africa has undergone a revolution recently replacing white minority rule with democratic rule. However, it has not changed the conditions of the great mass at the bottom of the system a great deal. It has allowed the growth of a black middle class that has joined whites in the suburbs. Will critical consciousness lead to liberal reform within the new system or another revolution? Perhaps this depends upon the reaction of the new black middle class and the old white middle class to the demands of the underclass. Of course this kind of speculation is predicated upon the success of peer counseling in creating a new consciousness in the black underclass. This new consciousness would demand a transformation of the political economy to allow people now at the bottom to gain control over their own lives, including control over their health. The implications of Freire's ideas are revolutionary, but perhaps necessary to dealing with the AIDS epidemic. It may be that social justice is the necessary precondition for dealing with the AIDS epidemic.

Earlier in this text we observed Merrill Singer's contention that HIV/AIDS was becoming a disease of the poor and powerless. We have since shown significant exceptions to this contention: the reckless behavior of wealthy men in East Africa and the severity of the disease among middle-class gays in America. However, what we have also seen is that these more powerful and affluent communities seem to have been able to adapt and change their behavior. Where the disease is expanding in America is among the most powerless minority residents of the inner city. Even within this category it is women, the most powerless of the powerless, that are now suffering the greatest increases in infection. Around the world the disease is expanding in the poorest corners of the planet. Africa is most hard hit, but Haiti, the poorest country in the Western Hemisphere, has an epidemic of near-African proportions and that shows no sign of abating. Russia, now sliding back into poverty as oil prices bottom out, is just at the beginning of the second stage of a drug-induced epidemic that promises to be on an African scale. In Eastern Europe, particularly the Ukraine, the epidemic, also driven by intravenous drug use, is now entering the second stage where it is exploding into the general population. This may also be happening in China, where in the past the government has been very lax in responding to the epidemic. These cases also make the point of those who advocate Freire's theory that we must have social justice growing from an awakened grassroots consciousness if we are going to change the conditions leading to AIDS.

It is too soon to know if the peer counseling approach to changing behavior in blighted communities will be successful. It does seem to be the approach that makes the greatest effort to understand and transform behaviors among the world's poor. Until there is a medical solution to the AIDS problem, our only recourse is to try to better understand the varieties of communities around the world and how and why they behave as they do. Behavioral change is now the only effective weapon against this disease. We have to learn how to help people to an understanding of themselves and their world so that they can act in a way that will be good for their own futures.

Summary

This chapter looks at HIV transmission through drug use and various prevention programs. In drug transmission the basic problem is sharing infected needles. The problem is two fold: first, poor judgment about the dangers of transmission between those with whom one is intimate; and second, the reluctance of society to provide clean needles for drug users because it is perceived as sanctioning immoral and illegal behavior. A second subject is the various social programs designed to change behavior. These programs fall into two general categories: the rational choice programs that emphasize education and information that will allow individuals, assumed to be rational, to make good choices, and behavior modification programs that recognize that when dealing with sex and drugs, people may not be as rational as they need to be.

Study Questions

1. What is the moral issue associated with resistance to public provision of clean needles to intravenous drug users?

2. What problems have been created by criminalizing drug use? Discuss the market phenomena.

3. Make an argument either for or against criminalization of drug use.

4. Make an argument either for or against the rational choice approach to fighting the drug-AIDS epidemic.

5. What irrational factors play a role in the decision by drug addicts to share needles?

6. Generally, how aware are drug addicts of the dangers of needle sharing? Do most addicts consider themselves to be at risk?

7. Explain the two stages of the AIDS epidemic unfolding in Russia. What role is government playing in combating the epidemic?

8. In the survey conducted in New York City who was more likely to demand the use of condoms of their male partners, sex workers or girlfriends?

9. Discuss the problems with abstinence-only education programs. What do you think is the balance between merits and faults?

10. For what demographic was the ad campaign designed by Saatchi and Saatchi? What problems did it encounter?

11. How does the South African Love-life program attempt to dissuade youth from risky behavior? What is your opinion of the efficacy of this approach?

12. Explain Paul Friere's concept of critical transivity. What are the difficulties of applying this in South African black townships?

13. How do calculations about the familiar and the other influence decisions about condom use and needle sharing?

14. In spite of the growth of the epidemic in Russia, what are the hopeful possibilities?

15. What role is the Orthodox church playing in Russia?

Selected Bibliography

Abdool, Karim S. S., Karim Abdool Q, and Sankar N Preston-Whyte. 1992. Reasons for lack of condom use among high school students. *South African Medical Journal* 82:107–10.

Adams, Vincanne, and Stacy Pigg. 2005. *Sex in development: Science, sexuality, and morality in global perspective.* Durham, NC: Duke University Press.

Adetunji, Jacob, and Dominique Meekers. 2003. Social marketing and communications for health consistency in condom use in the context of HIV/AIDS in Zimbabwe. PSI Research Division Working Paper No. 19. PSI (Population Services International), Washington, DC.

Agha, Sohail. 1997. Sexual activity and condom use in Lusaka, Zambia. PSI Research Division Working Paper No. 6. No. 19. PSI (Population Services International), Washington, DC.

Agha, Sohail, and Ronan Van Rossem. 2001. The impact of mass media campaigns on intentions to use the female condom in Tanzania. PSI Research Division Working Paper No. 44. No. 19. PSI (Population Services International), Washington, DC.

Ai, Pin. 2004. Aizi xiaotou panxing: Rendaodajizhihou de zhidukaoliang (Sentenced AIDS thieves: Measure of system after moral attack). *Fazhi yu xinwen* (*Law and News*) 4:34–36.

Amadora-Nolasco, Fiscalina, Renae Alburo, Elmira Judy Aguilar, and Wenda Trevathan. 2001. Knowledge, perception of risk for HIV, and condom use. *AIDS and Behavior* 5(4):319–30.

An, Ni. 2006. Anquantao yehui taozou nuxing jiankang (Condoms can strip a woman of health). *Qianlong Xinwen Wang,* April 10.

Anagnost, Ann. 1995. A surfeit of bodies: Population and the rationality of the state in post-Mao China. In *Conceiving the New World Order,* ed. Faye Ginsburg and Rayna Repp. Berkeley: University of California Press.

Andors, Phillis. 1983. *The unfinished liberation of Chinese women, 1949–1980.* Bloomington: Indiana University Press.

Anonymous. 1964. *Nongcun weisheng shouce* (*Hygiene handbook in the countryside*). Nanchang: Jiangxi Renmin Chubanshe.

______. 1991. Biyunhuan wenti (Questions on IUD). *Women of China* 10:42.

______. 2002. *Anquantao tuxian anquan wenti* (*The issue of safety of condoms*). http://www.jynk.com, August 32.

______. 2004a. 2004 wenjuan (Survey in 2004). *Dazhong wenzhai* (*Popular Digest*) 11(47):16–17.

______. 2004b. Xingqu shoucang (Sex interests). *Shenghuo yu jiankang* (*Life and Health*) 2:34.

______. 2005a. Publication Statistics (Faxing Tongji). *Bosom Friend* (*Zhiyin*) 3:12.

______. 2005b. Zhuanjia yuce: Zhongguo anquantao shichang qianli chao baiyiyuan (Experts predicted that the market potential of condoms in China exceeded tens of billions of yuan). http://info.china.alibaba.com, December 21.

______. 2006a. Jiankang shenghuo yidiantong (Help on health and life). *Dushi Zhufu* (*Hers*) 7:116.

______. 2006b. Lian aizibing renshu shangsheng 46.67% (HIV infection increasing rate is 46.67% in Dalian). *Dongbei Xinwen,* November 29.

______. 2006c. Zhongguo Aizibing Ershinian (1985–2005) (Twenty years of AIDS in China). Sohu.com.

Aral, Sevgi. O., and Janet S. St. Lawrence. 2002. The ecology of sex work and drug use in Saratov Oblast, Russia. *Sexually Transmitted Diseases* 29:789–805.

Baer, Hans A., Merrill Singer, and Ida Susser. 1997. *Medical anthropology and the world system.* Westport, CT: Bergin & Garvey.

Bandura, Albert. 1977. *Social learning theory.* Englewood Cliffs, NJ: Prentice Hall.

Bandura, Albert. 1997. *Self-efficacy: The exercise of control.* New York: W. H. Freeman.

______. 2005. Guide for creating self-efficacy scales. In *Self-efficacy beliefs of adolescents,* ed. Frank Pajares and Tim Urdan. Greenwich, CT: Information Age.

Bankole, Akinrinola. 1999. Book reviews. *Studies in Family Planning* 30:89–92.

Bankole, Akinrinola, G. Rodriguez, and C. F. Westoff. 1996. Mass media messages and reproductive behavior in Nigeria. *Journal of Biosocial Science* 28:227–39.

Barlow, Tani. 1994. Theorizing woman: Funu, Guojia, Jiating. In *Body, subject and power in China,* ed. Angela Zito and Tani E. Barlow. Chicago: University of Chicago Press.

Barme, Geremie. 1995. To screw foreigners is patriotic: China's avant-garde nationalist. *China Journal* 34:209–34.

Bastos, Cristiana. 1999. *Global response to AIDS.* Bloomington: Indiana University Press.

Basuki, Endang, Ivan Wolffers, Walter Deville, Noni Erlaini, Dorang Luhpuri, Rachmat Hargono, and Nuning Maskuri. 2002. Reasons for not using condoms among female sex workers in Indonesia. *AIDS Education Preview* 14:102–16.

Bin, Lang. 2003a. AIDS shiji youling (Century ghost). *Jiankang Guwen (Health Consultation)* 1–3(124):4–13.

______. 2003b. Butong renqun de yufang (Prevention for different groups). *Jiankang Guwen (Health Consultation)* 1–3(124):9.

______. 2003c. Shenmo shi Aizibing (What is AIDS). *Jiankang Guwen (Health Consultation)* 1–3(124):6–7.

Birkinshaw, Marie. 1989. *Social marketing for health.* Geneva: World Health Organization.

Blanc, Marie-Eve. 2004. Sex education for Vietnamese adolescents in the context of the HIV/AIDS epidemic: The NGOs, the school, the family and the civil society. In *Sexual cultures in East Asia,* ed. Evelyne Micollier, 241–62. New York: RoutledgeCurzon.

Blecher, Mark, M. Steinberg, W. Pick, M. Hennick, and N. Durcan. 1995. AIDS knowledge, attitudes, and practices among STD clinic attenders in the Cape Peninsula. *South African Medical Journal* 85(12):1261–86.

Bloor, Michael. 1995. *The sociology of HIV transmission.* London: Sage.

Bolton, Ralph, and Merrill Singer, eds. 1992. *Rethinking AIDS prevention: Cultural approaches.* Philadelphia: Gordon & Breach Science.

Bond, George C., John Kreniske, Ida Susser, and Joan Vincent. 1997. *AIDS in Africa and the Caribbean.* Boulder, CO: Westview.

Brandt, Allan. 1988. AIDS: From social history to social policy. In *AIDS: The burdens of history,* ed. Daniel Fox and Elizabeth Fee, 141–71. Berkeley: University of California Press.

Bray, Francesca. 1997. *Technology and gender: Fabrics of power in Late Imperial China.* Berkeley: University of California Press.

Brownell, Susan. 1995. *Training the body for China: Sports in the moral order of the People's Republic.* Chicago: University of Chicago Press.

______. 2000. Gender and nationalism in China at the turn of the millennium. In *China briefing 2000,* ed. Tyrene White. Armonk, NY: M. E. Sharpe.

Buckley, Sandra. 1997. The foreign devil returns: Packaging sexual practice and risk in contemporary Japan. In *Sites of desire: Economics of pleasure,* ed. Lenore Manderson and Margaret Jolly, 262–91. Chicago: University of Chicago Press.

Cai, Fang. 2000. *Zhongguo renkou wenti baogao (A report of the problem of the Chinese population).* Beijing: Shehui Kexue Wenxian Chubanshe.

Calves, Anne E. 1999. Condom use and risk perceptions among male and female adolescents in Cameroon. PSI Research Division Working Paper No. 22. PSI (Population Services International), Washington, DC.

Campbell, Carole. 1995. Male gender roles and sexuality: Implications for women's AIDS risk and prevention. *Social Science and Medicine* 41(2):197–210.

Campbell, Catherine. 2000. Selling sex in the time of AIDS: The psycho-social context of condom use by sex workers on a Southern African mine. *Social Science and Medicine* 50:479–94.

Campbell, Catherine, Zodwa Mzaidume, and B. Williams. 1998. Gender as an obstacle to condom use: HIV prevention amongst commercial sex-workers in a mining community. *Agenda* 39:50–59.

______, and Catherine MacPhail. 2001. I think condoms are good but, aai, I hate those things: Condom use among adolescents and young people in a Southern African Township. *Social Science and Medicine* 52:1613–27.

Cao, Xiaoyong. 2004. Jujue tongfang shi jiating baoli ma (Is refusal to have sex domestic violence). *Zhongguo Funu (Women of China)* 3(621):29.

Carrier, Joseph M. 1989. Sexual behavior and the spread of AIDS in Mexico. *Medical Anthropology* 10:129–42.

Carrier, Joseph M., and Rachel Magana. 1991. Use of ethnosexual data on men of Mexican origin for HIV/AIDS prevention programs. *Journal of Sexual Research* 28(2):189–202.

Carrillo, Hector. 2002. *The night is young.* Chicago: University of Chicago Press.

Chanpong, Gail Fraser, Maidy Putri, Sophal Oum, Ung Sam An, Mam Bunheng, Jeffrey Ashley, James R. Campbell, and Andrew L. Corwin. 2001. Prevalence of HIV infection in Cambodia: Implications for the future. *International Journal of STD and AIDS* 12(6):413–16.

Chatterjee, Partha. 1993. *The nation and its fragments.* Princeton, NJ: Princeton University Press.

Che, Yan, and John Cleland. 2003. Contraceptive use before and after marriage in Shanghai. *Studies in Family Planning* 34(1):44–52.

Chen, Jiali. 2002. Yangshi anquantao guanggao beipo linshi genggai (CCTV condom advertisements forced to be changed at the last minute). *Zhongxinwang* (*Chinese News Internet*), December 5.

Chen, Shi. 1958. Shengyu you jihua, shengchan jintou da (Planned birth, more energy for production). *Women of China* 5:30–31.

Chen, Yang. 2005. Shenmo shi anquan xingshenghuo (What is safe sex). *Jiankang Zhoubao* (*Health Weekly*) 1(18):C3.

Cheng, Sealing. 2005. Popularising purity: Gender, sexuality, and nationalism in HIV/AIDS prevention for South Korean Youths. *Asia Pacific Viewpoint* 46(1):7–20.

Chiang, Mai. 2004. Brief introduction of school HIV/AIDS prevention education in China. International seminar/workshop on learning and empowering key issues in strategies for HIV/AIDS prevention, Thailand, March 1–5.

Ch'iu Lyle, Katherine. 1980. Report from China: Planned birth in Tianjin. *China Quarterly* 83:551–67.

Chu, Zhaorui, and Suide Shao. 2005. AIzibing fangzhigongzuo keburonghuan (AIDS prevention work is pressing). In *Zhongguo Aizibing Fangzhi* (*Prevention of HIV/AIDS in China*). Beijing: Capital University of Medical Science.

Civic, Diane, and David Wilson. 1996. Dry sex in Zimbabwe and implications for condom use. *Social Science and Medicine* 42(1):91–95.

Clarke, Kamari Maxine. 1999. To reclaim Yoruba tradition is to reclaim our queens of Mother Africa: Recasting gender through mediated practices of the everyday. In *Feminist fields: ethnographic insights*, ed. Sally Cooper Cole, Rae Bridgman, and Heather Howard-Bobiwash. New York: Broadview Press.

Clatts, Michael. 1989. Ethnography and AIDS intervention in New York City: Life history as an ethnographic strategy. In *Community-based AIDS prevention, studies of intravenous drug users and their sexual partners*, ed. Michael Clatts. Rockville, MD: National Institute on Drug Abuse.

______. 1994. "All the king's horses and all the king's men": Some personal reflections on ten years of AIDS ethnography. *Human Organization* 53:93–95.

Cohen, Barney, and James Trussell. 1996. *Preventing and mitigating AIDS in sub-Saharan Africa: Research and data priorities for arresting AIDS in sub-Saharan Africa.* Washington, DC: National Academies Press.

Coleman, Patrick. 1988. Enter-educate: New word from Johns Hopkins. *JOICFP Review* 15:28–31.

Cook, James. 1996. Penetration and neocolonialism: The Shen Chong rape case and the anti-American Student Movement of 1946–47. *Republican China* 22(1):65–97.

Cusick, Linda. 1998. Female prostitution in Glasgow: Drug use and occupational sector. *Addiction Research* 6:115–30.

Day, Sophie. 1990. Prostitute women and the ideology of work in London. In *Culture and AIDS*, ed. Douglas A. Feldman, 93–110. New York: Praeger.

Day, Sophie, Helen Ward, and John Richard Harris. 1988. Prostitute women and public health. *British Medical Journal* 297:1585.

de Zalduondo Barbara, and Jean Maxius Bernard. 1995. Meanings and consequences of sexual-economic exchange. In *Conceiving sexuality: Approaches to sex research in a postmodern world*, ed. Richard G. Parker and John H. Gagnon, 155–80. New York: Routledge.

Dechamp, Jean-Francois, and Odilon Couzin. 2006. Access to HIV/AIDS treatment in China: Intellectual property rights, generics, and barriers to effective treatment. In *AIDS and social policy in China*, ed. Arthur Kleinman, Joan Kaufman, and Tony Saich, 125–51. Cambridge, MA: Harvard University Asia Center.

Dikotter, Frank. 1995. *Sex, culture, and modernity in China: Medical science and the construction of sexual identities in the Early Republican Period.* London: Hurst.

______. 2004. A history of sexually transmitted diseases in China. In *AIDS in Asia: The challenge ahead*, ed. Jal P. Narciin, 67–84. New Delhi: World Health Organization Regional Office for South-East Asia, Sage.

Dong, Bian. 1955. Zenyang renshi biyun wenti (How should we think about the problem of contraception). *Xin zhongguo funu* (*Women of New China*) 4(66):27.

______. 1965. Yingai quanmian de lijie jihua shengyu (We must understand family planning from all aspects). *Women of China* 12:30.

______. 1966a. Yinggaixiang laoren he nantongzhi xuanchuan jihuashengyu (We should broadcast family planning to the old and the men). *Women of China* 4:32.

______. 1966b. Zhege tou daidehao (It is great to take the lead). *Women of China* 1:25.

Dong, Jingmin. 2005. Shoudu jichang jianqi Aizibing Jiancedian (Surveillance was established at the capital airport). *Jiankang wenzhai bao* (*Health and Digest Newspaper*), April 3:8.

Dong, Tong. 1999. Xingbaojianpin dadande xianqi gaitoulai (Lifting the veil of sex health products). *Beijing Chenbao* (*Beijing Morning Newspaper*), November 30.

Dong, Xiaoci, and Ling Wang. 2003. Zhangfu Fubai laopo guan? "Furen geming" yinfa sikao (Husbands are corrupt, should the wives be responsible? "Wife revolution" induces thinking). *Zhongguo Funu* (*Women of China*), August(1):14.

Douglas, Mary. 1991. Witchcraft and leprosy: Two strategies for rejection. *Man* 26(4):723–36.

Du, Hailan. 2004. Aizibing fangzhi de zhengcefalu yudai gaishan (Room for improvement of AIDS policies and laws). *Fazhi ribao* (*Law Daily*), December 1:5.

Dube, N., and D. Wilson. 1996. Peer education programs among HIV-vulnerable communities in Southern Africa. In *HIV/AIDS management in southern Africa: Priorities for the mining industry*, ed. Brian Williams and Catherine Campbell, 107–10. Johannesburg: Epidemiology Research Unit.

Elias, Christopher. 1991. Sexually transmitted diseases and the reproductive health of women in developing countries. Working Paper No. 5. Population Council, New York.

Elifson, Kirk W., Jacqueline Boles, William Darrow, and Claire Sterk. 1999. HIV seroprevalence and risk factors among clients of female and male prostitutes. *Journal of Acquired Immune Deficiency Syndromes and Human Retrovirology* 20:195–200.

Epstein, Helen. 2003. AIDS in South Africa: The invisible cure. *New York Review of Books* 50(11).

Esu-Williams, Eka. 1995. Clients and commercial sex work. In *HIV and AIDS, the global interconnections*, ed. Elizabeth Reid, 91–99. West Hartford, CT: Kumarian Press.

Evans, Harriet. 1997. *Women and sexuality in China: Dominant discourse on female sexuality and gender since 1949.* London: Polity Press.

Evans, Harriet. 2002. Past, perfect or imperfect: Changing images of the ideal wife. In *Chinese femininities, Chinese masculinities*, ed. Jeffrey Wasserstrom and Susan Brownell, 335–60. Berkeley: University of California Press.

Fajans, Peter, Kathleen Ford, and Dewa Nyoman Wirawan. 1995. AIDS knowledge and risk behaviors among domestic clients of female sex workers in Bali, Indonesia. *Social Science and Medicine* 41:409–17.

Fan, Guiyu. 2001. *Zhonghua shengyu wenhua daolun* (*An introduction to Chinese birth culture*). Beijing: Zhongguo renkou chubanshe (China Population Publishing House).

Fan, Hui. 2002. Anquantao guanggao mingnian zhengshi fangkai? (Will condom ads be opened up next year?). *Zhongguo xinwen wang* (*China News Net*), December 6.

Fang, Gang. 1996 Aizibing bijin zhongguo (AIDS impending China). *Women of China* (*Zhongguo Funu*) 1:24–27.

Farmer, Paul. 1992. *AIDS and accusation: Haiti and the geography of blame.* Berkeley: University of California Press.

______. 1999. *Infections and inequalities: The modern plagues.* Berkeley: University of California Press.

______. 2006. A biosocial understanding of China. In *AIDS and social policy in China*, ed. Arthur Kleinman, Joan Kaufman, and Tony Saich, x–xxii. Cambridge, MA: Harvard University Asia Center.

Farmer, Paul, Margaret Connors, and Janie Simmons, eds. 1996. *Women, poverty, and AIDS: Sex, drugs, and structural violence.* Monroe, ME: Common Courage Press.

Farmer, Paul, Shirley Lindenbaum, and Mary-Jo Delvecchio Good. 1993. Women, poverty, and AIDS: An introduction. *Cultural Medical Psychiatry* 17(4):387–97.

Farquhar, Judith. 2002. *Appetites: Food and sex in post-Socialist China.* Durham, NC: Duke University Press.

Farquhar, Judith, and Qicheng Zhang. 2005. Biopolitical Beijing: Pleasure, sovereignty, and self-cultivation in China's capital. *Cultural Anthropology* 20(3):303–27.

Farrer, James. 2002. *Youth sex culture and market reform in Shanghai.* Chicago: University of Chicago Press.

Fausto-Sterling, Anne. 2000. *Sexing the body.* New York: Basic Books.

Feldman, Douglas A., ed. 1994. *Global AIDS policy.* Westport, CT: Bergin & Garvey.

Finnane, Antonia. 1996. What should Chinese women wear? *Modern China* 22(2):99–131.

Fisher, Jeffrey D., William A. Fisher, Stephen Misovich, Diane Kimble, and Thomas Malloy. 1992. Changing AIDS-risk behavior. *Psychological Bulletin* 111:453–74.

Fisher, Jeffrey D., and Stephen J. Misovich.1992. Impact of perceived social norms on adolescents' AIDS-risk behavior and prevention. In *Adolescents and AIDS: A generation in jeopardy*, ed. Ralph J. DiClemente, 117–36. Newbury Park, CA: Sage.

Fitzgerald, John. 1996. *Awakening China, politics, culture, and class in the Nationalist Revolution.* Stanford, CA: Stanford University Press.

Flowers, Nancy. 1988. The spread of AIDS in rural Brazil. In *AIDS 1988: AAAS symposia papers*, ed. Ruth Kulstad, 159–73. Washington, DC: American Association for the Advancement of Science.

Foucault, Michel. 1978. *History of sexuality.* Vol. 1. New York: Random House.

Frankenberg, Ronnie. 1994. The impact of HIV/AIDS on concepts relating to risk and culture within British community epidemiology: Candidates or targets for prevention? *Social Science and Medicine* 38(10):325–35.

Freire, Paulo. 1970. *Pedagogy of the oppressed.* New York: Herder and Herder.

Furth, Charlotte. 1992. Chinese medicine and the anthropology of menstruation in contemporary Taiwan. *Medical Anthropology Quarterly* 6(1):27–48.

______. 1994. Rethinking Van Gulik: Sexuality and reproduction in traditional Chinese medicine. In *Endangering China: Women, culture, and the state*, ed. Gail Hershatter, Christina K. Gilmartin, Lisa Rofel, and Tyrene White, 125–46. Cambridge, MA: Harvard University Press.

Gao, Dewei. 2000. *Qingchun renge yu xingjiankang jiaoyu* (*Youth personality and sex health education*). Beijing: Beijing Xingjiankang Jiaoyu Yanjiuhui (Beijing Sex Health Education Research Association).

Gao, Ersheng, Shaobo Xiao, Junqing Wu, and Wei Yuan. 2002. *Biyun jieyu youzhi fuwu yu zhiqing xuanze* (*Excellent contraceptive service and client-based choice*). Beijing: Zhongguo Renkou Chubanshe.

Gao, Tian. 1919. Xing zhi sheng wu xue (Biology of sex). *Xin Qing Nian* (*New Youth*) 8(6):1–12.

Gao, Yaowu. 1998. Funu hunnei xingquanli xuyao falu baohu (Women's sex rights in marriage needs legal protection). *Women of China* 8:50–51.

Ge, Zihong. 2006. Shenyang shouli Aizibing ganranzhe shinianlai shenghuo Zhengchang (The first AIDS inflected in Shenyang has led a normal life for ten years). China.com.cn.

Geng, Xuebao. 1964. Yao hezuo, yao jianchi (Necessary cooperation and resolution). *Women of China* 9:26.

Giffin, Karen, and Catherine M. Lowndes. 1999. Gender, sexuality, and the prevention of sexually transmissible diseases: A Brazilian study of clinical practice. *Social Science and Medicine* 48:283–92.

Gil, Vincent E., Marco Wang, Allen F. Anderson, and Guao Matthew Lin. 1994. Plum blossoms and pheasants: Prostitutes, prostitution, and social control measures in contemporary China. *International Journal of Offender Therapy and Comparative Criminology* 38(4):319–37.

Gill, Bates, Jennifer Chang, and Sarah Palmer. 2002. China's HIV crisis. *Foreign Affairs,* March–April:96–110.

Glick-Schiller, N. 1992. What's wrong with this picture? The hegemonic construction of culture in AIDS research in the United States. *Medical Anthropology Quarterly* 6(3):237–54.

Gomez, Cynthia A., and Barbara M. VanOss. 1996. Gender, culture, and power: Barriers to HIV-prevention strategies for women. *Journal of Sex Research* 33(4):355–62.

Goodkind, Daniel. 1997. Reasons for rising condom use in Vietnam. *International Family Planning Perspectives* 23:173–78.

Gordon, Linda, ed. 1979. *The struggle for reproductive freedom: Three stages of feminism.* New York: Monthly Review Press.

Gossett, Milton, and Jeremy Warshaw. 1992. The New York City campaign. In *AIDS: Prevention through education,* ed. Jaime Sepulveda et al., 283–96. New York: Oxford University Press.

Green, Edward, Janice A. Hogle, Vinand Nantulya, Rand Stoneburner, and John Stover. 2002. *What happened in Uganda? Declining HIV prevalence, behavior change, and the national response.* Washington, DC: U.S. Agency for International Development.

Greenhalgh, Susan, and Edwin A. Winckler. 2005. *Governing China's population.* Stanford, CA: Stanford University Press.

Gu, Sujuan. 1981. Tan jishu yuanyin (On technological reasons). *Women of China* 2:43.

Gu, Zhen. 1956a. Biyun yingxiang jiankang ma (Does contraception affect health). *Women of China* 7:26.

______. 1956b. Buyao suibian quzuo rengong liuchan (Don't do abortions casually). *Women of China* 6:24.

Guan, Shan. 2001. Buxiangxin Yanlei (I do not believe in tears). In *Yi lu ben zou* (*Marching on*), 18–143. Beijing: Huayi Chubanshe (Huayi Publishing House).

Guo, Huimin. 2002. Waiyu, ke raoshu de zui (Extramarital affairs are forgivable). *Zhongguo Funu* (*Women of China*) 8(2):28–29.

Gupta, Geeta Rao, and Ellen Weiss. 1993. Women's lives and sex: Implications for AIDS prevention. *Cultural Medical Psychiatry* 17(4):399–412.

Gutmann, Matthew. 2007. *Fixing men: Sex, birth control, and AIDS in Mexico.* Berkeley: University of California Press.

Guttmacher, Sally, et al. 1997. Condom availability in New York City Public high schools: Relationships to condom use and sexual behavior. *American Journal of Public Health* 87:1427–33.

Hammar, Lydia. 1996. Bad canoes and bafalo: The political economy of sex on Daru Island, Western Province, Papua New Guinea. *Gender* 23:212–43.

Handwerker, Lisa. 1995. The hen that can't lay an egg: Conceptions of female infertility in modern China. In *Deviant bodies: Critical perspectives on difference in science and popular culture,* ed. Jennifer Terry and Jacqueline Urla. Bloomington: Indiana University Press.

Hanenberg, R. S., W. Rojanapithayakorn, P. Kunasol, and D. C. Sokal. 1994. Impact of Thailand's HIV-control program as indicated by the decline of sexually transmitted diseases. *Lancet* 344(8917):243–45.

Hansen, Helena, Maria Margarita Lopez-Iftikhar, and Margarita Alegria. 2002. The economy of risk and respect: Accounts by Puerto Rican sex workers of HIV risk taking. *Journal of Sex Research* 39(4):292–301.

Hao, Baiyu. 2005. Wen jiabao tichufangzhi aizibing de jiuxiang cuoshi (Wenjiabao proposed nine measures). *Dalian Daily,* June 16:A6.

Hart, G. J., R. Pool, G. Green, S. Harrison, S. Nyanzi, and J. A. Whitworth. 1999. Women's attitudes to condoms and female-controlled means of protection against HIV and AIDS in south-western Uganda. *AIDS Care* 11(6):687–98.

He, Chisheng. 1964. Zhe shi zisi zili de si xiang (This is a selfish thought). *Women of China* 8:30.

He, Mu. 2003. Waiyuzhong de Xingyinsu (The element of sex in extramarital affairs). *Jiatingshenghuo zhinan* (*Direction to Family Life*) 8(218):52–53.

He, Sanwei. 2005. Aizinusheng de qiqie zhuiwen (The sad questions of an AIDS female student). *Nanfang zhoumo* (*Southern Weekend*), June 23:1.

Hearst, Norman, and Sanity Chen. 2004. Condom promotion for AIDS prevention in the developing world: Is it working? *Studies in Family Planning* 35(1):39–47.

Henrickson, Mark. 1990. A mobile HIV education, counseling, and testing unit: A pilot initiative. *AIDS Education Review* 2(2):137–44.

Henriot, Christian. 2001. *Prostitution and sexuality in Shanghai: A social history, 1849–1949.* Cambridge: Cambridge University Press.

Herdt, Gilbert, ed. 1996. *Third sex, third gender.* New York: Zone Books.

Herdt, Gilbert, and Andrew Boxer. 1991. Ethnographic issues in the study of AIDS. *Journal of Sexual Research* 28(2):171–87.

Herdt, Gilbert, and Shirley Lindenbaum. 1992a. Sexual identity and risk for AIDS among gay youth in Chicago. In *Sexual behavior and networking: Anthropological and socio-cultural studies on the transmission of HIV,* ed. Tim Dyson, 153–202. Liege: Derouaz-Ordina.

______, ed. 1992b. *The time of AIDS: Social analysis, theory, and method.* Newbury Park, CA: Sage.

Herdt, Gilbert, William L. Leap, and Melanie Sovine. 1991. Anthropology, sexuality and AIDS. *Journal of Sex Research* 28(2):167–69.

Hershatter, Gail. 1986. *The workers of Tianjin, 1900–1949*. Stanford, CA: Stanford University Press.

______. 1997. *Dangerous pleasures: Prostitution and modernity in twentieth-century Shanghai*. Berkeley: University of California Press.

Hershatter, Gail, and Emily Honig. 1988. *Personal voices: Chinese women in the 1980s*. Stanford, CA: Stanford University Press.

Hillier, Lynne, Lyn Harrison, and Deborah Warr. 1998. When you carry condoms all the boys think that you want it: Negotiating competing discourses about safe sex. *Journal of Adolescence* 21:15–29.

Himes, Norman E. 1963. *Medical history of contraception*. New York: Gamut Press.

Holland, Janet, Caroline Ramazanoglu, Sue Scott, Sue Sharpe, and Rachel Thomson. 1990. Sex, gender and power: Young women's sexuality in the shadow of AIDS. *Sociology of Health and Illness* 12:336–50.

______. 1991. Between embarrassment and trust: Young women and the diversity of condom use. In *AIDS: Responses, interventions, and care*, ed. Peter Aggelton, 127–48. London: Falmer Press.

______. 1992a. Pleasure, pressure, and power: Some contradictions of gendered sexuality. *Sociological Review* 40:645–74.

______. 1992b. Risk, power, and the possibility of pleasure: Young women and safer sex. *AIDS Care* 4(3):273–83.

______. 1994a. Achieving masculine sexuality: Young men's strategies for managing vulnerability. In *AIDS: Setting a feminist agenda*, ed. Tamsin Wilton. Southport: Taylor & Francis.

______. 1994b. Desire, risk, and control: The body as a site of contestation. In *AIDS: Setting a feminist agenda*, ed. Lesley Doyal and Tamsin Wilton, 61–79. Southport: Taylor & Francis.

Honig, Emily. 1986. *Sisters and strangers: Women in the Shanghai cotton mills, 1919–1949*. Stanford, CA: Stanford University Press.

Hsu, Mei-Ling, Wen-Chi Lin, and Tsui-Sung Wu. 2004. Representations of "Us" and "Others" in the AIDS news discourse: A Taiwanese experience. In *Sexual cultures in East Asia*, ed. Evelyne Micollier, 183–222. London: RoutledgeCurzon.

Hu, Xiaoyun. 2005. Xiaochu Aizibing qishi, luhai henyuan (A long road to eliminating prejudice against AIDS patient). *Jiankang wenzhai bao* (*Health Digest Newspaper*), May 10:1.

Huang, Shirlena, and Brenda S. A. Yeoh. 2008. Heterosexualities and the global(ising) city in Asia: Introduction. *Asian Studies Review* 32(March):1–6.

Hubbard, Philip. 2000. Desire/disgust: Mapping the moral contours of heterosexuality. *Progress in Human Geography* 24(2):191–17.

Hunt, Charles W. 1996. Social vs. biological: Theories on the transmission of AIDS in Africa. *Social Science and Medicine* 42(9):1283–96.

Hunter, Susan S. 2005. *AIDS in Asia: A continent in peril*. New York: Palgrave Macmillan.

Hyde, Sandra Teresa. 2007. *Eating spring rice: The cultural politics of AIDS in southwest China*. Berkeley: University of California Press.

Ibañez, Gladys E., Barbara Oss Marin, Cristina Villareal, and Cynthia Gomez. 2005. Condom use at last sex among unmarried Latino men: An event level analysis. *AIDS and Behavior* 9(4):433–41.

Inciardi, James A., Hilary L. Surratt, and Paulo R. Telles. 2000. *Sex, drugs, and HIV/AIDS in Brazil*. Boulder, CO: Westview Press.

Ingham, Roger, Alison Woodcock, and Karen Stenner. 1991. Getting to know you . . . young people's knowledge of their partners at first intercourse. *Journal of Community and Applied Social Psychology* 1(2):117–32.

International Council on Adolescent Fertility. 1989. Media as messengers: Shaping programs to entertain and educate. *Passages: International Council on Adolescent Fertility* 9(1):1–4.

Jeffrey, Leslie Ann. 2002. *Sex and borders: Gender, national identity, and prostitution policy in Thailand*. Vancouver: University of British Columbia Press.

Jeffreys, Elaine. 2004. *China, sex, and prostitution*. London: RoutledgeCurzon.

______, ed. 2006. *Sex and sexuality in China*. Abingdon: Routledge.

Ji, Xiangde. 2005. Hunnei qiangjian lilun de lilun yuandian (The theoretical base of marital rape). *Zhongguo Faxuewang* (*Chinese Law Net*), September 8.

Jian, Ping. 2001. Caifang shouji: Jingyan Dalian (Interview memoirs in Dalian). *Xinzhoukan* (*New Weekly*) 10:44.

Jiang, Deyuan, Shuquan Qu, Wei Liu, Kyung-Hee Choi, Rongjian Li, Deyuan Jiang, Yuejiao Zhou, et al. 2002. The potential for rapid sexual transmission of HIV in China: Sexually transmitted diseases and condom failure highly prevalent among female sex workers. *AIDS and Behavior* 6(3):267–75.

Jiang, Xiaoyuan. 2003. *Xing gan, Sex: Yizhong wenhua jieshi* (*Sexy, sex: One kind of cultural interpretations*). Haikou: Hainan chubanshe.

Jiang, Yunfei. 2005. Ezhi Aizi, lvxing chengnuo (Curbing AIDS infection, implementing promise). *Dalian Ribao* (*Dalian Daily*).

Jiang, Zongtao. 1966. Ta zhenshi ge guanxin sheyuan de haoganbu (She is a good cadre concerned about other members). *Women of China* 1:25.

Jin, Gege. 2003. Baozhu zhangfu de yanmian (Protecting the face of the husband). *Zhongguo Funu* (*Women of China*) 10(2):37.

Jin, Ying. 2002. Anquantao guanggao (Condom Ads). *Xinwen Zhoukan* (*News Weekly*), November 27.

Jing, Feng. 2004. Fafang anquantao juefei "Fang AI" quanbu (Issuing condoms is by no means the complete AIDS prevention). *Xinhuawang* (*Xinhua Net*), November 30.

Jing, Jun. 2006. The social origin of AIDS panics in China. In *AIDS and social policy in China*, ed. Arthur Kleinman, Joan Kaufman, and Tony Saich, 152–69. Cambridge, MA: Harvard University Asia Center.

Ju, Liya. 2006. *Diary of AIDS female university student*. Beijing: Beijing Publishing House.

Kaler, Amy. 2004. The moral lens of population control: Condoms and controversies in southern Malawi. *Studies in Family Planning* 35:105–15.

Kammerer, Cornelia Ann, Otome Klein Hutheesing, Ralana Maneeprasert, and Patricia V. Symonds. 1995. Vulnerability to HIV infection among three hill tribes in northern Thailand. In *Culture and sexual risk*, ed. Han ten Brummelhuis and Gilbert H. Herdt, 53–75. Amsterdam: Gordon & Breach.

Kapumba, Sipo, V. Manda, and R. Zambezi. 1991. *Focus group research on condom use for AIDS prevention*. Ndola: Planned Parenthood Association of Zambia.

Katende, Charles, Ruth Knight, Reeru Gupta, Rodney Knight, and Cheryl Lettenmaier. 2000. *Uganda delivery of improved services for health evaluation surveys 1999*. Chapel Hill, NC: Measure Evaluation.

Kaufman, Joan, and Jun Jing. 2002. China and AIDS—The time to act is now. *Science* 296(June 28):2339–40.

Kaufman, Joan, Arthur Kleinman, and Tony Saich, eds. 2006a. *AIDS and social policy in China*. Cambridge, MA: Harvard University Asia Center.

______. 2006b. Introduction: AIDS and social policy in China. In *AIDS and social policy in China*, ed. Arthur Kleinman Joan Kaufman, and Tony Saich, 3–14. Cambridge, MA: Harvard University Asia Center.

Kaufman, Joan, and Kathrine Meyers. 2006. AIDS surveillance in China: Data gaps and research for AIDS policy. In *AIDS and social policy in China*, ed. Arthur Kleinman, Joan Kaufman, and Tony Saich. Cambridge, MA: Harvard University Asia Center.

Kegeles, Susan M., R. Greenblatt, J. Catania, C. Cardenas, J. Gottlieb, and T. Coates. 1989. AIDS risk behavior among sexually active Hispanic and white adolescent females. Fifth International Conference on AIDS, Montreal.

Keller, Sarah N., and Jane Brown. 2002. Media interventions to promote responsible sexual behavior. *Journal of Sex Research* 39(1):67–72.

Kelly, J. A. 1992. AIDS prevention: Strategies that work. *The AIDS Reader*, July–August:135–41.

Kelly, Paula-Frances, ed. 2004. *What is known about gender, the constructs of sexuality, and dictates of behavior in Vietnam as a Confucian and socialist society and their impact on the risk of HIV/AIDS epidemic*. New York: RoutledgeCurzon.

Kerriga, Deanna, Jonathan Ellen, Luis Moreno, Santo Rosario, Joanne Katz, David Celentano, and Michael Sweat. 2003. Environmental-structural factors significantly associated with consistent condom use among female sex workers in the Dominican Republic. *AIDS* 17:415–23.

Kirby, Douglas, Nancy Brener, Nancy Brown, Nancy Peterfreund, Pamela Hillard, and Ron Harrist. 1998. The impact of condom distribution in Seattle schools on sexual behavior and condom use. *American Journal of Public Health* 89:182–87.

Klein, Megan. 2001. Social marketing and communications for health determinants of condom use among unmarried youth in Yaounde and Douala. PSI Research Division Working Paper No. 47. PSI (Population Services International), Washington, DC.

Klein, Megan, and Y. Coombes. 1999. *Trust and condom use: The role of sexual caution and sexual assurances for Tanzanian youth*. PSC Research Division Working Paper No. 64. PSI (Population Services International), Washington, DC.

Knodel, John, and Anthony Pramualratana. 1994. *Prospects for increased condom use in marital unions in Thailand*. PSC Research Report No. 95-337. PSC Research Division Working Paper No. 64. PSI (Population Services International), Washington, DC.

Ko, Dorothy. 1994. *Teachers of the inner chambers: Women and culture in seventeenth century China*. Stanford, CA: Stanford University Press.

Koetswang, Suporn, and N. J. Ford. 1999. *A self-esteem and personal future-focused intervention programme to promote condom use by female sex workers in Thailand*. Nakhon Pathom, Thailand: Institute for Population and Social Research, Mahidol University.

Ku, Andrzej. 2004. The sociocultural context of condom use within marriage in rural Lebanon. *Family Planning* 35141:246–60.

Kuang, Caiwei. 1979. Wei sihua zhisheng yige zinu guangrong (It is glorious to give birth to one child for four modernizations). *Women of China* 8:24.

Lamptey, Peter, and Gail A. W. Goodridge. 1991. Condom issues in AIDS prevention in Africa. *AIDS* 5(Suppl. 1):S183–S191.

Lan, Huaisi. 2006. Directing a perfect sex (Daoyan yichang wanmei xingai). *Hers* 2(20):182–84.

Lane, Sandra D. 1997. Television minidramas: Social marketing and evaluation in Egypt. *Medical Anthropology Quarterly* 11(2):164–82.

Lang, Jinghe. 1980. Yousheng de diyibu—Hunqian jiancha (The first step in eugenics: Premarital test). *Women of China* 8:46–47.

Lao, Yu. 2005. Tantao jinji biyunyao de daodewenti (On the moral issues of emergency contraceptives). *Xin zhoukan* (*New Weekly*), November 2.

Laqueur, Thomas. 1990. *Making sex: Body and gender from the Greeks to Freud.* Cambridge, MA: Harvard University Press.

Larson, Wendy. 2002. The self-loving the self: Men and connoisseurship in modern Chinese literature. In *Chinese femininities, Chinese masculinities,* ed. Jeffrey Wasserstrom and Susan Brownell, 175–94. Berkeley: University of California Press.

Lau, Joseph I. E., A. S. Tang, and H. Y. Tsui. 2003. The relationship between condom use, sexually transmitted diseases, and location of commercial sex transaction among male Hong Kong clients. *AIDS* 17:105–12.

Law, Lisa. 2000. *Sex work in Southeast Asia: The place of desire in a time of AIDS.* London: Routledge.

Lear, Dana. 1995. Sexual communication in the age of AIDS: The construction of risk and trust among young adults. *Social Science and Medicine* 41:1311–23.

Leclerc-Madlala, Suzanne. 2001. Virginity testing: Managing sexuality in a maturing HIV/AIDS epidemic. *Medical Anthropology Quarterly* 15:533–52.

Lee, Ching Kwan. 1998. *Gender and the South China miracle.* Berkeley: University of California Press.

Lei, Jieqiong. 1957. He nianqingren tan hunshi (Talking about marriage with young people). *Women of China* 4:24–25.

Lei, Zhenwu. 1979. Shouren kuazai de jieyu cuoshi (Applaudable birth control measures). *Women of China* 11:45.

Lewin, Kurt. 1958. The group reason and social change. In *Readings in social psychology,* ed. Eleanor Maccoby. London: Holt, Rinehart and Winston.

Li, Fei. 1958. *Xingzhishi wenda (Questions and answers of sex knowledge).* Baoding: Hebei Renmin Chubanshe.

Li, Jinxing. 2000. Jinanshi shouli HIV-1 ganranzhe diaochabaogao (Report of HIV-1 infected people in Jinan). *Zhongguo Xingbing Aizibing Fangzhi (Prevention of STI and AIDS in China)* 6(2):113.

Li, Qingshan. 2005. Guilin gongshang (Guilin industrial commerce). *Zhongguo Xiaofeizhe Bao (Chinese Consumer Newspaper),* July 25.

Li, Shunlai. 2000. Anquantao Guanggao Women Zai Dengdai (We are waiting for condom ads). *Zhongguo Funu bao (Chinese Women Newspaper),* April 11.

Li, Tong. 2001. Falu gaibugai gei anquantao yige mingfen? (Should the law give condom a name?). *Beijing Qingnian Bao (Beijing Youth Newspaper),* September 7.

Li, Xiaofeng, Li Ma, Xiaohong Gao, Cuili Zhang, Shu Zhang, and Chengzhi Lv. 2004. 1999, 2000 Nian Dalian shi xingbing liuxingbingxue fenxi (An epidemiological analysis of STIs in Dalian in 1999 and 2000). *Shiyong Yufang Yixue (Pragmatic Prevention Medicine)* 3:16–17.

Li, Xiongqiong. 1957. Woneng daying tade yaoqiu ma (Can I say yes to his request?). *Women of China* 3:14–15.

Li, Yali. 2002. Bamitude zhangfu daihuijia (Bring back the astraying husband). *Zhongguo Funu (Women of China)* 8(2):26–28.

Li, Yaling. 1999. Kaojin mingpai daxue liangcaizi bei xiaojie yinyou ranshang linbing (An outstanding student in a key university is seduced by a hostess and contracted a STD). *Chengdu Shangbao (Chengdu Commerce Newspaper),* 2.

Li, Yanchun. 2004. Anquantao anweibuliao posuidexin (Condom cannot comfort a broken heart). *Beijing Qingnianbao (Beijing Youth Newspaper),* November 29.

Li, Yinhe. 2002. Anquantao lunzheng de beihou (Behind the debate of condoms). *21 shiji huanqiu baodao (Report Around the World in the 21st Century),* December 26.

Li, Zengqing. 2003. Daxuesheng hunqian xingxingwei, tongju xianxiang sikao (Thoughts on cohabitation and sex conducts of college students). *Jiatingbaojian (Family Health)* 12:22–23.

Li, Zhongfeng. 2004. Wuyouwulu de ai diaocha: Anquantao Guanggao (Love without worries: Condom ads). *Shichang Bao (Market Newspaper),* July 11.

Li, Zhongmao. 2005. Zhongguo de sici xinggeming (Four sex revolutions in China). *Wenzhai Zhoubao (Digest Weekly Newspaper),* June 7:1.

Liang, Jun, and Kongling Xu. 1997. Jihuashengyu yu funushengyujiankang zhi libi (The drawback and benefit of family planning to women). In *Shengyu de Chuantong yu Xiandaihua (The tradition of reproduction and modernization),* ed. Xiaojiang Li, 42–54. Zhengzhou: Henan Renmin Chubanshe.

Liang, Qiusheng, and Che-Fu Lee. 2006. Fertility and population policy: An overview. In *Fertility, family planning, and population policy in China,* ed. Dudley L. Poston, Chiung-Fang Chang, Che-Fu Lee, Sherry L. McKibben, and Carol S. Walther, 8–20. London: Routledge.

Liang, Yong. 2003. Anquantao guanggao shang yangshi shiguanniande jinbu (It is ideological progress for condom ads to be on CCTV). *Xinhuawang (Xinhua Net),* November 28.

Liang, Zhao. 1957. Jihua shengyu bing bunan (It is not difficult to have family planning). *Women of China* 4:25.

Lin, Ho Swee. 2008. Private love in public space: Love hotels and the transformation of intimacy in contemporary Japan. *Asian Studies Review* 32(March):31–56.

Lin, Minduo. 2005. Ezhi gaoweirenqun aizibing chuanbo de sikao (Reflections on blocking HIV/AIDS high risk population). In *Zhongguo Aizibing fangzhi (Prevention of HIV/AIDS in China).* Beijing: Capital University of Medical Science.

Lin, Peng, and Hua Wang. 2000. Guangdongsheng HIV/AIDS jiancexitong de jianli jiqi xiaoguopingjia (Guangdong HIV/AIDS surveillance system). *Zhongguo Xingbing Aizibing Fangzhi (Prevention of STI and AIDS in China)* 6(3):133–34.

Lin, Quanyi. 2002. Training on condom social marketing conducted in Urumqi, Xinjiang. International Conference on AIDS, Manchester, July 7–12.

Lin, Wei. 1998. Biyuntao nengzuo guanggao ma? (Can condoms be advertised?). *Zhongguo Qingnian Bao (China Youth Daily),* December 4.

Lindan, Christina, S. Allen, M. Carael, F. Nsengumuremyi, P. Van de Perre, A. Serufilira, J. Tice, D. Black, et al. 1991. Knowledge, attitudes, and perceived risk of AIDS among urban Rwandan women: Relationship to HIV infection and behavior change. *AIDS* 5(8):993–1002.

Lindenbaum, Shirley. 1997. AIDS: Body, mind, and history. In *AIDS in Africa and the Caribbean*, ed. George C. Bond, John Kreniske, Ida Susser, and Joan Vincent, 191–94. Boulder, CO: Westview.

______. 1998. Images of catastrophe: The making of an epidemic. In *The political economy of AIDS*, ed. Merrill Singer, 33–58. Amityville, NY: Baywood.

Ling, Feng. 2004. Wuzhi jiaju "Kongai Zheng" (Ignorance exacerbate paranoid of AIDS). *Jiankang bao* (*Health Newspaper*), November 29:1.

Ling, Yun. 2003. Gaozhi fuqi tongshuo hunwaiqing (Speaking of extramarital affairs). Zhongguo Funu (*Women of China*) 1(2):34.

Little, J. 2003. Riding the rural love train: Heterosexuality and the rural community. *Sociologia Ruralis* 43(4):401–17.

Liu, Dalin, et al. 1997. *Sexual behaviour in modern China*. New York: Continuum.

Liu, Huizhen. 1966. Shishuo buru yizuo (Ten speeches speak lower than one deed). *Women of China* 1:24.

Liu, Jianlin. 1999. Sanpeinu chengwei fanzui gaofa qunti (The highest crime rate is found in the group of bar hostesses). In *Zhongguo Qingnianbao* (*Chinese Youth Newspaper*), 3.

Liu, Jianqiang. 2005 Zhongyang dangxiaoli de aizi guannian jiaofeng (Conflict of views on AIDS in central party schools). *Nanfang Zhoumo* (*South Weekend*), June 23:A6.

Liu, Jiansheng. 2004. Qieshijiaqiang aizibing fangzhi gongzuo (Strengthening AIDS prevention work). *Fazhi Ribao* (*Law Daily*), December 1:1.

Liu, Wei, and Zhou Yuejiao. 2001. Evaluation of an intervention designed to reduce risk behaviors among woman engaged in illegal commercial sex activities in frontier areas of Guangxi province. *Chinese Journal of STD/AIDS Prevention and Control* 4:223–25.

Liu, Xingyu, and Jiang Xu. 2005. Hunyin: Nurende quanli he zeren (Marriage: Women's rights and responsibilities). *Zhongguo Funu* (*Women of China*), April 2(647):32–33.

Liu, Yuanli, and Joan Kaufman. 2006. Controlling HIV/AIDS in China: Health system challenges. In *AIDS and social policy in China*, ed. Arthur Kleinman, Joan Kaufman, and Tony Saich, 75–95. Cambridge, MA: Harvard University Asia Center.

Liu, Zhen. 2002. Feifatongju: Weixiandeshishang (Illegal cohabitation: Dangerous style). *Zhongguo Funu* (*Women of China*) 6:18.

Liu, Zheng, and Cangping Wu. 1979. Funumen, zhengdang jihua shengyu gongzuo de cujin pai (Women, fight as the harbinger of family planning). *Women of China* 8:22–23.

Liu, Ziliang. 2004. Zhimian Aizi (Confronting AIDS). In *Mianduimian* (*Face to Face*), ed. Jianzeng Liang, 149–62. Changchun: Jilin Renmin Chubanshe.

Longfield, Kim, Megan Klein, and Joh Berman. 2002. *Criteria for trust and how trust affects sexual decision-making among youth*. Washington, DC: Population Services International.

Luo, Gang. 2005a. E zhu AIDS manyan de yanhou (Strangle the throat of AIDS transmission). *Jiankang Wenzhai Bao* (*Health and Digest Newspaper*), no. 709 (March 20):8.

______. 2005b. Wo jiu zai ni shenpao (I am right by your side). *Jiankang Bao* (*Health Newspaper*), April 20:7.

Lupton, Deborah. 1994. *Moral themes and dangerous desires: AIDS in the news media*. London: Taylor & Francis.

Lyttleton, Chris. 1996. Health and development: Knowledge systems and local practice in rural Thailand. *Health Transition Review* 6(1):25–48.

Ma, Jinyu. 2005. Yuaizibing nudaxuesheng mianduimian: Zai aiqingzhong shalu qingchun (Facing an AIDS female university student: Killing the youth in love). *Nanfang Renwuzhoukan* (*South Weekly*), June 3:4.

Ma, Qinghuai. 1954. Lenin talks about the issue of women, marriage and sex. *Xin Zhongguo Funu* (*New Women of China*) 51(1):6–7.

Macaluso, M., M. J. Demand, L. M. Artz, and E. W. Hook. 2000. Partner type and condom use. *AIDS* 14:537–46.

MacPhail, Catherine, and Catherine Campbell. 2001. I think condoms are good but, aai, I hate those things: Condom use among adolescents and young people in a Southern African township. *Social Science and Medicine* 52:1613–27.

Maharaj, Pranitha. 2001. Obstacles to negotiating dual protection: Perspectives of men and women. *African Journal of Reproductive Health* 5(3):150–61.

______. 2004. Perception of risk of HIV infection in marital and cohabiting partnerships. *African Journal of AIDS Research* 3(2):131–43.

Maharaj, Pranitha, and John Cleland. 2004. Condom use within marital and cohabitating partnerships in Kwa-Zulu-Natal, South Africa. *Studies in Family Planning* 35(2):116–24.

Mahler, K. 1996 Condom use increase in Norway appears related more to contraception than to disease prevention. *Family Planning Perspectives* 28(2):82–83.

Mann, Jonathan. 1996. *Human rights and AIDS: The future of the pandemic*. New York: Plenum.

Mann, Susan. 1997. *Precious records: Women in China's long eighteenth century*. Stanford, CA: Stanford University Press.

Marandu, Edward E., and Mbaki A. Chamme. 2004. Attitudes towards condom use for prevention of HIV infection in Botswana. *Social Behavior and Personality* 32(5):491–510.

Martin, Barbara Van Oss, and Cynthia A. Gomez. 1996. Latino culture and sex: Implications for HIV Prevention. In *Psychological interventions and research with Latino populations*, ed. Jorge G. Garcia Maria Cecilia Zea, 73–93. Needham Heights, MA: Allyn and Bacon.

Maticka-Tyndale, Eleanor. 1991. Sexual scripts and AIDS prevention: Variations in adherence to safer-sex guidelines by heterosexual adolescents. *Journal of Sex Research* 28:45–66.

______. 1992. Social construction of HIV transmission and prevention among heterosexual young adults. *Social Problems* 39:238–52.

Maticka-Tyndale, Eleanor, David Elkins, Melissa Haswell-Elkins, Darunee Rujkarakorn, Thicumporn Kuyyakanond, and Kathryn Stam. 1997. Contexts and patterns of men's commercial sexual partnerships in northeastern Thailand: Implications for AIDS prevention. *Social Science and Medicine* 44(2):199–213.

Matuszak, Sascha. 2003. Safe sex in China. Antiwar.com, June 13.

McGrath, Janet. 1993. Anthropology and AIDS. *Social Science and Medicine* 36(4):429–39.

McMahon, James M., Stephanie Tortu, Enrique R. Pouget, Rahul Hamid, and Alan Neaigus. 2006. Contextual determinants of condom use among female sex exchanges in East Harlem, NYC: An event analysis. *AIDS and Behavior*, June 16:731–41.

McMillan, Jo. 2006. Selling sexual health: China's emerging sex shop industry. In *Sex and sexuality in China*, ed. Elaine Jeffreys, 124–38. London: Routledge.

Meekers, Dominique. 1999. Patterns of use of the female condom in urban Zimbabwe. PSI Research Division Working Paper No. 28. PSI (Population Services International), Washington, DC.

Mehryar, Amir. 1995. Condoms: Awareness, attitudes, and use. In *Sexual behavior and AIDS in the developing world*, ed. John Cleland and Benoit Ferry, 124–56. London: Taylor & Francis.

Meng, Tie. 2006. Yeti anquantao neng shamie bingdu (Liquid condoms can kill viruses). *Hangzhou Ribao* (*Hangzhou Daily*), August 9.

Messersmith, Lisa J., Thomas T. Kane, Adetanwa I. Odebiyi, and Alfred A. Adewuyi. 2000. Who's at risk? Men's STD experience and condom use in southwest Nigeria. *Studies in Family Planning* 31(September):203–16.

Micollier, Evelyne. 2003. HIV/AIDS-related stigmatization in Chinese society: Bridging the gap between official responses and civil society: A cultural approach to HIV/AIDS prevention and care. UNESCO/UNAIDS Research Project No. 20. Paris: UNESCO.

______, ed. 2004a. *Sexual cultures in East Asia*. New York: RoutledgeCurzon.

______, ed. 2004b. Social significance of commercial sex work: Implicitly shaping a sexual culture? In *Sexual cultures in East Asia*, ed. Evelyne Micollier, 1–23. New York: RoutledgeCurzon.

______. 2005a. AIDS in China: Discourses on sexuality and sexual practices. *China Perspectives* 60:2–14.

______. 2005b. Collective mobilisation and transnational solidarity to combat AIDS in China: Local dynamics and visibility of groups sexual and social minorities. *Perspectives on Health* 7:30–38.

______. 2006. Sexualities and HIV/AIDS vulnerability in China, an anthropological perspective. *Sexologies* 15:192–201.

Middel, Anne. 2001. Interpretations of condom use and nonuse among young Norwegian gay men: A qualitative study. *Medical Anthropology Quarterly* 15(1):58–83.

Miller, Maureen, and Alan Neaigus. 2002. An economy of risk: Resource acquisition strategies of inner city women who use drugs. *International Journal of Drug Policy* 13(5):409–18.

Mills, Singh, P. Benjarattanaporn, A. Bennett, R. N. Pattalung, D. Sundhagul, P. Trongsawad, S. E. Gregorich, N. Hearst, and J. S. Mandel. 1997. HIV risk behavioral surveillance in Bangkok, Thailand: Sexual behavior trends among eight population groups. *AIDS* 11(Suppl. 1):S43–S51.

Mnyinka, K. S., G Kvale, and K. I. Klepp. 1995. Perceived function of and barriers to condom use in Arusha and Kilimanjaro regions of Tanzania. *AIDS Care* 7(3):295–305.

Mo, Yunshi. 1964. Xiading juexin, yangcheng xiguan (Make a determination, form a habit). *Women of China* 5(31).

Molm, Linda, Nobuyuki Takahashi, and Gretchen Peterson. 2000. Risk and trust in social exchange: An experimental test of a classical proposition. *American Journal of Sociology* 105:1396–1427.

Moore, Susan, and Doreen Rosenthal. 1992. The social context of adolescent sexuality: Safe sex implications. *Journal of Adolescence* 15:415–35.

Morris, Martina, Anthony Pramualratana, Chai Podhisita, and M. J. Wawer. 1995. The relational determinants of condom use with commercial sex partners in Thailand. *AIDS* 9(5):507–15.

Mosse, George L. 1985. *Nationalism and sexuality*. Madison: University of Wisconsin Press.

Mukasa, Rebecca, Janet W. McGrath, Charles B. Rwabukwali, Debra A. Schumann, Jonnie Pearson-Marks, Barbara Namande, Sylvia Nakayiwa, and Lucy Nakyobe. 1992. Cultural determinants of sexual risk behavior for AIDS among Baganda women. *Medical Anthropology Quarterly* 6(2):153–61.

Ngai, Pun. 2005. *Made in China: Women factory workers in a global workplace*. Durham, NC: Duke University Press.

Nie, Jing-bao. 2005. *Behind the silence: Chinese voices on abortion*. New York: Rowman & Littlefield.

Nie, Mao. 2004. *Aifengle, lefengle* (*Love is crazy*). Beijing: Minzu Chubanshe.

Obbo, Christine. 1995 Gender, age, and class: Discourses on HIV transmission and control in Uganda. In *Culture and sexual risk: Anthropological perspectives on AIDS*, ed. Han ten Brummelhuis and Gilbert Herdt, 79–95. Amsterdam: Gordon & Breach.

Oladosu, Muyiwa. 2001. Consistent condom use among sex workers in Nigeria. PSI Research Division Working Paper No. 39. PSI (Population Services International), Washington, DC.

O'Leary, Ann. 2000. Women at risk for HIV from a primary partner: Balancing risk and intimacy. *Annual Review of Sex Research* 11:191–234.

Pan, Jianqing. 2005. Qiantan "hunnei qiangjian" (Discussion of "marital rape"). *Jiaxing Sifa Xingzhengwang (Jianxing Law Executive)* 11:12–30.

Pan, Mingxin. 2004. Anquan tao-anquan fangbian kuaile (Condom—Safe, convenient, and happy). *Shenghuo yu Jiankang (Life and Health)* 2:51.

Pan, Suiming. 2006. Transformation in the primary life cycle: The origins and nature of China's sexual revolution. In *Sex and sexuality in China*, ed. Elaine Jeffreys, 21–42. London: Routledge.

______. 2007. HIV and FSWs. Seminar on HIV prevention and sex work, Beijing, UNDP. June 4.

Parish, William L., Edward O. Laumann, Myron S. Cohen, Suiming Pan, Heyi Zheng, Irving Hoffman, Tianfu Wang, and Kwai Hang Ng. 2003. Population based study of chlamydia infection in China: A hidden epidemic. *Journal of the American Medical Association* 289(10):1303–5.

Parish, William L., and Suiming Pan. 2006. Sexual partners in China: Risk pattern for infection by HIV and possible interventions. In *AIDS and social policy in China*, ed. Arthur Kleinman, Joan Kaufman, and Tony Saich, 190–213. Cambridge, MA: Harvard University Asia Center.

Parker, Andrew, Mary Russo, Doris Sommer, and Patricia Yaeger. 1992. Introduction. In *Nationalisms and sexualities*, ed. Andrew Parker, Mary Russo, Doris Sommer, and Patricia Yaeger, 1–18. New York: Routledge.

Parker, Richard G. 1987. Acquired immunodeficiency syndrome in urban Brazil. *Medical Anthropology Quarterly*, new series, 1:155–72.

______. 1988. Sexual culture and AIDS education in urban Brazil. In *AIDS 1988: AAAS symposia papers*, ed. Ruth Kulstad, 269–89. Washington, DC: American Association for the Advancement of Science.

______. 1991. *Bodies, pleasures, and passions: Sexual culture in contemporary Brazil.* Boston: Beacon Press.

______. 1994. Sexual cultures, HIV transmission, and AIDS prevention. *AIDS* 8(Suppl.):S309–S314.

______. 2001. Sexuality, culture, and power in HIV/AIDS research. *Annual Review of Anthropology* 30:163–79.

Parker, Richard G., Delia Easton, and Charles H. Klein. 2000. Structural barriers and facilitators in HIV prevention: A review of international research. *AIDS* 14(Suppl. 1):S22–S32.

Paxson, Heather. 2002. Rationalizing sex: Family planning and the making of modern lovers in urban Greece. *American Ethnologist* 29(2):307–34.

Perkins, Roberta, and Garrett Prestage. 1994. *Sex work and sex workers in Australia.* Sydney: University of New South Wales Press.

Pfeiffer, James. 2004. Condom social marketing, Pentecostalism, and structural adjustment in Mozambique: A clash of AIDS prevention messages. *Medical Anthropology Quarterly* 18(1):77–103.

Phoolcharoen, Wiput. 1998. HIV/AIDS prevention in Thailand: Success and challenges. *Science* 280(5371):1873–74.

Pigg, Stacy Leigh, and Simon Fraser. 2001. Languages of sex and AIDS in Nepal: Notes on the social production of commensurability. *Cultural Anthropology* 16(4):491–541.

Piot, Peter, and Marie Laga. 1991. Current approaches to sexually transmitted disease control in developing countries. In *Research issues in human behavior and sexually transmitted diseases in the AIDS era*, ed. Judith N. Wasserheit, Sevgi O. Aral, King K. Holmes, and Penelope J. Hitchcock, 281–95. Washington, DC: American Society for Microbiology.

Plant, Michael A. 1993. *AIDS, drugs, and prostitution.* London: Routledge.

Plummer, Mary L., Daniel Wight, Joyce Wamoyi, Gerry Mshana, Richard J. Hayes, and David A. Ross. 2006. Farming with your hoe in a sack: Condom attitudes, access, and use in rural Tanzania. *Studies in Family Planning* 37(1):29–40.

Porter, Doug. 1997. A plague on the borders: HIV, development, and traveling identities in the Golden Triangle. In *Sites of desire: Economies of pleasure*, ed. Lenore Manderson and Margaret Jolly, 212–32. Chicago: University of Chicago Press.

Porter, Robert W. 1994. AIDS in Ghana: Priorities and policies. In *Global AIDS policy*, ed. Douglas A. Feldman, 90–106. Westport, CT: Bergin & Garvey.

Preston-Whyte, Eleanor, and Maria Zondi. 1991. Adolescent sexuality and its implications for teenage pregnancy and AIDS. *Continuing Medical Education* 9(11):1389–94.

Pritchard, Annette, and Nigel Morgan. 2006. Hotel Babylon? Exploring hotels as liminal sites of transition and transgression. *Tourism Management* 27(5):762–72.

Pyett, Priscilla M., and Deborah J. Warr. 1997. Vulnerability on the streets: Female sex workers and HIV risk. *AIDS Care* 9:539–47.

Qu, Shuquan. 1997. 1996 nian zhongguo aizibing shaodian jiance baogao (Report of sentinel surveillance in China in 1996). *Zhongguo Xingbing Aizibing Fangzhi (Prevention of STI and AIDS in China)* 3(5):193–98.

______. 2001. National AIDS/HIV surveillance and current HIV epidemic status in China. National Workshop on HIV/STI Surveillance, Nanjing, China.

Qu, Shuquan, Wei Liu, Kyung-Hee Choi, Rongjian Li, Deyuan Jiang, Yuejiao Zhou, Fang Tian, et al. 2002. The potential for rapid sexual transmission of HIV in China: Sexually Transmitted Diseases and Condom Failure Highly Prevalent among Female Sex Workers. *AIDS and Behavior* 6(3).

Qu, Xuesong. 2005. Moba xingjiaoyu biancheng xingshanghai (Don't turn sex education to sexual abuse). *Zhongguo Funu* (*Women of China*), no. 2 (October):46.

Ramazanoglu, Caroline, and Janet Holland. 1993 Women's sexuality and men's appropriation of desire. In *Up against Foucault: Explorations of some tensions between Foucault and feminism*, ed. Caroline Ramazanoglu, 239–64. London: Routledge.

Reed, Dave, and Martin S. Weinberg. 1984. Premarital coitus: Developing and establishing sexual scripts. *Social Psychology Quarterly* 47:129–38.

Ren, Min. 2003. Yeti biyuntao queyou qishi (True liquid condoms). *Nanfang Dushi Bao* (*South City Newspaper*), February 3.

Ren, Qingyun. 1997. Yingxiang zhongyuan nongcun funu shengyu jiankang de ruogan yinsu (Elements that affect rural women's reproductive health). In *Shengyu: Chuantong yu xiandaihua* (*Reproduction: Tradition and Modernity*), ed. Xiaojiang Li, 153–54. Zhengzhou: Henan Renmin Chubanshe.

Ren, Xin. 1999. Prostitution and economic modernization in China. *Violence against Women* 5(12):1411–36.

Renaud, Michelle Lewis. 1997. *Women at the crossroads: A prostitute community's response to AIDS in urban Senegal.* New York: Routledge.

Roche, Brenda, Alan Neaigus, and Maureen Miller. 2005. Street smarts and urban myths: Women, sex work, and the role of storytelling in risk reduction and rationalization. *Medical Anthropology Quarterly* 19(2):149–70.

Rofel, Lisa. 2007. *Desiring China: Experiments in neoliberalism, sexuality, and public culture.* Durham, NC: Duke University Press.

Rogers, Everett, S. Aikat, S. Chang, P. Poppe, and P. Sopory. 1989. Proceedings from the Conference on Entertainment-Education for Social Change. Annenberg School of Communications and the University of Southern California, Los Angeles.

Rojanapithayakorn, Wiwat, and R. Hanenberg. 1996. The 100% condom program in Thailand. *AIDS* 10:1–7.

Rong, Dongyue. 1999. Anquantao daodi zenmo xuanchuan. *Beijing Wanbao* (*Beijing Evening Newspaper*), November 30.

Rossem, Ronan Van, Dominique Meekers, and Zacch Akinyemi. 2000. Condom use in Nigeria: Evidence from two waves of a sexual behavior and condom use survey. PSI Research Division Working Paper No. 31. PSI (Population Services International), Washington, DC.

Rou, Keming, Zunyou Wu, Sheena G. Sullivan, Fan Li, Jihui Guan, Jihui Xu, Dahua Liu, et al. 2007. A five-city trial of a behavioural intervention to reduce sexually transmitted disease/HIV risk among sex workers in China. *AIDS* 21(8):95–101.

Rowe, William T. 1984. *Hankow: Commerce and society in a Chinese city: 1796–1889.* Stanford, CA: Stanford University Press.

Ru, Xiaomei. 2006. Youth and HIV/AIDS in China. In *AIDS and social policy in China*, ed. Arthur Kleinman, Joan Kaufman, and Tony Saich, 232–42. Cambridge, MA: Harvard University Asia Center.

Ruan, Fangyu. 1991. *Sex in China: Studies in sexology in Chinese culture.* New York: Plenum.

Rwabukwali, Charles B., Janet McGrath, and Debra Schumann. 1991. Socioeconomic determinants of sexual risk behavior among Baganda women in Kampala, Uganda. Seventh International Conference on AIDS, Florence, Italy. June 16–21.

Sacks, Valerie. 1996. Women and AIDS: An analysis of media misrepresentations. *Social Science & Medicine* 42(1):59–73.

Saich, Tony. 2006. Social policy development in the era of economic reform. In *AIDS and social policy in China*, ed. Arthur Kleinman, Joan Kaufman, and Tony Saich, 15–46. Cambridge, MA: Harvard University Asia Center.

Sanders, Teela. 2004. The risks of street prostitution: Punters, police, and protesters. *Urban Studies* 41(9):1703–17.

Schoepf, Brooke. 1988. Women, AIDS, and economic crisis in Central Africa. *Canadian Journal of African Studies* 22(3):625–44.

______. 1991. Ethical, methodological, and political issues of AIDS research in Central Africa. *Social Science and Medicine* 33:749–63.

______. 1992. AIDS, sex, and condoms: African healers and the reinvention of tradition in Zaire. *Medical Anthropology* 14:225–42.

______. 1995. Culture, sex research, and aids prevention in Africa. In *Culture and sexual risk: Anthropological perspectives on AIDS*, ed. Han ten Brummelhuis and Gilbert Herdt, 29–51. Amsterdam: Gordon & Breach.

______. 2001. International AIDS research in anthropology: Taking a critical perspective on the crisis. *Annual Reviews of Anthropology* 30:335–61.

Schoepf, Brooke G. 1998. Inscribing the body politic: Women and AIDS in Africa. In *Women and biopower: What constitutes resistance?*, ed. Patricia Kaufert and Margaret Lock, 98–126. New York: Cambridge University Press.

Schoepf, Brooke G., Rukarangira-Wa Nkera, Claude Schoepf, Engundu Walu, and Payanzo Ntsomo. 1988. AIDS and society in Central Africa: A view from Zaire. In *AIDS in Africa: Social and policy impact*, ed. Richard C. Rockwell and Norman Miller, 211–35. Lewiston, ME: Edwin Mellen Press.

Schoepf, Brooke G., Claude Schoepf, and Joyce V. Milien. 2000. Theoretical therapies, remote remedies: SAPS and the political ecology of health in Africa. In *Dying for growth: Global inequality and the health of the poor*, ed. Jim Y. Kim and Joyce V. Millen, 91–125. Monroe, ME: Common Courage Press.

Schumann, Debra A., Janet W. McGrath, Charles B. Rwabukwali, Jonnie Pearson-Marks, Barbara Namande, Lucy Nakyobe, Sylvia Nakayiwa, and Rebecca Mukasa. 1991. Culture and the risk of AIDS: The social organization of sexual risk behavior in Uganda. American Association meetings, Chicago. November 20–24.

Scott, James. 1976. *The moral economy of the peasant: Rebellion and subsistence in Southeast Asia.* New Haven, CT: Yale University Press.

Seeley, Janet A., Sam S. Malamba, Andrew J. Nunn, Daan W. Mulder, Jan F. Kengeya-Kayondo, and Thomas G. Barton. 1994. Socioeconomic status, gender, and risk of HIV-1 infection in a rural community in south west Uganda. *Medical Anthropology Quarterly* 8(1):78–89.

Seidel, Gill. 1993. The competing discourses of HIV/AIDS in sub-Sahara Africa: Discourses of rights and empowerment vs. discourses of control and exclusion. *Social Science and Medicine* 36(3):175–94.

Sellers, Deborah, Sarah A. McGraw, and John B. McKinlay. 1994. Does the promotion and distribution of condoms increase teen sexual activity? Evidence from an HIV prevention program for Latino Youth. *American Journal of Public Health* 84:1952–58.

Serovich, Julianne, and Kathryn Greene. 1997. Predictors of adolescent sexual risk taking behaviors which put them at risk for contracting HIV. *Journal of Youth and Adolescence* 26:429–44.

Setel, Philip W. 1999. *A plague of paradoxes: AIDS, culture, and demography in northern Tanzania.* Chicago: University of Chicago Press.

Shao, Jing. 2006. Fluid labor and blood money: The economy of HIV/AIDS in rural central China. *Cultural Anthropology* 21(4):535–69.

Shen, Hsiu-Hua. 2008. The purchase of transnational intimacy: Women's bodies, transnational masculine privileges in Chinese economic zones. *Asian Studies Review* 32(March):57–75.

Shen, Jie, Kangmai Liu, Mengjie Han, and Fujie Zhang. 2004. The China HIV/AIDS epidemic and current response. In *AIDS in Asia: The Challenge Continues*, ed. Jai P. Narain, 171–90. Newbury Park, CA: Sage.

Shen, Wei. 2001. Gonggong zaiqu e'xi shi ci mousha momo (The malicious second wife attempts to murder her man's wife ten times). *Xin Shang Bao* (*New Commerce Newspaper*), 20.

Shen, Ying. 2007. Dalian nvxing Aizibing ganranzhe zengduo (Increasing rate of HIV infected women in Dalian). *Zhongguo Funv Bao* (*Chinese Women's Newspaper*), 3.

Sigley, Gary. 2001. Keep it in the family: Government, marriage, and sex in contemporary China. In *Borders of being: Citizenship, fertility, and sexuality in Asia and the Pacific*, ed. Margaret Jolly and Kalpana Ram, 118–53. Ann Arbor: University of Michigan Press.

Silva, Martha, Dominique Meekers, and Megan Klein. 2003. Determinants of condom use among youth in Madagascar. PSC Research Report No. 55. PSI (Population Services International), Washington, DC.

Singer, Merrill. 1994. AIDS and the health crisis of the U.S. urban poor: The perspective of critical medical anthropology. *Social Science and Medicine* 39(7):931–48.

______. 1998. *The political economy of AIDS.* Amityville, NY: Baywood.

Singer, Merrill, Candida Flores, Lani Davison, Georgine Burke, Zaida Castillo, Kelley Scalon, and Migdalia Rivera. 1990. SIDS: The economic, social, and cultural context of AIDS among Latinos. *Medical Anthropology Quarterly* 4(1):72–114.

Singer, Merrill, Zhongke Jia, Jean J. Schensul, Margare Weeks, and J. Bryan Page. 1992. AIDS and the IV drug user: The local context in prevention efforts. *Medical Anthropology* 14:285–306.

Singhal, Arvind, and Everett M. Rogers. 1999. *Entertainment-education: A communication strategy for social change.* Mahwah, NJ: Lawrence Erlbaum Associates.

Singhal, Arvind, and Everett Rogers. 1988. Television soap operas for development in India. *Gazette* 41:109–26.

Smith, Beverly. 1996. AIDS: Religion and medicine in rural Kenya. In *AIDS education: Interventions in multicultural societies*, ed. Inon I. Schenker, Galia Sabar-Friedman, and Francisco S. Sy, 239–49. New York: Plenum.

Smyth, Fiona. 1998. Cultural constraints on the delivery of HIV/AIDS prevention in Ireland. *Social Science and Medicine* 46(6):661–72.

Sobo, E. J. 1993. Inner-city women and AIDS: Psychosocial benefits of unsafe sex. *Cultural Medical Psychiatry* 17:454–85.

______. 1994. Attitudes towards HIV testing among impoverished urban African-American women. *Medical Anthropology* 16:1–22.

______. 1995a. *Choosing unsafe sex: AIDS-risk denial among disadvantaged women.* Philadelphia: University of Pennsylvania Press.

______. 1995b. Finance, romance, social support, and condom use among impoverished inner-city women. *Human Organization* 54:115–28.

______. 1998. Love, jealousy, and unsafe sex among inner-city women. In *The political economy of AIDS*, ed. Merrill Singer, 75–103. Amityville, NY: Baywood.

Solinger, Dorothy. 1999. *Contesting citizenship.* Berkeley: University of California Press.

Sontag, Susan. 1989. *AIDS and its metaphors.* Trans. Michael Henry Heim. New York: Farrar, Straus, and Giroux.

Stine, Gerald. 2007. *AIDS update 2007.* New York: Pearson.

Stoler, Ann Laura. 1991. Carnal knowledge and imperial power: Gender, race, and morality in colonial Asia. In *Gender at the crossroads of knowledge*, ed. M. de Leonardo. Berkeley: University of California Press.

Strand, David. 1989. *Rickshaw Beijing: City people and politics in the 1920s.* Berkeley: University of California Press.

Sun, Minghua. 2007. Dalian Aizibing yiqing shangsheng qushi mingxian 7 cheng chengwei xingchuanbo (Dalian AIDS infection rate is rapidly rising, more than 70% from sexual transmission). In *Zhong guang wang.* Beijing: Zhongguo Guangbowo (Chinese Broadcast Net).

T., F. 1977. Fertility control and public health in rural China: Unpublicized problems. *Population and Development Review* 3(4):482–85.

Taylor, Christopher C. 1990a. AIDS and the pathogenesis of metaphor. In *Culture and AIDS: The human factor*, ed. D. Feldman, 55–65. Westport, CT: Praeger.

______. 1990b. Condoms and cosmology: The "fractal" person and sexual risk in Rwanda. *Social Science and Medicine* 31(9):1023–28.

Thuy, Nguyen, Thi Thanh, Christina P. Lindan, Nguyen Hoan, John Barclay, and Khiem Ha. 2000. Sexual risk behavior of women in entertainment services. *AIDS and Behavior* 4:93–101.

Tien, H. Yuan. 1965. Sterilization, oral contraception, and population control in China. *Population Studies* 18(3):215–35.

______. 1973. *China's population struggle: Demographic decisions of the People's Republic, 1949–1969*. Columbus: Ohio State University Press.

Tierney, John. 1990. With "social marketing," condoms combat AIDS. Special to the *New York Times*, September 18.

Tong, Wei, and Dejun Li. 1996. Dalian shouci faxian HIV Ganranzhe (The first HIV infected people in Dalian). *Zhongguo Xingbing Aizibing Fangzhi* (*Prevention of STI and AIDS in China*) 4:15–16.

Tong, Wei, and Xiaoming Yang. 1998. Dalianshi shoulei jingwai yiyuanxing ganren HIV baogao (The first case of overseas origin of HIV infection in Dalian). *Zhongguo Xingbing Aizibing Fangzhi* (*Prevention of STI and AIDS in China*) 3:103.

Tran, Trung Nam, Roger Detels, and Hoang Phuong Lan. 2006. Condom use and its correlates among female sex workers in Hanoi, Vietnam. *AIDS and Behavior* 10(2):159–67.

Travers, Michele, and Lydia Bennett, eds. 1996. *AIDS, women, and power*. New York: Taylor & Francis.

Triechler, Paula. 1987. AIDS, homophobia, and biomedical discourse: An epidemic of signification. *Cultural Studies* 1(3):263–305.

Tu, Xiao. 2001. Wohe Aizibingren youge yuehui (I have an appointment with an AIDS patient). *Jia Ting* (*Family*) 1(251):20–24.

UNAIDS. 2003. *Join the fight against AIDS in China*. Geneva: Joint United Nations Programme on HIV/AIDS.

Vance, Carol. 1982. Pleasure and danger: Toward a politics of sexuality. In *Pleasure and danger: Exploring female sexuality*, ed. Carol S. Vance. London: Pandora.

Van den Hoek A., Y. L. Fu, N. H. T. M. Dukers, Z. H. Chen, J. T. Feng, L. N. Zhang, and X. X. Zhang. 2001. High prevalence of syphilis and other sexually transmitted diseases among sex workers in China: Potential for fast spread of HIV. *AIDS* 15(6):753–59.

Van den Hoek, J., Roel A. Coutinho, Harry J. A. van Haastrecht, Alt W. van Zadelhoff, and Jaap Goudsmit. 1988. Prevalence and risk factors of HIV infections among drug users and drug using prostitutes in Amsterdam. *AIDS* 2(1):55–60.

Van Gulik, R. H. 2003. *Sexual life in ancient China*. Trans. Li Ling and Guo Xiaohui. New York: Brill Academic.

Vanwesenbeeck, Ine, Ron De Graaf, Gertjan Van Zessen, Cees J. Starver, and Jan H. Visser. 1993. Protection styles of prostitutes' clients: Intention, behavior, and considerations in relation to AIDS. *Journal of Sex Education and Therapy* 19:79–92.

Vaughan, Peter W., and Everett M. Rogers. 2000. A staged model of communication effects: Evidence from an entertainment-education radio soap opera in Tanzania. *Journal of Health Communication* 5:203–27.

Waddell, Charles E. 1996a. HIV and the social world of female commercial sex workers. *Medical Anthropology Quarterly* 10:75–82.

______. 1996b. Female sex work, non-work sex and HIV in Perth. *Australian Journal of Social Issues* 31(4):410–24.

Waldby, Cathy, Susan Kippax, and June Crawford. 1993. Cordon sanitaire: "Clean" and "unclean" women in the AIDS discourse of young men. In *AIDS: Facing the second decade*, ed. Peter Davies Peter Aggleton and Graham Hart, 29–39. London: Falmer Press.

Walden, Vivien Margaert, Kondwani Mwangulube, and Paul Makhumula-Nkhoma. 1999. Measuring the impact of a behaviour change intervention for commercial sex workers and their potential clients in Malawi. *Health Education Research* 14(4):545–54.

Walters, Ian. 2004. Dutiful daughters and temporary wives: Economic dependency on commercial sex in Vietnam. In *Sexual cultures in East Asia: The social construction of sexuality and sexual risk in a time of AIDS*, ed. Evelyne Micollier, 76–97. London: RoutledgeCurzon.

Wang, Aili. 1995. Dangjin chengshi hunyin yanbian de jiben biaozheng jiqi zouxiang (The basic characteristics and trend of current city marriage changes). *Women of China* 2:20–21.

Wang, Changshan. 2005. Jianjue ezhi aizibing de liuxing he manyan (Insist in blocking the spread of AIDS). *Nanfang Zhoumo* (*South Weekend*), June 23:1.

Wang, Gan. 1999. Conspicuous consumption, business networks, and state power in a Chinese City. PhD diss., Yale University.

Wang, Jichuan, Baofa Jiang, Harvey Siegal, Russel Falck, and Robert Carlson. 2001a. Sexual behavior and condom use among patients with sexually transmitted diseases in Jinan, China. *American Journal of Public Health* 91(4):650–51.

______. 2001b. Level of AIDS and HIV knowledge and sexual practices among sexually transmitted disease patients in China. *Sexually Transmitted Disease* 28(3):171–75.

Wang, Jinling. 2006. *Zhongguo funu fazhan baogao No. 1* (*A report on Chinese women's development*). Beijing: Shehui Kexue Wenxian Chubanshe (Social Science Publishing House).

Wang, Lijuan. 2007. Condom promotion for HIV/AIDS prevention in China: The role of epistemic community. Eighth International Congress on AIDS in Asia and the Pacific, Colombo, August 19–23.

Wang, Longde. 2007. Overview of the HIV/AIDS epidemic, scientific research and government responses in China. *AIDS* 21(8):3–7.

Wang, Shancheng. 1956. Tan xingshenghuo (Talk about sex life). *Women of China* 8:30.

Wang, Wei. 2005. Dalian 1/4 yihun nuxing fanghuan biyun. In *Bandao Chenbao* (*Bandao Morning Newspaper*), June 13.

Wang, Wenbin, Zhiyi Zhao, and Mingxun Tan. 1956. *Xing de zhishi* (*Sexual knowledge*). Beijing: Renmin Weisheng Chubanshe (People's Hygiene Publishing House).

______. 1957. *Xing de zhishi* (*The knowledge of sex*). Beijing: Kexue Puji Chubanshe.

Wang, Yan. 2007. Anti-HIV/AIDS prevention within sex workers in Sichuan. Seminar on HIV Prevention and Sex Work, UNDP, Beijing. June 4.

Wang, Yuefeng. 2005. Qiantan weifa fanzui renyuanzhong ganran aizibingren de guanli (On the management of AIDS Criminals). In *Zhongguo Aizibing fangzhi* (*HIV Prevention in China*). Beijing: Capital University of Medical Science.

Wang, Zhenhua. 2003. Anquandai Yu anquantao (Safety belt and condoms). *Shandong Qingnian Bao* (*Shandong Youth Newspaper*), February 22.

Warr, Deborah J., and Priscilla M. Pyett. 1999. Difficult relations: Sex work, love, and intimacy. *Sociology of Health and Illness* 21:290–309.

Wawer, Maria J., Chai Podhisita, Uraiwan Kanungsukkasem, A. Pramualratana, and R. Mcnamara. 1996. Origins and working conditions of female sex workers in urban Thailand: Consequences of social context for HIV transmission. *Social Science and Medicine* 42:453–62.

Webb, Douglas. 1997. *HIV and AIDS in Africa*. Cape Town: David Philip.

Wei, Jingjing. 2002. "Yetibiyuntao" nengfou taolao jiankang he kuaile (Can liquid condom offer health and happiness). *Zhongguo Funu* (*Women of China*) 12(614):6.

Wei, Ping. 2005. Nuxingjiankang yao baowo sange zhuanxingqi (Caring female health should grasp three transitional period). *Jiankang Bao* (*Health News*) 7:7.

Weissman, Carol S., Constance A. Nathanson, Margaret Ensminger, Martha A. Teitelbaum, J. Courtland Robinson, and Stacey Plichta. 1989. AIDS knowledge, perceived risk, and prevention among adolescents of a family planning clinics. *Family Planning Perspectives* 21:213–17.

Wen, Chihua. 2002. No condoms, please, we're Chinese men. *Asia Times Online*, April 11.

Wen, Jin. 1958. Jieyu xuanchuan zai yuhuasha chang (Publicity of birth control in Yuhua Yarn Factory). *Women of China* 6:30–31.

Wen, Li. 2005a. Nuren, diode de zuihou shouhuzhe: Jiatingzhulian, dizhifubaizhufangxian (Women are the last defenders of ethics: Helping with the cleanness of the family, resisting corruption). *Zhongguo Funu* (*Women of China*), September 2:10–11.

______. 2005b. Nuren, diode de zuihou shouhuzhe: Jiatingzhulian, dizhifubaizhufangxian (Women are the last defenders of ethics: Helping with the cleanness of the family, resisting corruption). *Zhongguo Funu* (*Women of China*), October 2:51–52.

______. 2005c. Nuren, diode de zuihou shouhuzhe (Women are the last defenders of ethics). *Zhongguo Funu* (*Women of China*), July 2:52–53.

______. 2005d. Nuren, diode de zuihou shouhuzhe (Women are the last defenders of ethics). *Zhongguo Funu* (*Women of China*) no. 655 (August 2):52–53.

Wen, Zhenxiu. 2002. Social marketing to high risk groups in Yunnan and Sichuan, China. International Conference on AIDS, Manchester, July 7–12.

Werner, David. 1977. *Where there is no doctor: A village health care handbook*. Palo Alto, CA: Hesperian Foundation.

Wight, Daniel. 1994. "Boys" thoughts and talk in a working class locality of Glasgow. *Sociological Review* 42:703–37.

Williams, Sophie, and Lenore Lyons. 2008. It's about bang for your buck, bro: Singaporean men's online conversations about sex in Batam, Indonesia. *Asian Studies Review* 32(March):77–97.

Wilson, David, Babusi Sibanda, Lilian Mboyi, Sheila Msimanga, and Godwin Dube. 1990. A pilot study for an HIV prevention programme among commercial sex workers in Bulawayo, Zimbabwe. *Social Science and Medicine* 31:609–18.

Wilton, Tamsin, and Peter Aggleton. 1991. Condoms, coercion, and control: Heterosexuality and the limits to HIV/AIDS education. In *AIDS: Responses, interventions, and care*, ed. Peter Aggelton, Peter Davies, and Graham Hart, 149–56. London: Falmer Press.

Wiutehead, Tony L. 1997. Urban low-income African American men, HIV/AIDS, and gender identity. *Medical Anthropology Quarterly* 11(4):411–47.

Wojcicki, Janet, and Josephine Malala. 2001. Condom use, power, and HIV/AIDS risk: Sex-workers bargain for survival in Hillbrow/Joubert Park/Berea, Johannesburg. *Social Science and Medicine* 53:99–121.

Wolf, Margery. 1972. *Women and the family in rural Taiwan*. Stanford, CA: Stanford University Press.

Wong, M., I. Lubek, B. C. Dy, S. Pen, S. Kros, and M. Chhit. 2003. Social and behavioural factors associated with condom use among direct social workers in Siem Reap, Cambodia. *Sexually Transmitted Infections* 79:163–65.

Worth, Dooley. 1989. Sexual decision-making and AIDS: Why condom promotion among vulnerable women is likely to fail. *Studies in Family Planning* 20(6):297–307.

Wu, Bo. 2004. Jujue xingbing de fangshenshu (STI Prevention). *Baojian yu Shenghuo* (*Health and Life*) 7:38.

Wu, Yin. 1956. Zaibuneng youyi buding le (No longer hesitant). *Women of China* 7:26.

Wu, Zunyou, Keming Rou, Manhong Jia, Song Duan, and Sheena Sullivan. 2007. The first community-based sexually transmitted disease/HIV intervention trial for female sex workers in China. *AIDS* 21(8):89–94.

Wu, Zunyou, Rou Keming, and Cui Haixia. 2004. The HIV/AIDS epidemic in China: History, current strategies, and future challenges. *AIDS Education and Prevention* 16(Suppl. A):7–17.

Wulfert, Edelgard, and Choi K. Wan. 1995. Safer sex intentions and condom use viewed from a health belief, reasoned action, and social cognitive perspective. *Journal of Sex Research* 32(4):299–312.

Xi, Li. 2005. Liaojie AIDS yufang xinguannian (New views of prevention of AIDS). *Jiankang Wenzhai Bao* (*Health and Digest Newspaper*), no. 700 (February 20):8.

Xi, Zhu. 1964. Airen de sixiang kaile qiao (My husband's thought finally got straightened out). *Women of China* 8:30.

Xiao, Hua. 1965. Xinhun neng biyun ma (Can we proceed contraception as a newly married couple). *Women of China* 12:31.

Xiao, Liu. 2001. Siwang yinying longzhao "Xiaojie" qunti (Hostesses are shadowed by death). *Dalian Wanbao* (*Dalian Evening Newspaper*), 18.

Xie, Hanping. 1997. Buzhengchang de xingshenghuo weihaiduo (More harms of abnormal sex life). *Women of China* (*Zhongguo Funu*) 3:55.

Xin, Ren. 1999. Prostitution and economic modernization of China. *Violence against Women* 5(12):1411–36.

Xiwen, Zheng, Qu Shuquan, Kevin Yiee, and Jeffrey Mandel. 2000. HIV risk among patients attending sexually transmitted disease clinics in China. *AIDS and Behavior* 4(1).

Xu, Zongxiu. 1964. Zai jieshou le liangci jiaoxun yihou (After receiving two lessons). *Women of China* 5:30.

Yang, Chun. 2004a. He aizibingdu saipao (Racing AIDS virus). *Qingnian Shixun* (*Youth Express*), June 1(207):1.

______. 2004b. He aizibingdu saipao (Racing AIDS virus). *Qingnian Shixun* (*Youth Express*), no. 207 (July 22):1.

Yang, Junlan, and Yonggang Li. 1999. Liaoningsheng 1998 nian xingbing liuxing qingkuang ji fenxi (An epidemiological analysis of STI situation in Liaoning Province). *Zhongguo Xingbing Aizibing Fangzhi* (*Prevention of STI and AIDS in China*) 5(6):243–45.

Yang, Junlan, and Shibo Zhang. 1997. Liaoningsheng xingbing yiqing fenxi (An analysis of STI situation in Liaoning Province). *Zhongguo Xingbing Aizibing Fangzhi* (*Prevention of STI and AIDS in China*) 3(6):241–42.

Yang, Mayfair Mei-hui. 1999a. From gender erasure to gender difference: State feminism, consumer sexuality, and women's public sphere in China. In *Spaces of their own: Women's public sphere in transnational China*, ed. Mayfair Mei-hui Young, 35–67. Minneapolis: University of Minnesota Press.

______. 1999b. Introduction. In *Spaces of their own: Women's public sphere in transnational China*, ed. Mayfair Mei-hui Yang, 1–31. Minneapolis: University of Minnesota Press.

Yao, Ge. 2002. *Xinhun weisheng quanshu* (*Hygiene for newly married couple*). Fuzhou: Fujian Kexue Jishu Chubanshe.

Yeakley, Anna M., and Larry M. Gant. 1997. Cultural factors and program implications: HIV/AIDS interventions and condom use among Latinos. *Journal of Multicultural Social Work* 6:47–71.

Yi, Ming. 2001. Anquantao chulu hezai (Where is the outlet for condom). *Keji Ribao* (*Science Daily*), December 30.

Yin, Chengxi. 2006. Bieyaomohua Chongqingde anquantao xiangmu (Don't demonize Chongqing's condom program). *Xiandai Kuaibao* (*Modern Express Newspaper*), September 7.

Yip, Ray. 2006. Opportunity for effective prevention of AIDS in China: The strategy of preventing secondary transmission of HIV. In *AIDS and Social Policy in China*, ed. Arthur Kleinman, Joan Kaufman, and Tony Saich, 177–89. Cambridge, MA: Harvard University Asia Center.

You, Qing. 2000. Dangdai nudaxuesheng xingxingwei xintailu (A record of modern female university students' sex conduct and psyche). *Changjiang Ribao* (*Yangtsze River Daily*), October 26:4.

Yu, Dingzhen. 1957. Wode tongku cong helai (Where does my pain come from). *Women of China* 3:14–15.

Yu, Guangyuan. 1956. *Xing zhishi* (*Knowledge of sex*). Shanghai: Shanghai Weisheng Chubanshe.

Yu, Hushi. 2002. Pinglun: Woguo anquantao guanggao jiejin xiaoxiao de yige jinbu (Comments: A small progress of condom ads). *Fazhi Ribao* (*Law Daily*), December 3.

Yu, Muxia. 1935. Shanghai linzhao (Shanghai tidbits). Shanghai: Shanghai hubaoguan chubanbu (Shanghai Hubaoguan Publishing House).

Yu, Ping. 1957. Ku nao (Frustration). *Women of China* 3:14–15.

Yu, Sheng. 1958. Biyun geiwo dailai de haochu (Birth control brought me advantages). *Women of China* 4:31.

Yu, Xian. 1965. Fangle biyun huan buhui yingxiang shenti jiankang (IUD will not affect physical health). *Women of China* 10:31.

Yu, Ying. 2003. *Bi yun* (*Contraception*). Haikou: Nanhai Chuban Gongsi.

Yuan, Feng, and Jie Yun. 1990. Baohuzhencao de mijue (Secret to chastity). *Cha yu Fan Hou* (*After Tea and Meals*) 5:6.

Zeng, Liming. 2002. Zhongguo yanzhi chu neng shamie duozhong bingdu de yeti biyuntao (China has invented liquid condoms that can kill a plethora of viruses). *Beijing Qingnian Bao* (*Beijing Youth Newspaper*), October 18.

Zhang, Baichuan, D. Liu, X. Li, and T. Hu. 2001. A survey on HIV/AIDS related high risk behaviors and affecting factors of men who have sex with men in Mainland China. *Chinese Journal of Sexually Transmitted Infections* 1(1):7–16.

Zhang, Li. 2001. *Strangers in the city: Reconfigurations of space, power, and social networks within China's floating population*. Stanford, CA: Stanford University Press.

Zhang, Lizhi. 1966. Dui shehuizhuyi youli de shi won eng bu dai tou ma (Can't I lead others to help with socialism?). *Women of China* 1:24.

Zhang, L. Y., X. Gao, Z. W. Dong, Y. P. Tan, Z. L. Wu. 2002. Premarital sexual activities among students in a university in Beijing, China. *Sexually Transmitted Disease* 29(4):212–15.

Zhang, Qing. 2004. Nuxing ganranzhe bili you jiaoda fudu shangsheng (Rising ratio of the female infected). *Zhongguo Funubao* (*Chinese Women Newspaper*), December 6:5.

Zhang, Wei. 2006. Anquantao de zhunru yiyi (The meaning of entry of condoms). *Beijing Yule Xinbao* (*Beijing Entertainment Newspaper*), February 28.

Zhang, Youfang, and Lei Feng. 2001. *Abortion*. Beijing: Renmin Weisheng Chubanshe.

Zhang, Yujie. 1964. Yici meiyou jing zuzhi de zuotanhui (An unorganized seminar). *Women of China* 5:30–31.

Zhang, Zhongyuan, and Xun An. 2002. *Shengzhi jiankang zhinan* (*The handbook of biological health*). Chengdu: Sichuan Renmin Chubanshe.

Zhao, Jian. 2004. Yufang AIDS xuanchuan yu ganga (Embarrassment of advocating AIDS prevention). *Beijing Qingnian Bao* (*Beijing Youth Newspaper*), November 30.

Zhao, Pengfei. 2005. *Female condom consultation in China: Summer report of meeting*. Beijing: The Female Health Foundation. April 26.

Zhao, Ting. 2002. Zhangfu chuci "yuegui" shi (The first time when the husband went astray). *Zhongguo Funu* (*Women of China*) 6(2):32.

Zhao, Xueyi. 2006. Dalian "Fang Ai" zhaoer tingduo (Dalian has many AIDS-prevention means). *Liaoning Fazhi Bao* (*Liaoning Law Newspaper*).

Zhao, Zhiyi, and Hongzhao Song. 1955. *Biyun changshi* (*Common knowledge about contraception*). Beijing: Renmin Weisheng Chubanshe (People's Hygiene Publishing House).

Zhao, Zhongwei. 2006. Towards a better understanding of past fertility regimes: The ideas and practices of controlling family size in Chinese history. *Continuity and Change* 21(1):9–35.

Zhen, Yulan, and Longyin Mao. 2003. Chengshilide xin zhencao yundong (New chastity campaign in the city). *Shenzhen Qingnian* (*Shenzhen Youth*) 5(174):54–55.

Zheng, Lingqiao. 2004. Huanqi minzhong shi fangkong AIDS de dunpai (Mobilizing the populace is the shield against AIDS). *Jiankang Bao* (*Health Newspaper*), March 11:2.

Zheng, Tiantian. 2003. Consumption, body image, and rural-urban apartheid in contemporary China. *City and Society* 15(2):143–63.

______. 2004. From peasant women to bar hostesses: Gender and modernity in post-Mao Dalian. In *On the move: Women and rural to urban migration in contemporary China*, ed. Arianne Gaetano and Tamara Jacka, 80–108. New York: Columbia University Press.

______. 2006. Cool masculinity: Male clients' sex consumption and business alliance in urban China's sex industry. *Journal of Contemporary China* 15(46):161–82.

______. 2007. Claim for an equal social status: An ethnography of China's sex industry. In *Working in China: Ethnographies of labor and workplace transformation*, ed. Ching Kwan Lee, 124–44. New York: Routledge.

______. 2008a. Commodifying romance and searching for love: Rural migrant bar hostesses' moral vision in post-Mao Dalian. *Modern China* 35(4):442–76.

______. 2008b. Complexity of life and resistance: Informal networks of rural migrant karaoke bar hostesses in urban Chinese sex industry. *China: An International Journal* 6(1):69–95.

______. 2009. *Red lights: The lives of sex workers in postsocialist China*. Minneapolis: University of Minnesota Press.

Zheng, Xiwen, Kyung-Hee Choi, Xiwen Zheng, Shuquan Qu, Kevin Yiee, and Jeffrey Mandel. 2000. HIV risk among patients attending sexually transmitted disease clinics in China. *AIDS Behavior* 4(1):111–19.

Zhong, Xueping. 2000. *Masculinity besieged? Issues of modernity and male subjectivity in Chinese literature of the late twentieth century*. Durham, NC: Duke University Press.

Zhou, Efen. 1955. Biyun wenti daduzhe wen (Answer to the readers' questions on contraception). *Women of China* 12(74):26.

______. 1956. Tan zhongyao biyun (About contraceptive in Chinese medicine). *Women of China* 9:30–31.

Zhou, Huadong. 2005. Sancheng renliu nuxing wei zaixiao daxuesheng (Thirty percent of the women going through abortion are female college students). *Bandao Chenbao*, June 15:A13.

Zhu, Junlun, and Xiansong Li. 1993. *Xinhun bidu, fuqi biben* (*A must read for newly married couples and spouses*). Chengdu: Chengdu Keji Daxue chubanshe.

Zhu, Kun. 2002. Dang xing zaoyu aizi shashou (When sex encounters the killer of AIDS). *Xin Zhou Kan* (*New Weekly*), February 19.

CPSIA information can be obtained
at www.ICGtesting.com
Printed in the USA
LVHW060414221218
601155LV00005B/20/P

9 780757 590412